Advances in Intelligent Systems and Computing

Volume 1186

The series "Advances in Intelligent Systems and Computing" contains publications on theory, applications, and design methods of Intelligent Systems and Intelligent Computing. Virtually all disciplines such as engineering, natural sciences, computer and information science, ICT, economics, business, e-commerce, environment, healthcare, life science are covered. The list of topics spans all the areas of modern intelligent systems and computing such as: computational intelligence, soft computing including neural networks, fuzzy systems, evolutionary computing and the fusion of these paradigms, social intelligence, ambient intelligence, computational neuroscience, artificial life, virtual worlds and society, cognitive science and systems, Perception and Vision, DNA and immune based systems, self-organizing and adaptive systems, e-Learning and teaching, human-centered and human-centric computing, recommender systems, intelligent control, robotics and mechatronics including human-machine teaming, knowledge-based paradigms, learning paradigms, machine ethics, intelligent data analysis, knowledge management, intelligent agents, intelligent decision making and support, intelligent network security, trust management, interactive entertainment, Web intelligence and multimedia.

The publications within "Advances in Intelligent Systems and Computing" are primarily proceedings of important conferences, symposia and congresses. They cover significant recent developments in the field, both of a foundational and applicable character. An important characteristic feature of the series is the short publication time and world-wide distribution. This permits a rapid and broad dissemination of research results.

** Indexing: The books of this series are submitted to ISI Proceedings, EI-Compendex, DBLP, SCOPUS, Google Scholar and Springerlink **

More information about this series at http://www.springer.com/series/11156

Ewa Pietka · Pawel Badura ·
Jacek Kawa · Wojciech Wieclawek
Editors

Information Technology in Biomedicine

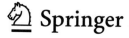 Springer

Editors
Ewa Pietka
Faculty of Biomedical Engineering
Silesian University of Technology
Gliwice, Poland

Pawel Badura
Faculty of Biomedical Engineering
Silesian University of Technology
Gliwice, Poland

Jacek Kawa
Faculty of Biomedical Engineering
Silesian University of Technology
Gliwice, Poland

Wojciech Wieclawek
Faculty of Biomedical Engineering
Silesian University of Technology
Gliwice, Poland

ISSN 2194-5357   ISSN 2194-5365 (electronic)
Advances in Intelligent Systems and Computing
ISBN 978-3-030-49665-4   ISBN 978-3-030-49666-1 (eBook)
https://doi.org/10.1007/978-3-030-49666-1

This Springer imprint is published by the registered company Springer Nature Switzerland AG
The registered company address is: Gewerbestrasse 11, 6330 Cham, Switzerland

Preface

The amount of available medical data constantly grows. The variety of multimodal content necessitates the demand for a fast and reliable technology, able to process the information and deliver results timely, in a user-friendly manner.

Multimodal acquisition systems, AI-powered applications, biocybernetic support of medical procedures, physiotherapy, and prevention give new meaning to optimization of the functional requirements of the healthcare system for the benefit of the patients. We give back to the readers the book, which includes chapters written by members of academic society. The book includes five parts that discuss various issues related to problem-dependent approaches in the area of signal and image analysis as well as new data analysis techniques including artificial intelligence and machine learning techniques. Special attention is paid to support of physiotherapy and physioprevention. More specifically, the scientific scope of particular parts includes the aspects listed below.

Artificial Intelligence part covers a broad range of deep learning approaches to the problems of atopic dermatitis in a chronic inflammatory cutaneous disease, detection of the tongue in speech disorder assessment, and segmentation of environmental microorganism in order to assist the microbiologists in their detection and identification.

Image Analysis part presents original studies reporting on scientific approaches to support the navigation in minimally invasive surgery, evaluation of the regeneration process of bone defects in micro-computed tomography, automated pancreas, and duodenum segmentation. An extraordinary effort has been devoted to develop a technique able to provide an insight into the morphology of historic specimens by the development of a transform in order to co-register histology images and facilitate a 3D visualization of microstructures of lung adenocarcinoma. A study on the correlation of age and the morphometric and texture of vertebrae in lateral cervical spine radiographs is a response to the need of the aging society.

Sound and Motion in Physiotherapy and Physioprevention part introduces an innovative support in physiotherapy by incorporating diagnosis prior to rehabilitation, real-time monitoring, and patient-related therapeutic activity. Metro-rhythmic stimulations and spontaneous activity become an important element. A novel, modern system (DISC4SPINE) of dynamic individual stimulation and control for spine and posture is presented. It is an outstanding example of combining professional knowledge and experience of experts in physiotherapy, medicine, and technical sciences. Prevention against hyperactivity and pain monitoring have been addressed in order to make the therapy safe and bearable to the patients.

Modeling and Simulation part presents studies that provide valuable solutions by giving clear insights into complex systems. Modeling the blood flow through the synthetic aortic valve with overset mesh as well as the flow in the myocardial bridge region are two interesting studies that address the coronary abnormality issue. The dehydration process in human skin has been simulated on an in-silico model in order to test measuring instrument that uses the electromagnetic waves. Simulation of electromagnetic field distribution inside a railway vehicle presents an analysis of its impact on the human head model.

Medical Data Analysis part highlights several interesting approaches including a study that introduces a method able to support the understanding of structural information by blind people, implementation of videoplethysmography to measure in a touchless way the pulse rate, and biomechanical methods of validating animations.

Editors would like to express their gratitude to the authors who have submitted their original research papers as well as all the reviewers for their valuable comments. Your effort has contributed to the high quality of the book that we pass on to the readers.

Gliwice, Poland   Ewa Pietka
June 2020

Contents

Artificial Intelligence

Deep Learning Approach to Subepidermal Low Echogenic Band Segmentation in High Frequency Ultrasound 3
Joanna Czajkowska, Wojciech Dziurowicz, Paweł Badura,
and Szymon Korzekwa

A Review of Clustering Methods in Microorganism Image Analysis 13
Chen Li, Frank Kulwa, Jinghua Zhang, Zihan Li, Hao Xu, and Xin Zhao

MRFU-Net: A Multiple Receptive Field U-Net for Environmental Microorganism Image Segmentation 27
Chen Li, Jinghua Zhang, Xin Zhao, Frank Kulwa, Zihan Li, Hao Xu,
and Hong Li

Deep Learning Approach to Automated Segmentation of Tongue in Camera Images for Computer-Aided Speech Diagnosis 41
Agata Sage, Zuzanna Miodońska, Michał Kręcichwost, Joanna Trzaskalik,
Ewa Kwaśniok, and Paweł Badura

Image Analysis

3-D Tissue Image Reconstruction from Digitized Serial Histologic Sections to Visualize Small Tumor Nests in Lung Adenocarcinomas 55
Bartłomiej Pyciński, Yukako Yagi, Ann E. Walts, and Arkadiusz Gertych

The Influence of Age on Morphometric and Textural Vertebrae Features in Lateral Cervical Spine Radiographs 71
Patrycja Mazur, Rafał Obuchowicz, and Adam Piórkowski

**Evaluation of Shape from Shading Surface Reconstruction Quality
for Liver Phantom**   81
Mateusz Bas and Dominik Spinczyk

Pancreas and Duodenum—Automated Organ Segmentation   95
Piotr Zarychta

**Evaluation of the Effect of a PCL/nanoSiO$_2$ Implant on Bone Tissue
Regeneration Using X-ray Micro-Computed Tomography**   107
Magdalena Jędzierowska, Marcin Binkowski, Robert Koprowski,
and Zygmunt Wróbel

Sound and Motion in Physiotherapy and Physioprevention

**Effect of Various Types of Metro-Rhythmic Stimulations
on the Variability of Gait Frequency**   121
Robert Michnik, Katarzyna Nowakowska-Lipiec, Anna Mańka,
Sandra Niedzwiedź, Patrycja Twardawa, Patrycja Romaniszyn,
Bruce Turner, Aneta Danecka, and Andrzej W. Mitas

Cross-Modal Music-Emotion Retrieval Using DeepCCA   133
Naoki Takashima, Frédéric Li, Marcin Grzegorzek,
and Kimiaki Shirahama

**Computer-Based Analysis of Spontaneous Infant Activity:
A Pilot Study**   147
Iwona Doroniewicz, Daniel Ledwoń, Monika N. Bugdol,
Katarzyna Kieszczyńska, Alicja Affanasowicz, Małgorzata Matyja,
Dariusz Badura, Andrzej W. Mitas, and Andrzej Myśliwiec

**Behavioral and Physiological Profile Analysis While
Exercising—Case Study**   161
Patrycja Romaniszyn, Damian Kania, Monika N. Bugdol, Anita Pollak,
and Andrzej W. Mitas

**Psychophysiological State Changes Assesment Based on Thermal
Face Image—Preliminary Results**   175
Marta Danch-Wierzchowska, Marcin Bugdol, and Andrzej W. Mitas

**Application of Original System to Support Specialist Physiotherapy
D4S in Correction of Postural Defects as Compared to Other
Methods—A Review**   187
Karol Bibrowicz, Tomasz Szurmik, Anna Lipowicz,
and Andrzej W. Mitas

**Methods of Therapy of Scoliosis and Technical Functionalities
of DISC4SPINE (D4S) Diagnostic and Therapeutic System**   201
Tomasz Szurmik, Karol Bibrowicz, Anna Lipowicz, and Andrzej W. Mitas

**Methods for Assessing the Subject's Multidimensional
Psychophysiological State in Terms of Proper Rehabilitation** 213
Anna Mańka, Patrycja Romaniszyn, Monika N. Bugdol,
and Andrzej W. Mitas

**Multimodal Signal Acquisition for Pain Assessment
in Physiotherapy** 227
Aleksandra Badura, Maria Bieńkowska, Aleksandra Masłowska,
Robert Czarlewski, Andrzej Myśliwiec, and Ewa Pietka

Classification of Heat-Induced Pain Using Physiological Signals 239
Philip J. Gouverneur, Frédéric Li, Tibor M. Szikszay,
Waclaw M. Adamczyk, Kerstin Luedtke, and Marcin Grzegorzek

Modeling and Simulation

**Flow in a Myocardial Bridge Region of a Coronary
Artery—Experimental Rig and Numerical Model** 255
Bartlomiej Melka, Marcin Nowak, Marek Rojczyk, Maria Gracka,
Wojciech Adamczyk, Ziemowit Ostrowski, and Ryszard Bialecki

**Numerical Model of the Aortic Valve Implanted Within Real
Human Aorta** 265
Marcin Nowak, Wojciech Adamczyk, Bartlomiej Melka,
Ziemowit Ostrowski, and Ryszard Bialecki

**Establishment of an In-Silico Model for Simulation of Dehydration
Process in Human Skin to Compare Output Parameter
with Clinical Study** 277
Jana Viehbeck, Alexandra Speich, Swetlana Ustinov, Dominik Böck,
Michael Wiehl, and Rainer Brück

**SAR Evaluation in Human Head Models with Cochlear Implant Near
PIFA Antenna Inside a Railway Vehicle** 289
Mariana Benova, Jana Mydlova, Zuzana Psenakova, and Maros Smondrk

Medical Data Analysis

**Methods Supporting the Understanding of Structural Information
by Blind People and Selected Aspects of Their Evaluation** 303
Michał Maćkowski, Katarzyna Rojewska, Mariusz Dzieciątko,
Katarzyna Bielecka, Mateusz Bas, and Dominik Spinczyk

**Videoplethysmographic Measurements of Pulse Wave Velocity
and Pulse Transit Time** 317
Anna Pająk and Piotr Augustyniak

Biomechanical Methods of Validating Animations 327
Filip Wróbel, Dominik Szajerman, and Adam Wojciechowski

**One 'Stop Smoking' to Take Away, Please! A Preliminary Evaluation
of an AAT Mobile App** 345
Tanja Joan Eiler, Tobias Forneberg, Armin Grünewald, Alla Machulska,
Tim Klucken, Katharina Jahn, Björn Niehaves, Carl Friedrich Gethmann,
and Rainer Brück

**The Classifier Algorithm for Recognition of Basic Driving
Scenarios** 359
Rafał Doniec, Szymon Sieciński, Natalia Piaseczna,
Katarzyna Mocny-Pachońska, Marta Lang, and Jacek Szymczyk

**Monitoring Temperature-Related Hazards Using Mobile Devices
and a Thermal Camera** 369
Mariusz Marzec

Author Index 385

Artificial Intelligence

Deep Learning Approach to Subepidermal Low Echogenic Band Segmentation in High Frequency Ultrasound

Joanna Czajkowska, Wojciech Dziurowicz, Paweł Badura, and Szymon Korzekwa

Abstract Atopic dermatitis is a chronic, pruritic, inflammatory cutaneous disease, which mainly occurrs in children and has a tendency to regress during childhood. The accurate therapy requires an objective method to examine the skin condition. However, there is a lack of standardization of diagnostic criteria using high-resolution, non-invasive methods. Therefore, we are faced with a need for accurate assessment and monitoring of treatment results. The newest clinical research mention the benefit of using high frequency ultrasound in skin condition analysis. With the use of high frequency ultrasound it is possible to segment and then measure the hypoechoic band below the echo entry (subepidermal low echogenic band), characteristic for atopic dermatitis. In this study we developed a two-step methodology consisting of the region of interest detection and segmentation based on convolutional neural network with a U-net architecture. The accuracy of the proposed framework was verified using 47 clinical images annotated by an expert, yielding mean Dice index value of 0.86 ± 0.04 and mean error of the hypoechoic band thickness estimation at 12.0 ± 9.3 µm.

Keywords High frequency ultrasound · Atopic dermatitis · SLEB segmentation · Deep learning

J. Czajkowska (✉) · W. Dziurowicz · P. Badura
Faculty of Biomedical Engineering, Silesian University of Technology, Roosevelta 40, 41-800 Zabrze, Poland
e-mail: joanna.czajkowska@polsl.pl

W. Dziurowicz
e-mail: pawel.badura@polsl.pl

S. Korzekwa
Division of Prosthodontics, Department of Temporomandibular Disorders, Poznan University of Medical Sciences, Poznań, Poland
e-mail: korzekwas@gmail.com

E. Piętka et al. (eds.), *Information Technology in Biomedicine*, Advances in Intelligent Systems and Computing 1186, https://doi.org/10.1007/978-3-030-49666-1_1

3

1   Introduction

Atopic dermatitis (AD) is nowadays most common eczema type. It is a chronic, pruritic, recurrent, inflammatory cutaneous disease, which mainly occurs in children (60% of all cases begin in the first year of life, and 90%—before the age of 5), with a tendency to regress during childhood (60–90% up to 15th year of life) [21]. It may persist in a chronic, recurrent course until adulthood. It is often resistant to any treatment strategy [9] coexisting with other IgE dependent atopic diseases. As reported in [7, 15] AD is the result of complex genetic, epigenetic, environmental and immunological interactions, coexisting with an epidermal barrier defect. The number of AD incidences increases worldwide and there is a lack of standardization of diagnostic criteria. Therefore, we are faced with a need for accurate assessment and monitoring of treatment results [9, 20]. There is no existing laboratory test which would determine the severity of the disease. An invasive skin biopsy does not show any specific histological characteristics either. The applied scoring indicators require subjective judgment and the result reproducibility seems to be poor [2]. The newest clinical research mention the benefit of using high frequency ultrasound (HFUS) to image inflammation of the skin [4]. A characteristic ultrasound feature of inflammatory dermatoses is the presence of a subepidermal low echogenic band (SLEB) below echo entry. It may represent an acute inflammatory process with an edema or infiltration of the upper dermis [1, 5]. Improvement of inflammatory skin conditions may be visualized as a decrease of the thickness of SLEB and an increase in the intensity of the dermis image [13]. There is a strong correlation between HFUS and histological features in the assessment of AD [13].

Ultrasound is defined as mechanical density waves with a frequency above 20 kHz, which represents the upper limit of human hearing frequency. As the frequency increases, the depth of penetration of ultrasonic waves decreases; for example, ultrasonic units using only 20 MHz penetrate up to 15 mm [16]. Due to the HFUS applications described above for imaging the epidermal barrier, the frequencies used in the present study allow for a visualisation of those areas with a higher resolution, allowing for measurements of the epidermis, at lower frequencies treated as an echo entry. The depth of penetration into the skin (4–6 mm of the 75 MHz applicator) is sufficient for the imaging of the epidermis, dermis, subcutaneous tissue and subcutaneous fat [16] (Fig. 1).

As HFUS gains popularity in dermatological diagnosis [5, 12, 13], more HFUS image processing methods are being developed [3, 4, 6, 17, 19]. For skin layers segmentation, active contours are the most commonly used technique [11, 19]. Active contours implemented to segment cancerous tumors in HFUS images [18] allowed achieving the Dice index value of 0.79. The active contour model described in [4] results in Dice index equal to 0.87 in SLEB segmentation. The algorithm described in [19] resulted in Dice index of 0.93 for dermis and epidermis segmentation, however the SLEB segmentation results have not been reported there. The use of convolutionary neural network (U-Net model) for psoriasis segmentation in skin biopsy images is described in [10]. The mean accuracy, estimated using Jaccard index in the best

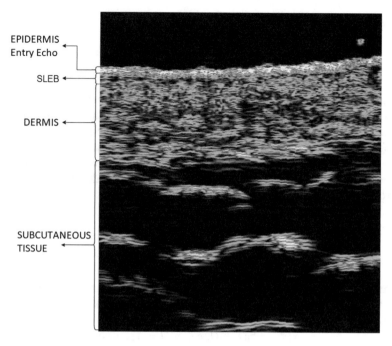

EPIDERMIS
Entry Echo

SLEB

DERMIS

SUBCUTANEOUS
TISSUE

Fig. 1 Illustration of skin layers in a HFUS image

case of dermis segmentation was equal to 0.77 and 0.78 for epidermis area. However the analysed there histopathological images significantly differ from the analysed HFUS data.

To meet the requirements for HFUS image analysis, the developed methodology is addressed at 75 MHz US image segmentation. This approach makes it possible to segment SLEB in an accurate and robust manner. The algorithm consists of two fully-automated steps: (1) region of interest (ROI) detection and (2) SLEB segmentation. The ROI detection algorithm makes it possible to divide the images into smaller sub-images and extract the image areas, which are then used as input data for the segmentation stage. The developed segmentation method employs the convolutional neural network (CNN) with the U-net architecture, which enables fast and accurate image segmentation [14]. The analysed data set consisted of 47 HFUS (75 MHz) annotated images of patients with diagnosed AD. The data set was randomly divided into training and testing subsets with a 3:1 ratio and the experiment was repeated 3 times. The obtained segmentation masks were compared to expert delineations using Dice index with a mean value of 0.86±0.04.

The paper is organized as follows. The developed methodology, divided into ROI detection and segmentation part is described in Sect. 2, followed by the experiments and obtained results presentation in Sect. 3. Section 4 summarizes the paper.

2   Materials and Methods

2.1   Region of Interest Detection

The automated SLEB segmentation in HFUS images starts with the ROI detection. The algorithm based on [4] detects the entry echo area. The detection algorithm uses an image $I = R + B$ as an input, being a linear combination of red (R) and blue (B) channels of the analysed chromatic HFUS scan of the $N \times M$ size, stored in the RGB format. First, the image I is partitioned into smaller non-overlapping sub-images of a width a (set up to 20). Then, a matrix I_m is determined, containing horizontal average of intensities within each sub-image of I:

$$I_m(i, d) = \sum_{j=1+a(d-1)}^{a+a(d-1)} \frac{I(i, j)}{a},$$ (1)

where $i = 1, \ldots, N, d = 1, \ldots, \lceil \frac{M}{a} \rceil$. I_m is analysed in a column-wise manner yielding a vector $\mathbf{x}$ containing indices of rows numbers with maximal elements in each column d in I_m:

$$\mathbf{x}(d) = \max_i I_m(i, d), \qquad i = 1, \ldots, N.$$ (2)

Finally, vector $\mathbf{x}$ is subjected to a smoothing median filtering with a window width of 11, yielding vector $\mathbf{x}'$. $\mathbf{x}'$ approximates the epidermis area throughout sub-images of a, and after back-interpolation—throughout the image I (Fig. 2).

With a given epidermis area, the image is partitioned into 100 ROIs of a 201×351 pixel size each, evenly spread from left-to-right and vertically centered along the detected line.

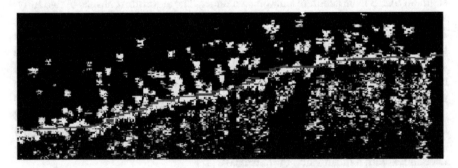

Fig. 2 Illustration of the entry echo area detection results (cropped image)

2.2 SLEB Segmentation

For the SLEB segmentation a fully convolutional neural network is applied [8, 14]. Thanks to their advantages in image recognition CNNs are now commonly introduced in many applications [22, 23], and also used for various image segmentation tasks [14]. Here, a U-Net [14] architecture is incorporated. It is based on a fully convolutional network described in [8] and modified to work with small training set [14]. The applied network consists of 2×4.5 blocks of layers, forming a characteristic U-shaped structure with a downsampling path on the left and an upsampling path on the right side (Fig. 3).

The network requires a 256×256 chromatic image as an input, so each ROI as described in Sect. 2.1 is resized using linear interpolation. Each full block in the

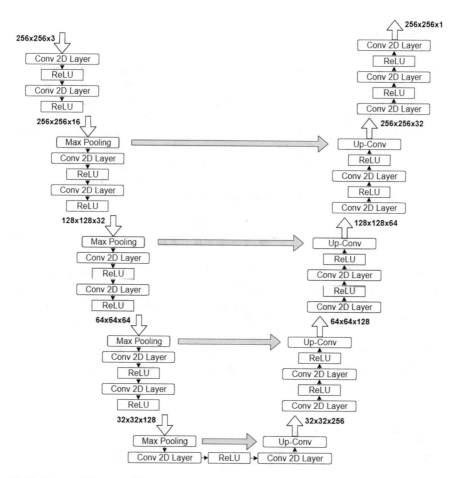

Fig. 3 U-net architecture of the segmentation network

downsampling path consists of two convolutional layers, each followed by a rectified linear unit (ReLU). The max pooling layer with a 2×2 pool size and stride connects each two blocks. The number of filters in each block doubles (starting with 16 in the first block), therefore the smallest feature map in the 4.5th block has a 16×16 size in 128 channels. In the upsampling block the feature map is processed using two convolutional layers with a ReLU, followed by a transverse concatenation with the feature map from corresponding downsampling block and transposed convolution a 2×2 stride. In the final layer a 1×1 convolution is used to map each feature vector to the desired number of classes (2). At the network output, a label matrix with the size of the input image is obtained as a result of a softmax operation and pixel classification. The adaptive moment estimation optimizer (ADAM) was used for training with the initial learning rate at 0.001.

3 Results

The HFUS images analysed in this study were acquired using a digital ultrasonic DUB Skinscanner (tpm GmbH, Germany) with a 75 MHz linear mechanical probe scanning depth of 4 mm and image resolution of 2067×1555 pixels. All the 47 images were delineated by an expert prior to network training and validation. The dataset was randomly divided into training (35 cases) and testing (12 cases) data. The experiment was repeated 3 times. Each analysed image (training or testing) was divided into 100 sub-images according to the ROI detection algorithm described in Sect. 2.1. It resulted in 3500 training and 1200 testing sub-images in each experiment.

The obtained segmentation results were verified using Dice index DI:

$$DI = \frac{2\cdot TP}{2\cdot TP + FP + FN},\tag{3}$$

where TP, FP, FN denote the number of true positive, false positive, and false negative pixels, respectively. The mean Dice index values for the set of 12 test images, 100 sub-mages each, are collected in Table 1. The maximum Dice index value was equal to 0.92, whereas the mean Dice index over all experiments was equal to 0.86 ± 0.04.

We also measured the segmentation error in terms of the mean absolute difference Δ_{th} between the SLEB thickness obtained using our segmentation framework and provided by the expert delineation:

Table 1 SLEB segmentation efficiency summary

Case	1	2	3	4	5	6	7	8	9	10	11	12	**Mean**
DI	0.85	0.83	0.81	0.86	0.89	0.85	0.89	0.90	0.82	0.92	0.90	0.78	**0.86±0.04**

Table 2 SLEB thickness errors

Case	1	2	3	4	5	6	7	8	9	10	11	12	**Mean**
Δ_{th} (μm)	4.3	5.2	5.4	11.6	14.1	4.4	29.9	15.4	2.7	9.1	12.7	29.8	**12.0±9.3**
δ_{th} (%)	7.3	15.4	10.2	4.6	11.6	5.7	11.7	12.7	1.2	8.9	7.6	27.2	**10.3±6.7**

$$\Delta_{th} = \left| \overline{th_s} - \overline{th_e} \right|, \tag{4}$$

where $\overline{th_s}$, $\overline{th_e}$ denote the mean SLEB thickness within the segmentation result and expert delineation, respectively. Obtained results are presented in Table 2 along with the relative SLEB thickness error δ_{th}:

$$\delta_{th} = \frac{\Delta_{th}}{\overline{th_e}} \cdot 100\%. \tag{5}$$

Exemplary segmentation results compared with the expert masks are shown in Fig. 4. The obtained segmentation metrics are comparable to the segmentation results described in [4], where the mean DI value for SLEB segmentation was equal to 0.87 (for 45 HFUS images). Moreover, in case of the developed algorithm, the future extension of the database could improve the obtained results and the tool reliability.

4 Conclusion

The paper presents a novel HFUS image segmentation technique. The study targets in subepidermal low echogenic band segmentation, which is typical for atopic dermatitis. The developed methodology is divided into two parts targeting in region of interest detection and SLEB segmentation. The dataset contains 47 HFUS images acquired using the 75 MHz linear mechanical US probe. The obtained segmentation results were compared with expert delineation resulting with mean Dice index equal to 0.86±0.04, what is comparable with the segmentation results described in literature. Moreover, the network architecture makes it possible to extend the dataset in the future, resulting in better accuracy.

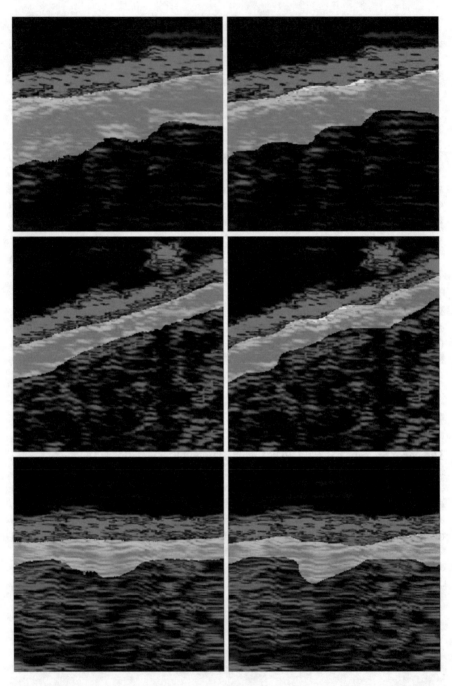

Fig. 4 Final SLEB segmentation results in three different cases of full test images (rows 1–3): left—fully automated segmentation result, right—expert mask; SLEB region indicated by brightened area

Acknowledgements This research is supported by the Polish National Science Centre (NCN) grant No.: 2016/21/B/ST7/02236. The funders had no role in study design, data collection and analysis, decision to publish, or preparation of the manuscript.

References

1. Borut, G., Jemec, E., Gniadecka, M., Ulrich, J.: Ultrasound in dermatology. Part I. High frequency ultrasound. Eur. J. Dermatol. **10**(6), 492–497 (2000)
2. Charman, C., Venn, A., Williams, H.: Measurement of body surface area involvement in atopic eczema: an impossible task? Br. J. Dermatol. **140**(1), 109–111 (1999). https://doi.org/10.1046/j.1365-2133.1999.02617.x
3. Czajkowska, J., Badura, P.: Automated epidermis segmentation in ultrasound skin images. In: Innovations in Biomedical Engineering, Advances in Intelligent Systems and Computing, vol. 925, pp. 3–11 (2019). https://doi.org/10.1007/978-3-030-15472-1_1
4. Czajkowska, J., Korzekwa, S., Pietka, E.: Computer aided diagnosis of atopic dermatitis. Comput. Med. Imaging Graph. **79**, 101,676 (2020). https://doi.org/10.1016/j.compmedimag.2019.101676
5. Danczak-Pazdrowska, A., Polanska, A., Silny, W., Sadowska, A., Osmola-Mankowska, A., Czarnecka-Operacz, M., Zaba, R., Jenerowicz, D.: Seemingly healthy skin in atopic dermatitis: observations with the use of high-frequency ultrasonography, preliminary study. Skin Res. Technol. **18**(2), 162–167 (2012). https://doi.org/10.1111/j.1600-0846.2011.00548.x
6. Gao, Y., Tannenbaum, A., Chen, H., Torres, M., Yoshida, E., Yang, X., Wang, Y., Curran, W., Liu, T.: Automated skin segmentation in ultrasonic evaluation of skin toxicity in breast cancer radiotherapy. Ultrasound Med. Biol. **39**(11), 2166–2175 (2013). https://doi.org/10.1016/j.ultrasmedbio.2013.04.006
7. Garmhausen, D., Hagemann, T., Bieber, T., Dimitriou, I., Fimmers, R., Diepgen, T., Novak, N.: Characterization of different courses of atopic dermatitis in adolescent and adult patients. Allergy **68**(4), 498–506 (2013). https://doi.org/10.1111/all.12112
8. Long, J., Shelhamer, E., Darrell, T.: Fully convolutional networks for semantic segmentation. In: 2015 IEEE Conference on Computer Vision and Pattern Recognition (CVPR), pp. 3431–3440 (2015). https://doi.org/10.1109/CVPR.2015.7298965
9. Napolitano, M., Megna, M., Patruno, C., Gisondi, P., Ayala, F., Balato, N.: Adult atopic dermatitis: a review. G Ital. Dermatol. Venereol. **151**(4), 403–411 (2016)
10. Pal, A., Garain, U., Chandra, A., Chatterjee, R., Senapati, S.: Psoriasis skin biopsy image segmentation using deep convolutional neural network. Comput. Meth. Programs Biomed. **159**, 59–69 (2018). https://doi.org/10.1016/j.cmpb.2018.01.027
11. Pereyra, M., Dobigeon, N., Batatia, H., Tourneret, J.: Segmentation of skin lesions in 2-D and 3-D ultrasound images using a spatially coherent generalized rayleigh mixture model. IEEE Trans. Med. Imaging **31**(8), 1509–1520 (2012). https://doi.org/10.1109/TMI.2012.2190617
12. Polańska, A., Dańczak-Pazdrowska, A., Jałowska, M., Żaba, R., Adamski, Z.: Current applications of high-frequency ultrasonography in dermatology. Adv. Dermatol. Allergol. **34**(6), 535–542 (2017). https://doi.org/10.5114/ada.2017.72457
13. Polanska, A., Danczak-Pazdrowska, A., Silny, W., Wozniak, A., Maksin, K., Jenerowicz, D., Janicka-Jedynska, M.: Comparison between high-frequency ultrasonography (dermascan c, version 3) and histopathology in atopic dermatitis. Skin Res. Technol. **19**(4), 432–437 (2013). https://doi.org/10.1111/srt.12064
14. Ronneberger, O., Fischer, P., Brox, T.: U-net: Convolutional networks for biomedical image segmentation. In: Navab, N., Hornegger, J., Wells, W.M., Frangi, A.F. (eds.) Medical Image Computing and Computer-Assisted Intervention—MICCAI 2015, pp. 234–241. Springer International Publishing, Cham (2015)

15. Schlapbach, C., Simon, D.: Update on skin allergy. Allergy **69**(12), 1571–1581 (2014). https://doi.org/10.1111/all.12529
16. Schmid, W., Monika, H., Burgdorf, W.: Ultrasound scanning in dermatology. Arch. Dermatol. **141**(2), 217–224 (2005). https://doi.org/10.1001/archderm.141.2.217
17. Sciolla, B., Ceccato, P., Cowell, L., Dambry, T., Guibert, B., Delachartre, P.: Segmentation of inhomogeneous skin tissues in high-frequency 3D ultrasound images, the advantage of non-parametric log-likelihood methods. Phys. Proc. **70**, 1177–1180 (2015). https://doi.org/10.1016/j.phpro.2015.08.253. Proceedings of the 2015 ICU International Congress on Ultrasonics, Metz, France
18. Sciolla, B., Cowell, L., Dambry, T., Guibert, B., Delachartre, P.: Segmentation of skin tumors in high-frequency 3-D ultrasound images. Ultrasound Med. Biol. **43**(1), 227–238 (2017). https://doi.org/10.1016/j.ultrasmedbio.2016.08.029
19. Sciolla, B., Digabel, J.L., Josse, G., Dambry, T., Guibert, B., Delachartre, P.: Joint segmentation and characterization of the dermis in 50 MHz ultrasound 2D and 3D images of the skin. Comput. Biol. Med. **103**, 277–286 (2018). https://doi.org/10.1016/j.compbiomed.2018.10.029
20. Silvestre Salvador, J., Romero-Perez, D., Encabo-Duran, B.: Atopic dermatitis in adults: a diagnostic challenge. J. Investig. Allergol. Clin. Immunol. **27**(2), 78–88 (2017). https://doi.org/10.18176/jiaci.0138
21. Spergel, J.M.: From atopic dermatitis to asthma: the atopic march. Ann. Allergy Asthma Immunol. **105**(2), 99–106 (2010). https://doi.org/10.1016/j.anai.2009.10.002
22. Zhang, X., Xiong, H., Zhou, W., Lin, W., Tian, Q.: Picking deep filter responses for fine-grained image recognition. In: The IEEE Conference on Computer Vision and Pattern Recognition (CVPR) (2016)
23. Zheng, H., Fu, J., Mei, T., Luo, J.: Learning multi-attention convolutional neural network for fine-grained image recognition. In: The IEEE International Conference on Computer Vision (ICCV) (2017)

A Review of Clustering Methods in Microorganism Image Analysis

Chen Li, Frank Kulwa, Jinghua Zhang, Zihan Li, Hao Xu, and Xin Zhao

Abstract Clustering plays a great role in microorganism image segmentation, feature extraction and classification, in all major application areas of microorganisms (medical, environmental, industrial, science and agriculture). Clustering methods are used for many years in microorganism image processing because they are simple algorithms, easy to apply and efficient. Thus, in order to clarify the potential of different clustering techniques in different application domains of microorganisms, we survey related works from the 1990s till now, while pinning out the specific challenges on each work (area) with the corresponding suitable clustering algorithm.

Keywords Microorganism image · Unsupervised learning · Image clustering · Feature extraction · Image segmentation

C. Li · F. Kulwa · J. Zhang · Z. Li · H. Xu
Microscopic Image and Medical Image Analysis Group, MBIE College, Northeastern University, Shenyang, China
e-mail: lichen201096@hotmail.com

F. Kulwa
e-mail: frank.kulwa@gmail.com

J. Zhang
e-mail: zhangjingh@foxmail.com

Z. Li
e-mail: 531801723@qq.com

H. Xu
e-mail: 154617829@qq.com

X. Zhao (✉)
Environmental Engineering, Northeastern University, Shenyang, China
e-mail: zhaoxin@mail.neu.edu.cn

E. Piętka et al. (eds.), *Information Technology in Biomedicine*, Advances in Intelligent Systems and Computing 1186, https://doi.org/10.1007/978-3-030-49666-1_2

1 Introduction

Microorganisms are very small living organisms which can appear as unicellular, multicellular and acellular types [20]. Some are beneficial and others are harmful to human [17]. Therefore, a depth understanding of microorganisms and their living habitat is of paramount importance, so as to leverage the beneficial ones. Microorganisms find roles in many areas such as agriculture [2], food [14], environments [34], industries [27], medical [12], water-borne [21] and science [7]. Figure 1. shows example of microorganisms in different application areas. In recent years, automatic image techniques have been used in identification, classification, segmentation and analysis of microorganisms, due to their advantage over traditional ways such as being consistent, accurate, fast and realiable [13, 19, 38].

Clustering methods plays an important role in microorganism image tracking, monitoring, segmentation, feature extraction and classification [8, 15]. Clustering methods are very useful in all microorganism application areas, because they are suitable in many image challeges such as uneven background noise on images [36]. Moreover, they are unsupervised or semi-supervised, and capable of capturing correlation between multiple objects in the image depending on subjected constraints (features) [9]. Clustering is the process of automatically classifying image dataset into a number of disjoint groups or clusters [37].

Because of the role and advantage of clustering methods in image (data) correlation and mining, a countable number of researches have been done on microorganisms using clustering methods, in all application areas of microorganisms (medical, industrial, water-bone, agriculture, food, environmental and science) [3, 11, 18]. Thus, in order to give light to upcoming researchers, we write this review on application and importance of clustering techniques in microorganisms image segmentation, in all application areas. The general development trend of clustering methods on segmentation of microorganisms since 1995 is given in Fig. 2.

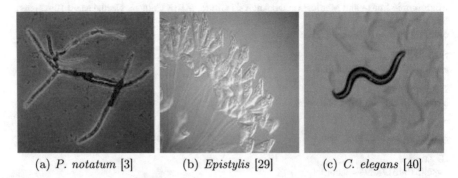

(a) *P. notatum* [3]   (b) *Epistylis* [29]   (c) *C. elegans* [40]

Fig. 1 Example of microorganisms (**a**) industrial microorganism used for fermentation, (**b**) water-borne microorganisms for water quality monitoring, (**c**) for biological genome studies

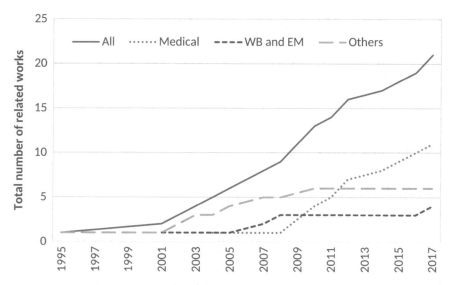

Fig. 2 The general trend on the use of image clustering techniques on different microorganisms application areas. Medical: indicates trend of clustering in medical microorganisms, "WB" and "EM" indicates water-borne and environmental microorganisms, and "Others" include agricultural, food, industrial and science microorganisms

Different microorganisms within their application areas have different clustering challenges which might not be the same in other areas but common within. In order to help the reader grasp which particular technique is suitable in particular microorganism application area, we categorize reviewed works into different application areas of microorganisms (medical, industrial, water-bone, agriculture, food, environmental and science).

To the best of our knowledge, there is no survey work which has been done particularly on clustering of microorganisms. Thus, we attempt to fill this gap by review of related works from the 1990s till now. This review is structured as follows, Sect. 2 discusses clustering works in medical area and a brief summary is given at the end. In Sect. 3, clustering works in environmental and water-borne microorganisms are well described. Section 4 gives detailed elaboration of clustering works in other application areas of microorganisms, with a brief summary at the end. Finally, Sect. 5 gives a general summary of clustering methods, and highlights common challenges in clustering works and the corresponding clustering techniques for remedy. Lastly, a short conclusion is also given in this section.

2 Clustering of Medical Microorganisms

Related works on application of clustering methods in medical microorganisms are discussed below and a brief summary on the most prominent techniques is given at the end.

2.1 Related Works

A semi-automatic clustering based segmentation scheme for multi-colour bacteria from images containing noisy background is proposed in [35]. Since the pixels of the foreground have variable colours, for perfect segmentation the RGB color separation is done first, then each channel is converted to gray image and finally segmented separately using adaptive neighbourhood similarity comparison clustering algorithm. In the experiments, 16 RGB images containing different kind of bacteria are used. The final segmentation accuracy of 96.70% is achieved.

In [30, 31], for automatic diagnosis of TB from tissue, a segmentation algorithm is designed, which uses k-means to cluster C-Y colour mode images. k-means separate the TB bacilli which normally occupy the higher saturation value, from the background pixels with the lower saturation value. Then to remove noise the 5×5 median filter is applied, followed by region growing to get the final segmented image. During experiment 100 RGB images of pixel size 600×800 are used. The results after each step during segmentation are shown in Fig. 3. Moreover, the segmentation results above are used in extraction of Zemike moments features in [28], then used in hybrid multi-layered perception network for classification TB or non-TB images. The final classification accuracy of 97.58% is achieved.

In [11], a clustering based algorithm for segmentation of *Plasmodium vivax* is presented, where RGB to CMYk color conversion is performed and only C channel is selected as it is found to give better presentation of the parasite in blood smear. After filtering, the images are segmented by modified fuzzy divergence clustering method which is based on Cauchy membership function. Finally, RGB color reconstruction

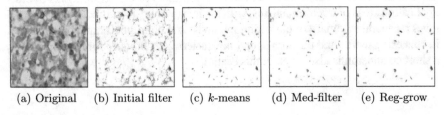

    (a) Original   (b) Initial filter   (c) k-means   (d) Med-filter   (e) Reg-grow

Fig. 3 Visual results after each segmentation step: (**a**) Original image, (**b**) result of initial filtering, (**c**) result of k-means, (**d**) result of median filter, (**e**) result of seed region growing [31]

is performed to get the segmented RGB image. 150 RGB images with a 2048 × 1536 pixel size are used for experiments.

In [5], an algorithm is designed for quantification of medical microorganisms. Bacteria images stained as positive gram and negative gram, are binarized using histogram thresholding, then free chain contour algorithm is applied for edge detection. Then the images are subjected to feature extraction in which 81 features are extracted. Finally, these features are used for clustering the images into two classes using k-means and self-organizing maps (SOM). The results show that SOM outperforms k-means by having lower clustering quality value because of its ability to embed the clusters in a low dimensional space right from the beginning and proceeds in a way that places related clusters close together. 500 RGB images are used during experiments. Cluster parameters, such as compactness, intra-cluster homogeneity and inter cluster separation, are used to get insight to the severity of disease during medical examination.

In [29], a comparison of performance between clustering and thresholding techniques on images containing TB bacilli from tissue is presented. First, RGB images are converted to C-Y colour mode, then the saturation component is used as input to all algorithms which are k-means, moving k-means, fuzzy c-means, and two adaptive thresholding algorithms, Otsu and iterative thresholding. During experiments 100 RGB captured from tissue containing TB bacilli are used for segmentation. The results show k-means outperforms with an accuracy of 99.49%.

In order to automate the promastigote parasite detection, from low contrast fluorescent images, an algorithm is proposed in [32]. Due to the capability of k-means to distinguish classes of data within low contrast images. It used to separate pixels into three classes ($k = 3$) from the fluorescent colour images. The resulted image which is having foreground, background and noise is subjected to Otsu thresholding for binarization. Finally, the removal of noise is done using region-props operation. 40 2D RGB images, captured under fluorescent microscope containing the parasite are used for experiments. Comparing with fuzzy c-means, the proposed algorithm over performs with precision of 85.50%.

A segmentation system for tuberculosis bacteria is introduced in [36]. In order to avoid local minima problem during training, images are divided into small patches of equal size, then k-means clustering is applied on each patch. The segmented patches are stored in dictionary, then reconstructed to form the whole segmented image. During experiments 400 RGB images of size 640 × 360 pixels are used. The final segmentation result of 97.68% accuracy is achieved.

In [25], a system is presented for automatic diagnosis of malaria parasites from images of blood smear containing four species of plasmodium. Firstly, images are converted to Lab color space, then k-means is applied on **a–b** component to separate infected blood containing malaria parasites from uninfected. Then, morphological parasite features are extracted and applied to kNN classifier, to classify between infected and non-infected images, among 300 RGB images. Finally, the classification results above 90.00% sensitivity are achieved for each parasite (*Plasmodium falciparum, Plasmodium vivax, Plasmodium malariae* and *Plasmodium ovale*).

In [24], an automatic image processing system is proposed for fast analysis of bright field microscopic images of TB bacterium, from sputum samples. Due to its efficiency, robust to noise parameters (corrupted pixels), fuzzy local information c-means (FLICM) is applied for segmentation. Then Hu moments and SIFT features are extracted for classification using least square support vector machines (LSSVM). During experiments 299 images with pixel size of 512×512 are used. The segmentation accuracy of 95.10% is achieved by the proposed algorithm.

In order to segment poor contrast microscopic images of stained TB sputum sample images in [23]. An improved fuzzy local information c-means (IFLICM) clustering is used for segmentation. It is capable of combining both local spatial and gray level information in a fuzzy way to preserve robustness and noise insensitiveness. During experiments, 29 images of pixel size 512×512 are used for training while 70 images are used for testing. The final segmentation accuracy of 96.05% is achieved.

2.2 Summary

From the review above, fuzzy and k-means related techniques are the most frequently applied ones. This is due to the that they are simple algorithms to implement and their general functions are embedded in most programming (development) tools like Matlab and python. Detailed explanation of their technical advantages on different challenges in microorganisms image analysis are given in Sect. 5.

3   Clustering of Environmental and Water-Borne Microorganisms

Since environmental and water-borne microorganism fields are closely related, the related works in both areas are discussed below.

3.1 Related Works

In [1], due to the nature of bacterioplankton frequently to form communities, sub-grouping them seem to be promising level for idea analysis, thus an automatic tool is designed for clustering the samples containing bacteria and algae. First, images are converted into gray scale and smoothed by low pass filter with a 7×7 kernel, then a constant value of 1 is subtracted to remove small isolated areas within black background. To form clusters, regional maxima are detected as canters of subgroups

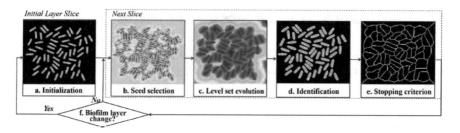

Fig. 4 Workflow for Bact-3D algorithm [41]

then borders between subgroups (clusters) are formed using watershed algorithm. During experiments, RGB images with a 256×256 pixel size are used.

To be able to segment bacterial cells in fluorescence in situ hybridization, which is subjected to inconsistent counting results when using thresholding techniques, a clustering approach is designed as a remedy in [42]. Due to its ability to give a percentage existence of one data into existing clusters, fuzzy c-means clustering is applied for segmentation. Each image from 15 images of pixel size 1388×1040, taken from soil and manure samples containing bacteria and archaea are binarized using entropy algorithm, then overlapping cells are separated using a watershed algorithm. Finally, morphological features are extracted and used for clustering. The count of cells is compared with manual results a and an accuracy of more than 90.00% is achieved.

In order to determine the biofilms structural growth characteristics from low resolution images under different external shear stresses in [22]. Firstly, spatial gray level dependence matrices (SGLDM) is applied on biofilm images for extraction of texture features, then 14 textural descriptors from each image are used to cluster biofilms into six growth phases, using k-means algorithm. During the experiments 5000 images are used.

A clustering algorithm capable of segmenting 3D images containing bacteria biofilms is introduced in [41], where each layer of 3D image is segmented differently using Bact-3D clustering algorithm then reconstruction of the segmented 3D volume is done to get the final segmented 3D image as shown in Fig. 4. During experiments 3D biofilm images are used, and a segmentation accuracy of 99.81% is achieved.

3.2 Summary

Due to the ability of clustering techniques to cluster data in unsupervised manner, they keep gaining more application in environmental and water-borne microorgansisms. A detailed explanation and a table showing the superiority of different clustering methods on specific segmentation challenges is given in Sect. 5.

4   Clustering of Microorganisms in Other Areas

Different related works in other microorganism application areas, such as agriculture, food, science and industry are discussed in this section.

4.1   Related Works

To assess the growth and differentiation of filamentous *Penicillium chrysogenum* in structured biofilm. An automatic image tool which can work on both monochrome and colour image is implemented in [39]. In one branch, binary image is formed using top-hat transform, in the other branch the same image is passed through watershed process to form lines of maxima local intensity, then binary and lined images are merged to form tessellation small areas on image. Finally, a fuzzy c-means (6-classes) is applied to cluster tessellation areas in segments which present morphological parts of the microorganisms. The experiments is done using 40 images (monochrome and colour images) of size 512×512 pixels. The results are compared with manual ground truth and an accuracy of more than 85.00% is achieved. Visual results at each stage are shown in Fig. 5.

To be able to assess similarities and differences of *C. elegans* mutants in [9, 10], firstly, the principal component analysis (PCA) is applied to find the pattern of selected features in the feature space graph. To find the optimal number of clusters within the data, gap statistics, information theoretic method and PCA are applied, then the k-means clustering is used to observed the correlation in classes of 8 mutants. It is observed that using $k = 6$, pairs of mutants which share close related features are grouped together while when $k = 8$, the discrimination between mutants increases. During experiments, 797 images from 8 mutants of *C.elegans* are used.

In [18], a clustering based model, self organising tree map (SOTM) neural network is investigated as a means of segmenting microorganisms from confocal microscopic images. From the extracted features, such as phase congruency, position and grey value. The significance of individual features on final results is investigated, and it

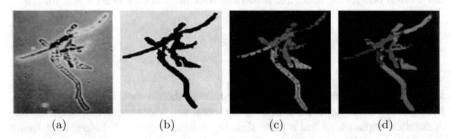

(a)   (b)   (c)   (d)

Fig. 5 Results of (**a**) original image, (**b**) top-hat transform, (**c**) tessellation small areas followed by colour matching, (**d**) fuzzy c-means clustering into 6-classes [39]

is proposed that, within the context of micro-biological image segmentation, better object delineation can be achieved if certain features are more dominant in the initial stages of learning.

The segmentation algorithms which are capable of segmenting multi-resolution images are proposed in [3]. Before application of multi-resolution border extraction for identification of individual clusters on the image, images are converted from RGB to HSV colour, then clustering is done using fuzzy c-means followed by self organising map (SOM) or learning vector quantization neural networks (LVQNN) to improve segmentation results. 15 images (which are taken at different resolution 512×512 and 256×256 pixel sizes) containing two types of biofilm of *E. coli* (ampicillin-resistant and an ampicillin-sensitive strain) are used during experiments. Finally, impressive visual segmentation results are obtained after experiments.

A segmentation system to identify individual *C. elgans* from clusters of worms is presented in [40], where clustering is performed first using local adaptive thresholding and morphological opening followed by watershed and extensive merging. Then probabilistic model, which is based on single worm to cluster area ratio and predefined path model, is applied to identify single worms from clusters. In the experiments, 56 images each containing approximately 15 worms are used.

4.2 Summary

Due to its capability to embed the clusters in low dimension right from the beggining of learning and being unsupervised, SOM gain uses in all microorganisms application areas. A more detailed analysis and a general application summary table are given in Sect. 5.

5 Methodology Analysis and Conclusion

Table 1 gives an overview and summary of different segmentation challenges in all reviewed works, the particular dataset, microorganisms application area and a suitable clustering technique for a particular challenge.

From Table 1, we can find that particular challenges on microorganism image analysis in different application areas, parallel with the suitable clustering technique for each challenge. It can be observed that, most challenges existing in microorganism images can get suitable solution for segmentation from clustering techniques. However, among the applied technique "fuzzy" related technique have been frequently used because of their ability to combine both local and gray level information in a fuzzy way which preserve robustness and noise insensitivity (which is exhibited by IFLICM) [23, 24]. Moreover, they have capability to segment images with no distinct histogram valleys between the classes [11] and they give percentage of

Table 1 The use of image clustering techniques on microorganisms application areas (APA), which are medical (MM), water-borne (WB), environmental (EM), industrial (IM), science (SM) and agriculture (AM), on specific microorganism type (MT)

Time	Author	Related Work	APA	MT	Clustering	
					Challenge	Technique
2004	R. Chandan	[35]	MM	Bacteria	Multicolored microbes with complex noisy background.	Adaptive neighbourhood similarity comparison algorithm
2010	M. Osman	[28, 30, 31]	MM	TB bacilli	Segmentation of TB bacteria from tissue images.	k-means clustering
2011	M. Ghosh	[11]	MM	*Plasmodium*	Low contras between foreground (microorganisms) and background	Modified fuzzy divergence
2012	M.Chayadevi	[5]	MM	Bacteria	Quantification of microorganisms (bacteria) for measuring severity of the disease	Self Organising Map (SOM)
2012	M. Osman	[29]	MM	TB bacilli	Segmentation of TB bacteria from tissue images	k-means clustering
2014	F. Ouertani	[32]	MM	*Leishmania*	Low contrast images	k-means clustering
2015	R. Rulaningtyas	[36]	MM	TB bacilli	Background noise on images due to uneven staining of samples.	Image patches and k-means clustering
2016	A. Nanoti	[25]	MM	*Plasmodium*	Low contrast image from blood smear	Lab color mode and k-means clustering
2017	K. Mithra	[24]	MM	TB bacilli	Bright field microscopic images of microorganisms	Fuzzy local information c-means (FLICM)
2017	K. Mithra	[23]	MM	TB bacilli	Low contrast stained microscopic images	Improved fuzzy local information c-means (IFLICM)
2001	S. Andreatta	[1]	WB	*P. notatum*	Analysis of bacterioplank in communities (bound in groups)	Watershed algorithm
2007	Z. Zhou	[42]	EM	Bacteria, *Archaea*	Overlapping bacteria	Watershed algorithm and fuzzy c-means clustering
2008	K. Milferstedt	[22]	WB	Bacteria	Identification of structural state of biofilm images using texture features	k-means clusterinng
2017	J. Wang	[41]	EM	Biofilm	3D multi-layered high resolution images of biofilm	Batch-3D algorithm

(continued)

Table 1 (continued)

Time	Author	Related Work	APA	MT	Clustering Challenge	Technique
1995	B. Vanhoutte	[39]	IM	*P. notatum*	Structural assessment of filamentious fungi in structured biofilm	Fuzzy *c*-means clustering
2003	W. Geng	[9, 10]	SM	*C. elegans*	Differences and similarities between groups of microorganisms (grouped data)	*k*-means clusterinng
2003	W. Geng	[10]	SM	*C. elegans*	Identification of behavioural pattern of multidimentional data (features)	Principle component analysis (PCA)
2005	K. Matthew	[18]	AM	Biofilm	Confocal microscopic images	Self Organising Tree Map (SOTM)
2007	S. Belkasim	[3]	SM	*E. coli*	Multi-resolution images	Fuzzy *c*-means clustering and SOM
2010	C. Wählby	[40]	SM	*C. elegans*	Clustering of overlapping microoganisms	Thresholding and watershed algorithms

existence of data into existing clusters which is perfect for confident classification (clustering) [42].

k-means and self organising map (SOM) have also been used in most of the reviewed works. This is due to the capability of *k*-means algorithm to discriminate data classes in the low contrast images [32]. Moreover they are simple to use and ready made function of *k*-means can be found in most of pragrammming tools such as matlab and python [4, 33]. The frequent use of SOM is due to the ability of SOM to embed the clusters in low dimensional space right from the beginning and proceeds in a way that places related classes of data close together.

All the aforementioned properties of the clustering techniques make them suitable for most of image segmentation and classification challenges found in all microorganisms application areas. Conclusively, due to their capability, the clustering techniques cannot only be suitable in segmentation of microorganisms but also in other areas which share similar challenges, such as sperm cells image classification and segmentation.

Acknowledgements We thank the "National Natural Science Foundation of China" No. 61806047 and the "Fundamental Research Funds for the Central Universities" No. N2019003. We thank B.Sc. Frank Kulwa, due to his contribution is considered as important as the first author in this paper. We also tank Miss Zixian Li and Mr. Guoxian Li, for their important advice and discussion.

References

1. Andreatta, S., Wallinger, M., Posch, T., Psenner, R.: Detection of subgroups from flow cytometry measurements of heterotrophic bacterioplankton by image analysis. Cytometry: J. Int. Soc. Anal. Cytol. **44**(3), 218–225 (2001)
2. Bagyaraj, D., Rangaswami, G.: Agricultural microbiology (2007)
3. Belkasim, S., Derado, G., Aznita, R., et al.: Multiresolution border segmentation for measuring spatial heterogeneity of mixed population biofilm bacteria. Comput. Med. Imaging Graph. **32**(1), 11–16 (2008)
4. Blanchet, G., Charbit, M.: Digital Signal and Image Processing Using MATLAB, vol. 4. Wiley, Hoboken (2006)
5. Chayadevi, M., Raju, G.: Data mining, classification and clustering with morphological features of microbes. Int. J. Comput. Appl. **52**(4), 1–5 (2012)
6. Chew, Y., Walker, D., Towlson, E., et al.: Recordings of caenorhabditis elegans locomotor behaviour following targeted ablation of single motorneurons. Sci. Data **4**, 170156 (2017)
7. Fields, S., Johnston, M.: Whither model organism research? Science **307**(5717), 1885–1886 (2005)
8. Forero, M., Sroubek, F., Cristobal, G.: Identification of tuberculosis bacteria based on shape and color. Real-time Imaging **10**(4), 251–262 (2004)
9. Geng, W., Cosman, P., Baek J., et al.: Image feature extraction and natural clustering of worm body shapes and motion characteristics. In: Proceedings of IAESTED, pp. 342–347 (2003)
10. Geng, W., Cosman, P., Baek, J., et al.: Quantitative classification and natural clustering of caenorhabditis elegans behavioral phenotypes. Genetics **165**(3), 1117–1126 (2003)
11. Ghosh, M., Das, D., Chakraborty, C., Ray, A.: Plasmodium vivax segmentation using modified fuzzy divergence. In: Proceedings of the ICIIP, pp. 1–5 (2011)
12. Gillespie, S., Bamford, K.: Medical Microbiology and Infection at a Glance (2012)
13. Haryanto, S., Mashor, M., Nasir, A., Jaafar, H.: A fast and accurate detection of schizont plasmodium falciparum using channel color space segmentation method. In: Proceedings of the CITSM, pp. 1–4 (2017)
14. Jay, J., Loessner, M., Golden, D.: Modern Food Microbiology (2008)
15. Koren, Y., Sznitman, R., Arratia, P., et al.: Model-independent Phenotyping of *C. elegans* locomotion using scale-invariant feature transform. PLoS One **10**(3), e0122326 (2015)
16. Kosov, S., Shirahama, K., Li, C., Grzegorzek, M.: Environmental microorganism classification using conditional random fields and deep convolutional neural networks. Patt. Recogn. **77**, 248–261 (2018)
17. Kulwa, F., Li, C., Zhao, X., et al.: A state-of-the-art survey for microorganism image segmentation method and future potential. IEEE Access **7**, 100243–100269 (2019)
18. Kyan, M., Guan, L., Liss, S.: Refining competition in the self organising tree map for unsupervised biofilm image segmentation. Neural Netw. **18**(5–6), 850–860 (2005)
19. Li, C., Wang, K., Xu, N.: A survey for the applications of content-based microscopic image analysis in microorganism classification domains. Artif. Intell. Rev. **51**(4), 577–646 (2019)
20. Madigan, M., Martinko, J., Parker, J., et al.: Brock Biology of Microorganisms, vol. 11. Pearson Education, London (1997)
21. Mara, D., Horan, N.J.: Handbook of Water and Wastewater Microbiology (2003)
22. Milferstedt, K., Pons, M., Morgenroth, E.: Textural fingerprints: a comprehensive descriptor for biofilm structure development. Biotechnol. Bioeng. **100**(5), 889–901 (2008)
23. Mithra, K., Emmanuel, W.: An efficient approach to sputum image segmentation using improved fuzzy local information c-means clustering algorithm for tuberculosis diagnosis. In: Proceedings of the of ICICI, pp. 126–130 (2017)
24. Mithra, K., Emmanuel, W.: Segmentation and classification of mycobacterium from ziehl neelsen stained sputum images for tuberculosis diagnosis. In: Proceedings of the ICCSP, pp. 1672–1676 (2017)

25. Nanoti, A., Jain, S., Gupta, C., Vyas, G.: Detection of malaria parasite species and life cycle stages using microscopic images of thin blood smear. In: Proceedings of the ICICT, pp. 1–6 (2016)
26. Nasir, A., Mashor, M., Mohamed, Z.: Segmentation based approach for detection of malaria parasites using moving k-means clustering. In: Proceedings of the IEEE-EMBS, pp. 653–658 (2012)
27. Okafor, N.: Modern Industrial Microbiology and Biotechnology. Enfield, New Hampshire (2007)
28. Osman, M., Mashor, M., Jaafar, H.: Detection of mycobacterium tuberculosis in ziehl-neelsen stained tissue images using zernike moments and hybrid multilayered perceptron network. In: Proceedings of the of ICSMC, pp. 4049–4055 (2010)
29. Osman, M., Mashor, M., Jaafar, H.: Performance comparison of clustering and thresholding algorithms for tuberculosis bacilli segmentation. In: Proceedings of the CITS, pp. 1–5 (2012)
30. Osman, M., Mashor, M., Saad, Z., Jaafar, H.: Colour image segmentation of tuberculosis bacilli in ziehl-neelsen-stained tissue images using moving k-means clustering procedure. In: Proceedings of the AICM/AMCS, pp. 215–220 (2010)
31. Osman, M., Mashor, M., Saad, Z., Jaafar, H.: Segmentation of tuberculosis bacilli in ziehl-neelsen-stained tissue images based on k-means clustering procedure. In: Proceedings of the ICIAS, pp. 1–6 (2010)
32. Ouertani, F., Amiri, H. Bettaib J. et al.: Adaptive automatic segmentation of leishmaniasis parasite in indirect immunofluorescence images. In: Proceedings of the EMBC 2014, pp. 4731–4734 (2014)
33. Pedregosa, F., Varoquaux, G., Gramfort, A., et al.: Scikit-learn: Machine learning in Python. J. Mach. Learn. Res. **12**, 2825–2830 (2011)
34. Pepper, I., Gerba, C.: Aeromicrobiology. Environ. Microbiol. **2015**, 89–110 (2015)
35. Reddy, C., Dazzo, F.: Computer-assisted segmentation of bacteria in color micrographs. Microsc. Anal. **18**, 5–8 (2004)
36. Rulaningtyas, R., Suksmono, A., Mengko, T., Saptawati, P.: Multi patch approach in k-means clustering method for color image segmentation in pulmonary tuberculosis identification. In: Proceedings of the ICICI-BME, pp. 75–78 (2015)
37. Sathya, B., Manavalan, R.: Image segmentation by clustering methods: performance analysis. Int. J. Comput. Appl. **29**(11), 27–32 (2011)
38. Sieracki, M., Reichenbach, S., Webb, K.: Evaluation of automated threshold selection methods for accurately sizing microscopic fluorescent cells by image analysis. Appl. Environ. Microbiol. **55**(11), 2762–2772 (1989)
39. Vanhoutte, B., Pons, M., Thomas, C., et al.: Characterization of penicillium chrysogenum physiology in submerged cultures by color and monochrome image analysis. Biotechnol. Bioeng. **48**(1), 1–11 (1995)
40. C. Waehlby, T. Riklin-Raviv, V. Ljosa and et al. Resolving Clustered Worms via Probabilistic Shape Models. In: Proc. of ISBI, 2010, pp. 552–555
41. Wang, J., Sarkar, R., Aziz, A., et al.: Bact-3D: A level set segmentation approach for dense multi-layered 3d bacterial biofilms. In: Proceedings of the ICIP, pp. 330–334 (2017)
42. Zhou, Z., Pons, M., Raskin, L., Zilles, J.: Automated image analysis for quantitative fluorescence in situ hybridization with environmental samples. Appl. Environ. Microbiol. **73**(9), 2956–2962 (2007)

MRFU-Net: A Multiple Receptive Field U-Net for Environmental Microorganism Image Segmentation

Chen Li, Jinghua Zhang, Xin Zhao, Frank Kulwa, Zihan Li, Hao Xu, and Hong Li

Abstract In this paper, we propose a *Multiple Receptive Field U-Net* (MRFU-Net) for an *Environmental Microorganism* (EM) image segmentation task to assist microbiologists to detect and identify EMs more effectively. The MRFU-Net is an improved deep learning structure based on U-Net and Inception. In the experiment, in contrast to the original U-Net, the overall segmentation performance of Dice, Jaccard, recall and accuracy increases from 85.24%, 77.42%, 82.27% and 96.76% to 87.23%, 79.74%, 87.65% and 97.30%, respectively. The overall volume overlap error (VOE) reduces from 22.58% to 20.26%. Thus, MRFU-Net shows its effectiveness and potential in the practical field of EM segmentation.

Keywords Environmental miroorganisms · Image segmentation · Deep convolutional neural networks · Multiple receptive field · U-net

C. Li · J. Zhang · F. Kulwa · Z. Li · H. Xu · H. Li (✉)
Microscopic Image and Medical Image Analysis Group, MBIE College, Northeastern University, Shenyang 110169, People's Republic of China
e-mail: lihong@bmie.neu.edu.cn

C. Li
e-mail: lichen201096@hotmail.com

J. Zhang
e-mail: zhangjingh@foxmail.com

F. Kulwa
e-mail: frank.kulwa@gmail.com

Z. Li
e-mail: 531801723@qq.com

H. Xu
e-mail: 154617829@qq.com

X. Zhao
Environmental Engineering Department, Northeastern University, Shenyang 110169, People's Republic of China
e-mail: zhaoxin@mail.neu.edu.cn

27

E. Piętka et al. (eds.), *Information Technology in Biomedicine*, Advances in Intelligent Systems and Computing 1186, https://doi.org/10.1007/978-3-030-49666-1_3

1   Introduction

In many countries, pollution has been threatening the environments, so methods of eliminating pollution are being established. These methods include three major categories: Chemical, physical, and biological approaches. By contrast, the biological method is harmless and efficient [1]. *Environmental Microorganisms* (EMs) are microscopic organisms living in the environments, which act as natural decomposers and indicators of pollution. For example, *Rotifera* can decompose rubbish in water and reduce the level of eutrophication. Therefore, the research of EMs plays a significant role in the management of pollution [2], and the identification of EMs is the basic step for related researches.

Generally, there are four types of EM identification methods. The first is the chemical method, which is highly accurate but often results in secondary pollution of chemical reagent [3]. The second is the physical method. It also has high accuracy but requires the expensive equipment [3]. The third is molecular biological method which distinguishes EMs by sequence analysis of genome [4]. This method needs expensive equipments, lots of time and professional researchers. The fourth is morphological observation which needs an experienced operator to observe EMs under a microscope and give the EM identities by their shape characteristics [1]. Hence, these methods have their respective disadvantages in practical work.

Due to the drawbacks of the traditional methods mentioned above and the excellent performance on segmentation tasks of deep learning methods, the widely used U-Net [5] is firstly considered in our work. However, the adaptability of U-Net is limited by its single receptive field setting. To solve this problem, we propose a *Multiple Receptive Field U-Net* (MRFU-Net) for the EM image segmentation task. The MRFU-Net is an improved deep learning structure based on U-Net [5] and Inception [6]. The main contribution of this paper is: The MRFU-Net for EM image segmentation is proposed to assist biologists, which achieves an overall better segmentation result than the original U-Net in this task. The workflow is shown in Fig. 1.

In Fig. 1, (a) denotes the 'Training Images': The training set contains 21 categories of EM images and their corresponding ground truth (GT) images. (b) shows the 'Data Augmentation': To solve a small training set problem, the size of dataset is increased. (c) is the 'Training Process': MRFU-Net is trained to perform the segmentation task and generate a segmentation model. (d) denotes the 'Test Images': The test set contains 21 categories of EM images.

The structure of this paper is as follows: Section 2 is the related work about existing EM segmentation methods. Section 3 gives a detailed description on our proposed method. Section 4 introduces the details about the experiment. Section 5 closes this paper with a brief conclusion.

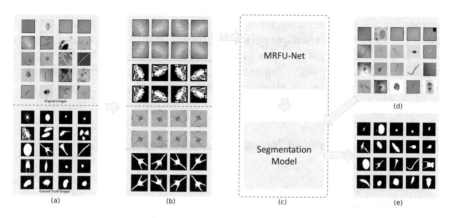

Fig. 1 The workflow of the proposed MRFU-Net based EM image segmentation method: **a** training images, **b** data augmentation, **c** training process, **d** test images, and **e** results

Table 1 The existing microorganism image segmentation methods

Category	Subcategory	Related work
Classical methods	Threshold based methods	[8–10]
	Edge based methods	[11–13]
	Region based methods	[14, 15]
Machine learning based methods	Unsupervised methods	[16–18]
	Supervised methods	[2, 19–21]

2 Related Work

Related works about microorganism image segmentation are briefly summarized in Table 1. For more details, please refer to our previous survey in [7].

2.1 Classical EM Image Segmentation Methods

As shown in Table 1, classical methods include threshold based methods, edge based methods and region based methods. One of the most representative threshold based methods is Otsu. Canny is the most famous edge based method. Watershed is noted in region based methods.

In [8–10], different threshold based methods are used for microorganism image segmentation. For instance, different algorithms which are based on Otsu thresholding are applied for segmentation of floc and filaments to enhance monitoring of actived sludge in waste water treatment plants in [9]. The related works [11–13] are concerned with edge based microorganism segmentation methods. For example, a segmentation and classification work is introduced to identify individual microorganism from a group of overlapping (touching) bacteria in [11]. Canny is used as the basic step of the segmentation part in [11]. The related works [14, 15] use region based methods in their works. For example, in [14], the segmentation is performed on gray level images using marker controlled watershed method.

2.2 Machine Learning Based EM Image Segmentation Methods

Machine learning methods can be categorised as unsupervised or supervised learning. Some typical examples of unsupervised methods are Markov random fields (MRFs) and k-means, while U-Net [5] is one of the most famous supervised learning methods.

The work [16–18] use unsupervised methods in their works. For example, the work of [16] makes an evaluation about clustering and threshold segmentation methods on tissue images containing TB Bacilli. The final result shows that k-means clustering ($k = 3$) achieves outstanding performance. In [17], a comparison between condition random fields and region based segmentation methods is presented. The final result shows that these two kinds of methods for microorganism segmentation have the average recognition rate above 80%. The related works [2, 19–21] use supervised methods in their works. For example, in [20], a segmentation system is designed to monitor the algae in water bodies. Its main thought is image enhancement (sharpening) is applied first by using Retinex filtering technique, then segmentation is done by using support vector machine. In [21], Rift Valley virus is segmentation subject. Because of the insufficient data, data augmentation is used to assist U-Net to perform the segmentation task.

3   MRFU-Net Based EM Image Segmentation Method

MRFU-Net is a deep learning structure based on U-Net [5] and Inception [6] for EM image segmentation.

3.1 Basic Knowledge of U-Net

U-Net is a convolutional neural network, which is initially used to perform the task of biomedical microscopic image segmentation. There are two important contributions of U-Net. First, data augmentation is used to solve the small training dataset problem. Then, end-to-end structures retrieve the spatial information of the network. With the outstanding performance, U-Net is widely used in tasks of semantic segmentation. The network structure of the original U-Net is shown in Fig. 2.

3.2 Basic Knowledge of Inception

The original Inception is proposed in GoogleNet [6], where different sizes of filters are jointly used, including 1×1, 3×3 and 5×5 convolution filters. Due to the utilization of these filters, Inception has the capacity to adapt to multi-scale objects in images.

3.3 The Structure of MRFU-Net

There are multi-scale objects in EM images. The examples are shown in Fig. 3.

Considering that U-Net is difficult to adapt to the situation of multi-scale objects in EM images as shown in Fig. 3, we propose the MRFU-Net to overcome this

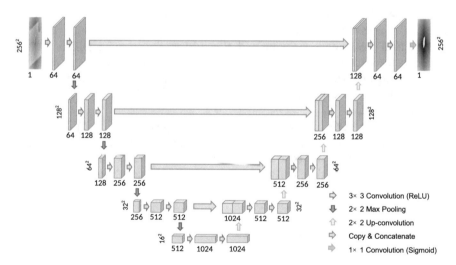

Fig. 2 The network structure of U-Net

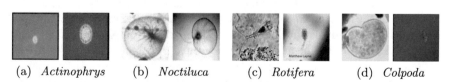

(a) *Actinophrys*   (b) *Noctiluca*   (c) *Rotifera*   (d) *Colpoda*

Fig. 3 An example of EM images with multiple scales

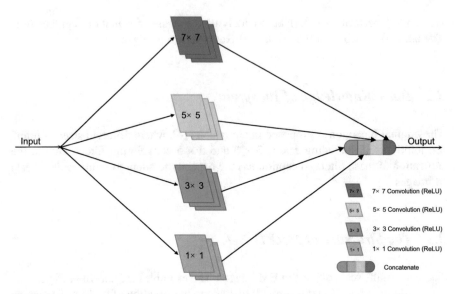

Fig. 4 The structure of BLOCK-I

problem. As the U-Net structure shown in Fig. 2, there is a sequence of two 3×3 convolution operations before each polling operation, each up-convolution operation and the final convolution operation with Sigmoid, so the receptive field is limited. In contrast, convolution filters of different sizes are used to obtain various receptive fields in Inception. Hence, we propose a new Inception based structure "BLOCK-I" as shown in Fig. 4, which incorporates 1×1, 3×3, 5×5 and 7×7 convolution filters in parallel.

Based on the BLOCK-I shown in Fig. 4, we propose the novel MRFU-Net as shown in Fig. 5. Besides, we add a batch normalization layer after each convolution layer and convolution transpose layer to reduce the internal covariate shift [22] in the MRFU-Net. In addition, the details of the MRFU-Net are shown in Table 2.

3.4 Evaluation Metric

In our previous work [2], Recall and Accuracy are used to measure the segmentation results. Besides that, we further employ Dice, Jaccard and VOE (volumetric overlap error) to evaluate the segmentation results in this paper. The definitions of these evaluation metrics are provided in Table 3. V_{pred} represents the foreground that predicted by the model. V_{gt} means the foreground in a ground truth image.

From the metrics shown in Table 3, the higher the values of the first four metrics (Dice, Jaccard, Recall and Accuracy) are, the better the segmentation results are. On the contrary, the lower the value of the final metric (VOE) is, the better the segmentation result is.

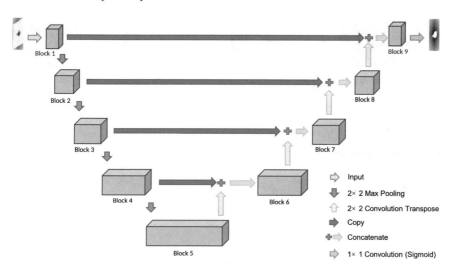

Fig. 5 The network structure of the MRFU-Net

Table 2 The detailed setting of the MRFU-Net. Cv2D is a 2D convolution operation provided in Keras

Block	Filter	Filter number	Block	Filter	Filter number	Block	Filter	Filter number
Block 1 & Block 9	Cv2D(3,3) Cv2D(5,5) Cv2D(7,7) Cv2D(1,1)	16	Block 2 & Block 8	Cv2D(3,3) Cv2D(5,5) Cv2D(7,7) Cv2D(1,1)	32	Block 3 & Block 7	Cv2D(3,3) Cv2D(5,5) Cv2D(7,7) Cv2D(1,1)	64
Block 4 & Block 6	Cv2D(3,3) Cv2D(5,5) Cv2D(7,7) Cv2D(1,1)	128	Block 5	Cv2D(3,3) Cv2D(5,5) Cv2D(7,7) Cv2D(1,1)	256			

Table 3 The definitions of evaluation metrics for image segmentation. TP (True Positive), FN (False Negative), FP (False Positive) and TN (True Negative)

Metric	Definition	Metric	Definition
Dice	$\frac{2 \times |V_{\text{pred}} \cap V_{\text{gt}}|}{|V_{\text{pred}}| + |V_{\text{gt}}|}$	Jaccard	$\frac{|V_{\text{pred}} \cap V_{\text{gt}}|}{|V_{\text{pred}} \cup V_{\text{gt}}|}$
Recall	$\frac{\text{TP}}{\text{TP}+\text{FN}}$	Accuracy	$\frac{\text{TP}+\text{TN}}{\text{TP}+\text{FN}+\text{FP}+\text{TN}}$
VOE	$1 - \frac{|V_{\text{pred}} \cap V_{\text{gt}}|}{|V_{\text{pred}} \cup V_{\text{gt}}|}$		

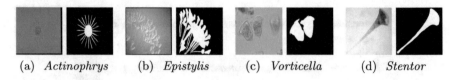

(a) *Actinophrys*   (b) *Epistylis*   (c) *Vorticella*   (d) *Stentor*

Fig. 6 Examples of the original and GT images in EMDS-5

4 Experiments

4.1 *Experimental Setting*

4.1.1 Data Setting and Augmentation

In our work, we use *Environmental Microorganism Dataset 5th Version* (EMDS-5), which is a newly released version of EMDS series [23], containing 21 classes of EMs, as shown in Fig. 6. Each EM class contains 20 original microscopic images and their corresponding ground truth images. Owing to the EM images have multiple scales, we convert all the image sizes into 256×256 pixels, uniformly.

We randomly divide each class of EMDS-5 images into training, validation and test datasets in a ratio of 1:1:2. In the training process, data augmentation can effectively make up the lack of training images. Considering the method proposed in [21] and our pre-tests, we augment the 105 training images with rotations of 0, 90, 180, 270 degrees and mirroring, which results in 840 images for training.

4.1.2 Experiment Environment

The experiment is conducted by Python 3 in Windows 10 operation system. The models we used in our experiment are implemented by Keras framework with Tensorflow as backend. In our experiment, we use a workstation with Intel(R) Core(TM) i7-8700 CPU with 3.20GHz, 32GB RAM and NVIDIA GEFORCE RTX 2080 8GB.

4.1.3 Parameter Setting

The task of the segmentation is to predict the individual pixels whether they represent a point of foreground or background. Thus, the task can be seen as a pixel-level binary classification. Hence, as the loss function of the network, we simply take the binary cross-entropy function and minimize it. The binary cross-entropy loss for the image is defined as Eq. 1.

$$L_1(X, Y, \hat{Y}) = -\sum_{i \in X}(y_i \log(\hat{y}_i) + (1 - y_i) \log(1 - (\hat{y}_i)) \tag{1}$$

In Eq. 1, for the image X, Y is the corresponding ground truth image, and $\hat{Y}$ represents the predicted segmentation result. For pixel i in image X, the network predicts $\hat{y}_i$, whereas, the ground truth value in the model is y_i.

For a batch with N images inside, the loss function J_1 is defined by Eq. 2.

$$J_1 = \frac{1}{N} \sum_{i=1}^{N} L_1(X_i, Y_i, \hat{Y}_i) \tag{2}$$

Besides, we use Adam optimizer with 1.5×10^{-4} learning rate in our training process. The models are trained for 50 epochs using Adam optimizer. Because the models have converged after 50 epochs.

4.2 Evaluation of the MRFU-Net Based Segmentation Method

In order to prove the effectiveness of the proposed MRFU-Net for EM image segmentation, we compare its segmentation results with other classical and state-of-the-art methods mentioned in Sect. 2, which include U-Net, Otsu, Canny, Watershed, k-means and MRF. So we provide the average evaluation indexes of the segmentation results generated by these methods in Fig. 7.

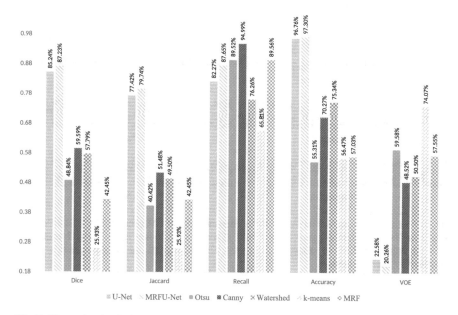

Fig. 7 The evaluation indexes of U-Net, MRFU-Net, Otsu, Canny, Watershed, k-means and MRF based segmentation methods

From Fig. 7, we can find that U-Net achieves a good performance, but the results of MRFU-Net are even better. Compared with U-Net, the average Dice value of MRFU-Net is increased around 2%; the value of average Jaccard of MRFU-Net makes 2.32% improvement; the improvement of the average Recall values made by MRFU-Net is 5.38%; for the average Accuracy, the improvement of MRFU-Net is 0.54%; the average VOE of MRFU-Net is reduced by 2.32%. Hence, from these evaluation indexes by MRFU-Net, the overall segmentation performance is effectively improved.

Compared with other methods, we can find from Fig. 7 that the results of MRFU-Net are better than that of these methods. But the recall values generated by these methods are higher than the recall values generated by U-Net and MRFU-Net. This is because some of the segmentation results generated by these methods have a lot of background parts partitioned into the foreground. What is more serious is that the whole picture is partitioned into the foreground. We can find this situation easily from Fig. 8. From the definition of Recall shown in Table 3, we can realize that as long as the foreground in the segmentation result contains the entire real foreground in ground truth, the value of recall is 1 regardless of whether the over-segmentation problem is existing or not [2]. Therefore, when we evaluate the EM image segmentation results, we should not judge them by the value of Recall alone. From the above, we should consider multiple indexes when we evaluate the segmentation results.

In order to observe the performance of these methods better, we provide part of the detailed indexes of the segmentation results of different EM category under these methods in Table 4. Besides, we also provide the examples of the segmentation results under these methods in Fig. 8.

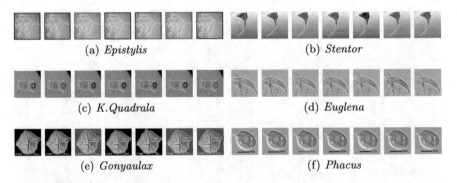

(a) *Epistylis*   (b) *Stentor*

(c) *K.Quadrala*   (d) *Euglena*

(e) *Gonyaulax*   (f) *Phacus*

Fig. 8 An example of segmentation results for each category of EM generated by U-Net, MRFU-Net, Otsu, Canny, Watershed, k-means and MRF (From the left to the right). The yellow outlines show the regions of EMs in ground truth images. The red regions are the segmentation results generated by these methods

Table 4 The average indexes for several EM categories generated by U-Net, MRFU-Net, Otsu, Canny, Watershed, *k*-means and MRF methods (In %)

EM	Methods	Evaluation metrics				
		Dice	Jaccard	Recall	Accuracy	VOE
Epistylis	U-Net	55.43	40.56	50.04	89.00	59.44
	MRFU-Net	68.38	52.90	70.82	90.67	47.10
	Otsu	24.72	14.75	90.01	22.98	85.25
	Canny	36.87	23.56	99.25	39.81	76.44
	Watershed	30.75	19.25	81.74	39.34	80.75
	k-means	24.72	14.75	90.01	22.99	85.25
	MRF	23.95	14.40	80.01	32.32	85.60
K.Quadrala	U-Net	93.06	87.23	91.36	97.38	12.77
	MRFU-Net	93.07	87.34	93.66	97.46	12.66
	Otsu	81.89	72.00	91.81	86.40	28.00
	Canny	82.68	84.44	96.10	96.33	15.56
	Watershed	86.87	77.41	87.17	95.14	22.59
	k-means	53.16	45.87	61.56	77.84	54.13
	MRF	78.00	68.09	97.83	83.00	31.91
Gonyaulax	U-Net	93.08	87.27	88.16	95.07	12.73
	MRFU-Net	95.23	90.96	92.84	96.47	9.04
	Otsu	73.25	63.89	93.31	68.78	36.11
	Canny	93.34	87.71	91.57	95.46	12.29
	Watershed	90.56	83.16	90.27	93.60	16.84
	k-means	44.09	35.65	64.40	57.64	64.35
	MRF	71.04	59.07	74.37	77.65	40.93
Stentor	U-Net	88.76	80.63	84.50	97.25	19.37
	MRFU-Net	91.02	83.78	91.03	97.67	16.22
	Otsu	51.66	41.92	93.14	60.62	58.08
	Canny	72.96	59.94	98.60	89.60	40.06
	Watershed	58.66	45.73	66.26	86.71	54.27
	k-means	32.19	24.88	66.89	63.76	75.12
	MRF	46.34	37.67	63.34	70.34	62.33
Euglena	U-Net	89.80	82.23	84.41	97.59	17.77
	MRFU-Net	92.89	87.08	88.93	98.27	12.92
	Otsu	58.89	48.05	77.64	75.02	51.95
	Canny	65.46	54.89	97.17	77.66	45.11
	Watershed	83.95	76.86	89.09	88.97	23.14
	k-means	35.76	29.06	52.81	73.97	70.94
	MRF	72.88	62.65	86.65	82.23	37.35

(continued)

Table 4 (continued)

EM	Methods	Evaluation metrics				
		Dice	Jaccard	Recall	Accuracy	VOE
Phacus	U-Net	91.56	85.20	85.43	98.37	14.80
	MRFU-Net	95.03	90.82	92.17	98.94	9.18
	Otsu	40.28	33.47	81.99	48.48	66.53
	Canny	57.15	50.79	97.16	61.44	49.21
	Watershed	63.62	56.80	75.32	81.57	43.20
	k-means	40.64	33.98	80.83	49.76	66.02
	MRF	53.15	48.06	95.29	52.46	51.94

4.3 Comparison with Local-Global CRF Segmentation

In our previous work of Local-global CRF [2], we use EMDS-4 dataset with 20 categories of EMs. In contrast to EMDS-4, EMDS-5 has one more EM category (*Gymnodinium*). Therefore, we evaluate the segmentation results obtained by MRFU-Net without *Gymnodinium* here. Futhermore, there are six models for segmentation in [2] to compare: Per-pixel RF (noEdges), CRF with Potts pairwise potentials (Potts), CRF with contrast-sensitive Potts model (PottsCS), fully connected CRF with Gaussian pairwise potentials (denseCRF), fully connected CRF on segmentation results by the original DeepLab method (denseCRForg), fully convolutional network (FCN). Considering the evaluation metrics used in our previous work, we use Average Recall and Overall Accuracy (OA) to evaluate the performance of the segmentation results in [2]. The Average Recall and OA values of MRFU-Net and our previous models are shown in Fig. 9.

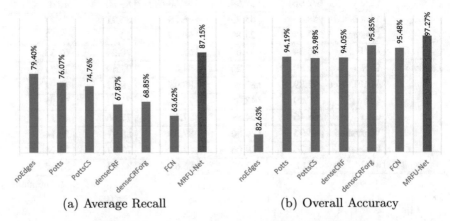

(a) Average Recall   (b) Overall Accuracy

Fig. 9 The comparison of MRFU-Net and Local-global CRF segmentation [2]

From Fig. 9, compared with the previous models, the Average Recall is improved by more than 7%, and the Overall Accuracy increases by at least 1%. Thus, the proposed MRFU-Net performs better than the models in our previous work [2].

5   Conclusion and Future Work

In this paper, we propose MRFU-Net for the EM segmentation task. MRFU-Net is a deep learning structure based on U-Net and Inception. In the evaluation of segmentation results, the values of evaluation indexes Dice, Jaccard, Recall, Accuracy and VOE (volume overlap error) are 87.13%, 79.74%, 87.12%, 96.91% and 20.26%, respectively. Compared with U-Net, the first four indexes are improved by 1.89%, 2.32%, 4.84% and 0.14%, respectively, and the last index is decrease by 2.32%. In addition, compared with our previous Local-global CRF model in [2], the performance of segmentation results is significantly improved, and the details of indexes are shown in Fig. 9. In our future work, we plan to increase the amount of data in the dataset in order to improve the performance. Meanwhile, we will propose an approach to optimize the memory and time costs.

Acknowledgements   We thank the "National Natural Science Foundation of China" No. 61806047 and the "Fundamental Research Funds for the Central Universities" No. N2019003. We also thank B.E. Jinghua Zhang, due to his great contribution is considered as important as the first author in this paper.

References

1. Maier, R., Pepper, I., Gerba, C.: Environmental Microbiology. Academic Press (2015)
2. Kosov, S., Shirahama, K., Li, C., Grzegorzek, M.: Environmental microorganism classification using conditional random fields and deep convolutional neural networks. Pattern Recognit. **77**, 248–261 (2018)
3. Li, C., Wang, K., Xu, N.: A survey for the applications of content-based microscopic image analysis in microorganism classification domains. Artif. Intell. Rev. **51**(4), 577–646 (2019)
4. Yamaguchi, T., Kawakami, S., Hatamoto, M., et al.: In situ DNA-hybridization chain reaction (HCR): a facilitated in situ HCR system for the detection of environmental microorganisms. Environ. Microbiol. **17**, 2532–2541 (2015)
5. Ronneberger, O., Fischer, P., Brox, T.: U-Net: convolutional networks for biomedical image segmentation. In: Proceedings of MICCAI 2015, pp. 234–241 (2015)
6. Szegedy, C., Liu, W., Jia, Y., et al.: Going deeper with convolutions. In: Proceedings of CVPR 2015 (2015), pp. 1–9
7. Kulwa, F., Li, C., Zhao, X., et al.: A state-of-the-art survey for microorganism image segmentation methods and future potential. IEEE Access **7**, 100243–100269 (2019)
8. Rojas, D., Rueda, L., Ngom, A., et al.: Image segmentation of biofilm structures using optimal multi-level thresholding. Int. J. Data Min. Bioinf. **5**(3), 266–286 (2011)
9. Khan, M., Nisar, H., Ng, C., et al.: Local adaptive approach toward segmentation of microscopic images of activated sludge flocs. J. Electron. Imaging **24**(6), 061102 (2015)

10. Khan, M., Nisar, H., Aun, N., Lo, P.: Iterative region based Otsu thresholding of bright-field microscopic images of activated sludge. In: Proceedings of IECBES 2016, pp. 533–538 (2016)
11. Dubuisson, M., Jain, A., Jain, M.: Segmentation and classification of bacterial culture images. J. Microbiol. Methods **19**(4), 279–295 (1994)
12. Forero, M., Cristobal, G., Alvarez-Borrego, J.: Automatic identification techniques of tuberculosis bacteria. In: Proceedings of SPIE 2003, pp. 71–81 (2003)
13. DaneshPanah, M., Javidi, B.: Segmentation of 3D holographic images using bivariate jointly distributed region snake. Opt. Express **14**(12), 5143–5153 (2006)
14. Hiremath, P., Bannigidad, P., Hiremath, M.: Automated identification and classification of rotavirus-a particles in digital microscopic images. In: Proceedings of RTIPPR 2010, pp. 69–73 (2010)
15. Long, F., Zhou, J., Peng, H.: Visualization and analysis of 3D microscopic images. PLoS Comput. Biol. **8**(6), e1002519 (2012)
16. Osman, M., Mashor, M., Jaafar, H.: Performance comparison of clustering and thresholding algorithms for tuberculosis bacilli segmentation. In: Proceedings of CITS 2012, pp. 1–5 (2012)
17. Kemmler, M., Fröhlich, B., Rodner, E., Denzler, J.: Segmentation of microorganism in complex environments. Pattern Recognit. Image Anal. **23**(4), 512–517 (2013)
18. Rulaningtyas, R., Suksmono, A., Mengko, T., Saptawati, P.: Multi patch approach in K-means clustering method for color image segmentation in pulmonary tuberculosis identification. In: Proceedings of ICICI-BME 2015, pp. 75–78 (2015)
19. Nie, D., Shank, E., Jojic, V.: A deep framework for bacterial image segmentation and classification. In: Proceedings of ACM BCB 2015, pp. 306–314 (2015)
20. Dannemiller, K., Ahmadi, K., Salari, E.: A new method for the segmentation of algae images using retinex and support vector machine. In: Proceedings of EIT 2015, pp. 361–364 (2015)
21. Matuszewski, D., Sintorn, I.: Minimal annotation training for segmentation of microscopy images. In: Proceedings of ISBI 2018, pp. 387–390 (2018)
22. Ioffe, S., Szegedy, C.: Batch Normalization: Accelerating Deep Network Training by Reducing Internal Covariate Shift (2015). arXiv: 1502.03167
23. Zou, Y., Li, C., Shirahama, K., et al.: Environmental microorganism image retrieval using multiple colour channels fusion and particle swarm optimisation. In: Proceedings of ICIP 2016, pp. 2475–2479 (2016)

Deep Learning Approach to Automated Segmentation of Tongue in Camera Images for Computer-Aided Speech Diagnosis

Agata Sage, Zuzanna Miodońska, Michał Kręcichwost, Joanna Trzaskalik, Ewa Kwaśniok, and Paweł Badura

Abstract This paper describes an approach for automated segmentation of tongue in camera images for computer-aided speech diagnosis and therapy. Speech disorders are often related to non-normative position of articulators. One of common pathologies in Polish pronunciation is interdentality, when the tongue protrudes between the front teeth. Segmentation and possible parametrization of tongue in camera images could support speech diagnosis. Presented system is based on images captured by two cameras directed at speaker's mouth at different angles on the left and right side. A convolutional neural network was designed and trained for semantic segmentation of tongue. Three datasets of input data were examined, two taken from each camera separately and one combined from both cameras. The mean Jaccard index reached 74.01% over the combined dataset with the corresponding accuracy at 96.09%.

Keywords Computer-aided speech diagnosis and therapy · Tongue segmentation · Convolutional neural network

---

A. Sage (✉) · Z. Miodońska · M. Kręcichwost · P. Badura
Faculty of Biomedical Engineering, Silesian University of Technology,
Roosevelta 40, 41-800 Zabrze, Poland
e-mail: agata.sage@polsl.pl

Z. Miodońska
e-mail: zuzanna.miodonska@polsl.pl

M. Kręcichwost
e-mail: michal.krecichwost@polsl.pl

P. Badura
e-mail: pawel.badura@polsl.pl

J. Trzaskalik
Jesuit University Ignatianum in Krakow, Kopernika 26, 31-501 Kraków, Poland
e-mail: joanna.trzaskalik@ignatianum.edu.pl

E. Kwaśniok
"Sluchmed" Hearing Therapy Center, Zabrzańska 72, 41-700 Ruda Śląska, Poland

---

E. Piętka et al. (eds.), *Information Technology in Biomedicine*, Advances in Intelligent
Systems and Computing 1186, https://doi.org/10.1007/978-3-030-49666-1_4

1 Introduction

The tongue is crucial for speech generation. Dependent of its position and cooperation with other articulators, different sounds might be produced. Non-normative movement patterns of a tongue are a reason of many speech disorders. One of common pathologies in Polish pronunciation is interdentality, when the tongue protrudes between the front teeth. In that case, visibility of tongue during speech is pathologically increased [6]. Detection, segmentation, and possible feature-based description of the tongue in images might be considered an important support for the therapists in speech pathology diagnosis.

In recent years, the popularity of deep learning techniques in image segmentation increased rapidly. Specifically, due to their efficiency and reliability, convolutional neural networks (CNN) were employed for various medical image processing problems [8]. Taking into consideration the general problem of tongue segmentation, several approaches were proposed involving deep learning techniques. Some studies were performed in RGB images for the purposes of Traditional Chinese Medicine (TCM) [7, 10, 14, 15, 17, 18]. The segmentation was incorporated into computer-aided diagnosis systems with certain assumptions and examination protocols. A large part of the tongue was clearly visible sticking out of the mouth. Due to the diagnostic purposes of segmentation, the tongues under investigation featured different properties, e.g. color, texture, pose, teeth or lips visibility and adjacency. Training and validation of designed deep learning models involved databases with the number of images varying between 552 [14] and 5616 [15].

The TCM studies employed images of tongue visible in positions unnatural for speech (Fig. 1a). Thus, their applicability to tongue segmentation in speech assessment, also for the diagnosis and therapy, is highly questionable. Possible tongue visibility during pronunciation depends on the individual speaker, speech disorder nature, or phone type. In most cases, the tongue is rather hidden behind teeth or lips than visible (Fig. 1b). For that reason, tongue segmentation for pronunciation assessment support can be considered a challenging task. Not many scientific reports can be found in this area so far. Bílková et al. [2] prepared a computer system for automated evaluation of speech therapy exercises based on web camera video recording. The paper focuses mainly on detection and tracking of lips movements, yet it introduces an idea for tongue segmentation based on a U-Net CNN. However, no quantitative

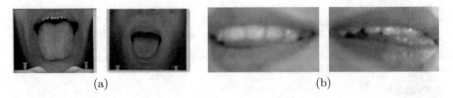

(a)   (b)

Fig. 1 Typical images used in studies addressing Traditional Chinese Medicine [10] (**a**) and recorded during speech (**b**)

evaluation was performed; presented illustrations show segmentation results with tongue in open mouth. Older studies rarely employed advanced image processing techniques for tracking tongue in images. Hassanat [4] described a visual speech recognition for, e.g., lip reading, yet his works concentrated mainly on face and lips detection techniques. The tongue appearance was assessed only based on a red channel level inside the detected mouth region. Zhang et al. [16] designed a visual speech feature extraction system for automatic speech recognition (ASR). Again, the possible tongue presence inside the mouth was detected using intensity constraints only as an additional information to precise lips area analysis.

Automated tongue segmentation and analysis is our idea to support and develop previous research on computer-aided speech diagnosis based on acoustic analysis of speech signal [5, 12, 13]. In the current study, we took preliminary steps in the process of creating an image analysis tool, which could eventually be employed to build a multi-modal computer-aided speech diagnosis tool, concerning both speech signal and vision.

The aim of the study presented in this paper was to design a prototype of a video recording system and to conduct a semantic segmentation of tongue in images recorded during speech. For segmentation, we prepared a multi-level methodology consisting of a preprocessing stage for tongue region of interest (ROI) detection and a SegNet-like architecture convolutional neural network [1]. Three datasets were used to validate the designed algorithm. Images of mouth area were acquired during specially prepared speech-like exercises, normal speech, and interdental speech simulation using two side-cameras directed at different angles.

2 Materials and Methods

2.1 Materials

Video data were acquired using a prototype experimental setup (Fig. 2) with two Logitech HD 720p cameras located on two sides of the speaker's face and a LED matrix for the mouth area illumination. Elements were mounted on a tripod. The distance between each camera and speaker's mouth was approximately 12.5 cm.

Collected database consisted of 27 893 RGB images of size 640×480. The images were obtained during specific exercises, normal speech, and simulated abnormal speech from 10 speakers (13 920 left images, 13 973 right images). Images were extracted from a video sequence with a frame rate of 30 frames per second. Due to specifics of mouth movement during pronunciation, the tongue visibility level was diversified, with most of the images showing small pieces of the tongue (ca. 55% of images vs. 30% with a relatively large tongue object). Multiple images did not contain the tongue at all (ca. 15% of the dataset). Expert delineation of the tongue was then prepared in each image, yielding a ground-truth database.

Fig. 2 Experimental setup
with two side cameras and a
LED matrix

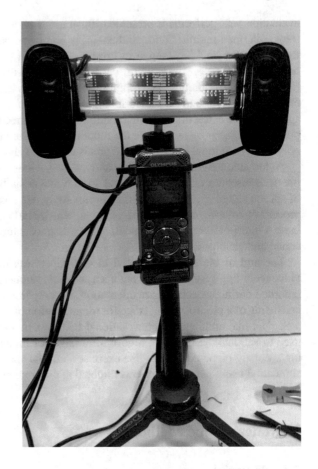

2.2 Methods

2.2.1 Preprocessing

Before reaching the main segmentation procedure, a preprocessing stage was performed for mouth area ROI detection (Fig. 3). Two auxiliary images were extracted
from the original 640×480 RGB image: (1) the image with attenuated blue channel
within the RGB color space [3]:

$$I_{-B} = \frac{2G - R - \frac{B}{2}}{4},\qquad(1)$$

where G, R and B denote green, red, and blue channels of RGB color space, respectively, and (2) saturation channel obtained according to the NTSC color gamut. The
idea was to differentiate the lips area and other parts of the speaker's face. The blue

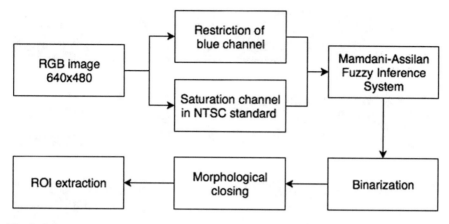

Fig. 3 Scheme of the preprocessing stage

RGB channel is considered less significant for the lip color, and as a result of its restriction, lips had higher intensity than skin and other objects. On the other hand, mouth presence in the NTSC saturation channel was reflected in lower intensity. Both channels constituted the input to the pixel-wise Mamdani–Assilan fuzzy inference system (FIS) [9]. A knowledge base with nine fuzzy rules was designed based on linguistic variables defined over intensity sets in both input images. Later, morphological operations were performed on the binary FIS outcome and the mouth area ROI was limited to the bounding-box covering the largest binary object of a given image, corresponding to the lips region. Resulting ROIs (Fig. 4) were then inputs to the convolutional neural network.

2.2.2 CNN Design

A directed acyclic graph (DAG) CNN was designed in order to perform tongue segmentation (Fig. 5). Parameters of the CNN architecture were chosen experimentally. The neural network's encoder path consisted of three convolutional layers, each including 64 filters of size 3×3. We decided to use cascade filters of a smaller kernel size (3×3) in order to prevent system from increased computational cost related to the use of larger kernels (e.g. 5×5) without loss of accuracy [11]. Each convolutional layer was followed by a rectified linear unit (ReLU) and a max pooling layer with a 2×2 stride over a 2×2 pool. The input image size was set to 32×64, thus the raw ROIs had to be properly resized. Smaller input image size unacceptably decreased image quality, whereas increased size caused unnecessary growth of computational cost and training time without significant gain of segmentation accuracy. Also, three transposed convolution layers followed by ReLU layers were prepared in the decoder path. The final layer was the pixel classification layer assigning a categorical label (*background* or *tongue* label) to each ROI pixel.

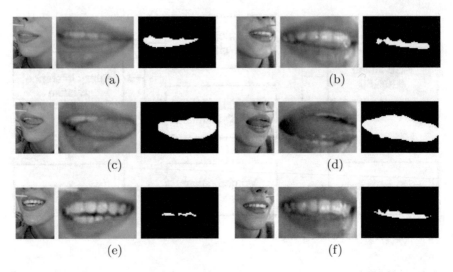

Fig. 4 Sample images and processing results. Each subplot presents the original image (left), detected mouth area ROI (middle), and corresponding expert tongue delineation (right). Images present different tongue positions captured by both cameras

Training was performed using stochastic gradient descent with momentum (SGDM) optimizer. The ratio of dataset partition to training, test, and validation subsets was equal to 80%:10%:10% in a speaker-wise manner. Image augmentation was applied with the input data rotation, scaling, and translation. Training involved a batch size of 64 samples. The maximum number of epochs was set to 150. Training process terminated when the validation loss did not decrease in recent 20 epochs. Weighting was used to stabilize distribution of classes in the training data.

3 Results and Discussion

Three datasets were used for the segmentation process. Datasets #1 and #2 consisted of images taken by individual cameras (left and right, respectively), whereas dataset #3 included all images presenting mouth area (i.e. captured by either left or right camera). In order to increase the assessment reliability, each network training & testing experiment was repeated 5 times. All reruns differed in the division of dataset into training, validation, and test subsets. The evaluation was performed by means of two segmentation quality measures: accuracy Acc and Jaccard index (or Intersection over Union) J (Table 1). Figure 6 presents examples of segmentation results.

The proposed segmentation tool worked relatively efficient. The tongue segmentation accuracy exceeded 96% for Datasets #1 and #3. Nevertheless, due to a significant overrepresentation of background pixels, the spatial overlap measures had to be taken into consideration. The highest value of the Jaccard index was obtained

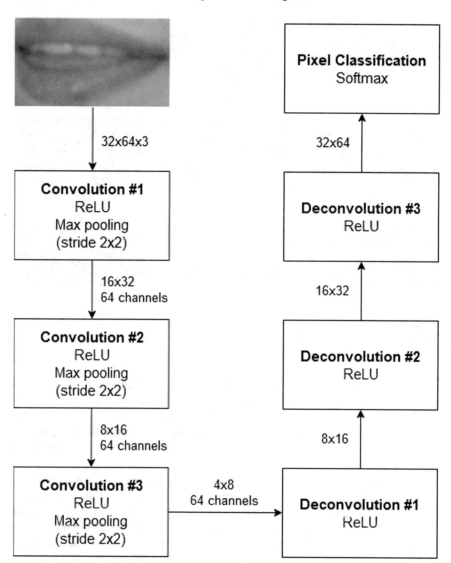

Fig. 5 Architecture of the convolutional neural network for tongue segmentation

Table 1 Tongue segmentation efficiency metrics in individual experiments

	Dataset #1	Dataset #2	Dataset #3
Acc (%)	96.60	88.65	96.09
J (%)	72.97	73.13	74.01

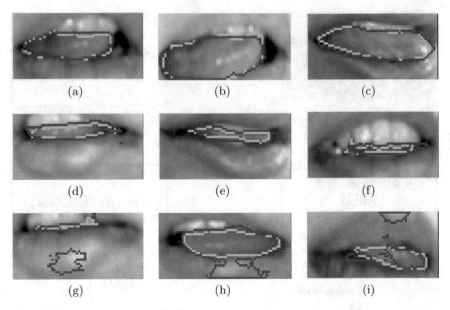

Fig. 6 Examples of segmentation results (red) versus the ground truth (green): **a–f** cases with $J > 85\%$, **g–i** missegmentations

for Dataset #3 (74.01%), while the lowest for Dataset #1 (72.97%). We have noticed a relatively high correlation between the tongue object area within the image and segmentation accuracy. Efficiency of segmentation process increases with the size of an object. This effect is presented in Fig. 7. However, for each experiment the number of Jaccard index values under 50% was significantly lower and mainly concerned segmentations of small parts of tongue.

Taking into account the fact of diversity of images within the datasets, obtained outcomes might be considered as relatively satisfying. Most of missegmentations occurred in case of barely visible tongue, its presence nearby lips, or superimposition of lips and tongue which are often characterized by similar colour and blurred contours. Based on presented results it may be assumed that the use of multiple image sources slightly increases effectiveness of segmentation process. Possible steps for improving the analysis include development of the preprocessing stage, CNN architecture, and stereoscopy processing involvement.

The state-of-the-art presented in Sect. 1 indicated a problem with possible comparative analysis of our approach to existing tongue segmentation frameworks. Studies concerning TCM [7, 10, 14, 15, 17, 18] were performed on images, where tongue visibility is drastically different than during speech. Therefore, obtained results are hardly possible to compare. In this paper, our motivation was to prepare a prototype segmentation workflow able to handle way more difficult and diversified tongue appearances related to mouth motion during pronunciation. Relatively large number of images did not contain any part of the tongue, in multiple others the tongue was

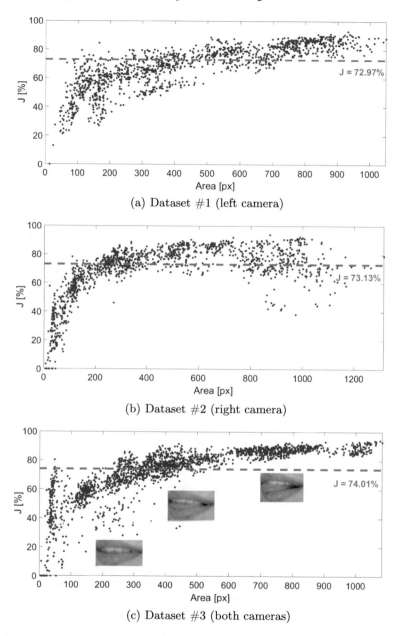

Fig. 7 Jaccard index as a function of tongue area in different datasets. In each case, blue line indicates the corresponding mean value of J. Images featuring different tongue areas are shown for illustration in adequate locations in (**c**)

barely visible. Thus, our preliminary segmentation model holds more information on different possibilities of the tongue appearance and the obtained efficiency metrics seem encouraging for further research concerning each of the following aspects: acquisition device design, methodology development including CNN adaptation, and image database extension (note that our current database size is almost five times greater than the largest database used by the tongue segmentation studies so far [15]).

4 Conclusion

The aim of presented study was to prepare and validate a prototype of a framework for tongue segmentation during pronunciation. A two-camera system was designed in order to overcome the problem of limited visibility of the tongue during speech therapy exercises. The designed CNN-based method is fast and applicable in real time. The mean accuracy and Jaccard index over a set of significantly different tongue shapes and sizes reaching 96% and 74%, respectively. The results give a good start for the system, concerning measurement equipment as well as processing methods.

Acknowledgements This research was supported by the National Science Centre, Poland (NCN) project No. 2018/30/E/ST7/00525.

References

1. Badrinarayanan, V., Kendall, A., Cipolla, R.: SegNet: a deep convolutional encoder-decoder architecture for image segmentation. IEEE Trans. Pattern Anal. Mach. Intell. **39**(12), 2481–2495 (2017). https://doi.org/10.1109/TPAMI.2016.2644615
2. Bílková, Z., Novozámský, A., Domínec, A., Greško, Š., Zitová, B., Paroubková, M.: Automatic evaluation of speech therapy exercises based on image data. In: Karray, F., Campilho, A., Yu, A. (eds) Image Analysis and Recognition. ICIAR 2019. Lecture Notes in Computer Science, vol. 11662, pp. 397–404. Springer, Cham (2019). https://doi.org/10.1007/978-3-030-27202-9_36
3. Canzlerm, U., Dziurzyk, T.: Extraction of non manual features for video based sign language recognition. In: Proceedings of IAPR Workshop, pp. 318–321 (2002)
4. Hassanat, A.B.: Visual speech recognition. Speech Lang. Technol. **1**, 279–303 (2011)
5. Krecichwost, M., Miodonska, Z., Badura, P., Trzaskalik, J., Mocko, N.: Multi-channel acoustic analysis of phoneme /s/ mispronunciation for lateral sigmatism detection. Biocybern. Biomed. Eng. **39**(1), 246–255 (2019). https://doi.org/10.1016/j.bbe.2018.11.005
6. Lebrun, Y.: Tongue thrust, tongue tip position at rest, and sigmatism: a review. J. Commun. Disord. **18**(4), 305–312 (1985)
7. Lin, B., Xie, J., Li, C., Qu, Y.: Deeptongue: tongue segmentation via resnet. In: 2018 IEEE International Conference on Acoustics, Speech and Signal Processing (ICASSP), pp. 1035–1039, Calgary (2018). https://doi.org/10.1109/ICASSP.2018.8462650
8. Litjens, G., Kooi, T., Bejnordi, B.E., Adiyoso Setio, A.A., Ciompi, F., Ghafoorian, M., van der Laak, J., van Ginneken, B., Sanchez, C.I.: A survey on deep learning in medical image analysis. Med. Image Anal. **42**, 60–88 (2017). https://doi.org/10.1016/j.media.2017.07.005

9. Mamdani, E.H., Assilan, S.: An experiment in linguistic synthesis with a fuzzy logic controller. Int. J. Man-Mach. Stud. **20**(2), 1–13 (1975)
10. Qu, P., Zhang, H., Zhuo, L., Zhang, J., Chen, G.: Automatic Tongue Image Segmentation for Traditional Chinese Medicine Using Deep Neural Network. Lecture Notes in Computer Science, pp. 247–259 (2017). https://doi.org/10.1007/978-3-319-63309-1_23
11. Szegedy, Ch., Vanhoucke, V., Ioffe, S., Wojna, Z.: Rethinking the inception architecture for computer vision. In: 2016 IEEE Conference on Computer Vision and Pattern Recognition (CVPR), pp. 2818–2826 (2015)
12. Woloshuk, A., Krecichwost, M., Miodonska, Z., Badura, P., Trzaskalik, J., Pietka, E.: CAD of sigmatism using neural networks. In: Pietka, E., Badura, P., Kawa, J., Wieclawek, W. (eds) Information Technology in Biomedicine. ITIB 2018. Advances in Intelligent Systems and Computing, vol. 762, pp. 260–271. Springer, Cham (2019). https://doi.org/10.1007/978-3-319-91211-0_23
13. Woloshuk A., Krecichwost M., Miodonska Z., Korona, D., Badura P.: Convolutional neural networks for computer aided diagnosis of interdental and rustling sigmatism. In: Pietka, E., Badura, P., Kawa, J., Wieclawek, W. (eds) Information Technology in Biomedicine. ITIB 2019. Advances in Intelligent Systems and Computing, vol. 1011, pp. 179–186. Springer, Cham (2019). https://doi.org/10.1007/978-3-030-23762-2_16
14. Xue, Y., Li, X., Wu, P., Li, J., Wang, L., Tong, L.: Automated tongue segmentation in Chinese medicine based on deep learning. In: 25th International Conference, ICONIP 2018, Siem Reap (2018). https://doi.org/10.1007/978-3-030-04239-4_49
15. Yuan, W., Liu, C.: Cascaded CNN for real-time tongue segmentation based on key points localization. In: 2019 IEEE 4th International Conference on Big Data Analytics (ICBDA), pp. 303–307, Suzhou (2019). https://doi.org/10.1109/ICBDA.2019.8712834
16. Zhang, X., Mersereau, R.M., Clements, M., Broun, C.C.: Visual speech feature extraction for improved speech recognition. In: 2002 IEEE International Conference on Acoustics, Speech, and Signal Processing, vol. 2, pp. II-1993 (2002). https://doi.org/10.1109/ICASSP.2002.5745022
17. Zhou, C., Fan, H., Li, Z.: Tonguenet: accurate localization and segmentation for tongue images using deep neural networks. IEEE Access **7**, 148779–148789 (2019). https://doi.org/10.1109/ACCESS.2019.2946681
18. Zhou, J., Zhang, Q., Zhang, B., Chen, X.: TongueNet: a precise and fast tongue segmentation system using U-Net with a morphological processing layer. Appl. Sci.-Basel **9**, 3128 (2019). https://doi.org/10.3390/app9153128

Image Analysis

3-D Tissue Image Reconstruction from Digitized Serial Histologic Sections to Visualize Small Tumor Nests in Lung Adenocarcinomas

Bartłomiej Pyciński, Yukako Yagi, Ann E. Walts, and Arkadiusz Gertych

Abstract 3-D histology has become an attractive technique providing insights into morphology of histologic specimens. However, existing techniques in generating 3-D views from a stack of whole slide images are scarce or suffer from poor co-registration performance when displaying diagnostically important areas at sub-cellular resolution. Our team developed a new scale-invariant feature transform (SIFT)-based workflow to co-register histology images and facilitate 3-D visualization of microstructures important in histopathology of lung adenocarcinoma. The co-registration accuracy and visualization capacity of the workflow were tested by digitally perturbing the staining coloration seven times. The perturbation slightly affected the co-registration but overall the co-registration errors remained very small when compared to those published to date. The workflow yielded accurate visualizations of expert-selected regions permitting confident 3-D evaluation of the clusters. Our workflow could support the evaluation of histologically complex tumors such as lung adenocarcinomas that are currently routinely viewed by pathologists in 2-D on slides, but could benefit from 3-D visualization.

Keywords Lung adenocarcioma · Image co-registration · 3-D image reconstruction · 3-D visualization · Tumor histology

B. Pyciński (✉) · A. Gertych
Faculty of Biomedical Engineering, Silesian University of Technology, Zabrze, Poland
e mail: bartlomiej.pycinski@polsl.pl

A. Gertych
e-mail: arkadiusz.gertych@cshs.org

Y. Yagi
Department of Pathology, Memorial Sloan Kettering Cancer Center, New York, USA
e-mail: yagiy@mskcc.org

A. E. Walts · A. Gertych
Department of Pathology and Laboratory Medicine, Cedars-Sinai Medical Center, Los Angeles, CA 90048, USA
e-mail: ann.walts@cshs.org

A. Gertych
Department of Surgery, Cedars-Sinai Medical Center, Los Angeles, CA 90048, USA

E. Piętka et al. (eds.), *Information Technology in Biomedicine*, Advances in Intelligent Systems and Computing 1186, https://doi.org/10.1007/978-3-030-49666-1_5

55

1 Introduction

Pathology has become digital as a result of the wide-spread availability and utilization of whole slide scanners that can convert the entire tissue section on a glass slide into a high-resolution image. Likewise, whole slide images (WSI) have enabled the development of numerous software tools for diagnostic and prognostic tasks that can serve as adjuncts to decision-making in pathology and oncology [14]. Slide digitization has also played a major role in enabling three-dimensional (3-D) histology by delivering WSIs generated from serial two-dimensional (2-D) tissue sections for stacking, alignment and subsequent visualization in 3-D as one piece of tissue [5, 10, 11, 24]. The high-speed of pathology slide scanners and the high-resolution of WSIs have made 3-D histology an attractive alternative to other 3-D scanning techniques (such as confocal microscopy or microtomography) by providing insights into the morphology of histologic specimens at sub-cellular resolution.

According to the 2015 World Health Organization (WHO) classification, spread through air spaces in lung adenocarcinoma is defined as "micropapillary clusters, solid nests, or single cells spreading within air spaces beyond the edge of the main tumor" [21]. Tumor spread through air spaces is a recently recognized histologic pattern and appears to have significant prognostic implications [6]. However, the concept of tumor spreading through the air spaces is currently controversial and the underlying mechanism is unclear [22, 23]. Original investigations into this pattern were based on evaluations of single sections (2-D pathology) showing cellular islands situated in the air spaces separated from the main tumor. Recent studies have demonstrated that the identification of tumor spread through air spaces in lung adenocarcinoma would benefit from 3-D visualization generated from a stack of consecutive histologic sections [12, 25, 26] stained with hematoxylin and eosin (H&E). In [12] the authors analyzed paraffin embedded sections from four cases and visualized clusters of tumor cells with interconnections between one another, as well as with the main tumor in two of these cases. Essentially, this 3-D visualization which involved an alignment of a stack of serial WSI sections revealed the details of spatial distribution and structural interaction of the tumor cell clusters that would be very difficult to assess in 2-D.

Accurate alignment of H&E stained WSIs organized into a stack is difficult and has been recognized as an unmet need in the 3-D reconstruction and visualization pipelines [2, 3, 15]. The process of aligning the images—often referred to as image co-registration—is one of the key components responsible for the quality and usefulness of tissue image reconstruction for 3-D visualization. The portfolio of co-registration approaches in digital pathology includes those developed to align pairs of WSIs [20] or pairs of images extracted from WSIs with tissues stained using different immunohistochemical panels [9]. These tools have low computational complexity and employed affine co-registration or a machine learning approach to align images. Unlike co-registration of two WSIs, the co-registration of an image stack comprising multiple WSIs is far more challenging due to the large amount of data and morphological heterogeneity of tissue at different levels in the WSI stack. The heterogeneity includes deformations introduced during paraffin embedding and sectioning, and differences in the placement and orientation of tissue in the WSIs that can be further exacerbated by slide-to-slide differences in staining coloration thereby negatively affecting the WSI stack co-registration performance [5, 7, 15]. When co-registering whole slide images in a stack, most existing 3-D reconstruction approaches optimize the co-registration globally [5, 7]—errors that are measured during the reconstruction are factored into the reconstruction procedure that aims to keep the errors small. Although this approach is robust for a variety of histological specimens and does not require manual input from a user, it often yields sub-optimal performance in applications that necessitate alignments at a single-cell level. Nevertheless this level of accuracy would be required in applications that aim to visually evaluate small anatomical objects such as glomeruli [15], capillaries [24], or isolated clusters of tumor cells defined as spread through air spaces [12, 13] in 3-D.

The limited body of literature addressing performances of 3-D reconstruction of lung tumors from WSIs motivated us to develop a new co-registration workflow. We also investigate whether a highly accurate alignment is achievable and how co-registration is impacted by H&E image coloration. The objectives of this study are as follows: (1) to develop an efficient co-registration and 3-D reconstruction framework to visualize sectioned tumor and isolated tumor nests in a stack of WSIs from tissue slides stained with H&E; (2) to investigate whether color normalization affects 3-D co-registration error when compared to the co-registration performed on original images (without color normalization), and (3) to evaluate whether color normalization can enhance visualization of tumor nest morphology in 3-D. Our studies were performed using a stack of slides prepared from a lung adenocarcinoma.

2 Materials

A formalin fixed paraffin embedded block of an excised tumor previously diagnosed as adenocarcinoma of the lung with solid architecture was sectioned using the Kurabo AS-200S robotic tissue cutting system (Kurabo Industries, Osaka, Japan). This system can generate tissue sections with thickness ranging between 3 μm and 8 μm and then fix them on glass slides for staining. As previously reported [13], the automated process of tissue sectioning yields slides with well-preserved tissue histomorphology and quality of sectioning that is comparable or exceeds that provided by an experienced histology technician.

The tissue cutting system was set-up to cut 5 μm thick sections. From a single tissue block, a set of 38 consecutive re-cuts was generated. After immediate fixation of the re-cuts on glass slides and staining with H&E, the slides were digitized on Panno-ramic Scan II (3DHistech, Budapest, Hungary) slide scanner equipped with a × 20 magnification objective. Each digital slide outputted by the scanner was encoded as an RGB 24bit color image matrix (*.mrxs format) with $0.369 \times 0.369 \, \mu m/px$ resolution, contained approximately $58,800 \times 82,100$ pixels and occupied in compressed form approximately 450 MB of hard drive space. The stack of WSIs was

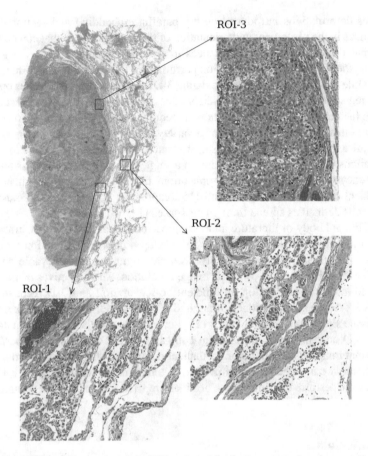

Fig. 1 Top WSI from the stack and the ROIs selected for further processing show small nests of tumor cells in the center of ROI-1 and ROI-2, and at the tumor border in ROI-3

made available by the Pathology Imaging Lab at the Memorial Sloan Kettering Cancer Center in New York. The tissue sectioning, staining and scanning was performed at Massachusetts General Hospital in Boston.

The first WSI from the stack was presented to the pathologist who was asked to mark rectangular regions comprising heterogeneous tissue. Two of the three regions that were marked represented isolated clusters of tumor cells situated within air spaces surrounded by normal lung tissue (ROI-1 and ROI-2). The third region was captured at the border of the tumor mass with some adjacent normal lung tissue (ROI-3, Fig. 1).

3   Methods

3.1   Image Co-registration

Each ROI is a rectangle parallel to the edges of the WSI. The largest ROI measured approximately 2000×2000 pixels, which is less than 5% of the height or width of the WSI. Subsequently, ROI coordinates were propagated down through the stack and region stacks were extracted for visual evaluation. Unfortunately, due to extensive rotations and shifts of the tissue on glass slides, the stacked images in each ROI were severely misaligned, hence prohibiting a reliable 3-D rendering and visualization of all selected ROIs. This motivated us to develop a custom co-registration workflow that can be guided by positions of ROIs selected by the user. The main objective was to deliver well aligned images for 3-D visualization of the ROI.

The co-registration was performed in three steps and instead of RGB images we utilized deconvoluted images of hematoxylin staining. Images were digitally separated into monochromatic images of hematoxylin and eosin stains using the color deconvolution algorithm [18]. Subsequently, the hematoxylin images were used to extract [8] features for image co-registration. The SIFT technique identifies key landmarks in which strongly differentiable areas are detected, filtered, and matched based on their features. We chose hematoxylin images for this task because hematoxylin labels cell nuclei that are good landmark candidates for SIFT feature extraction (Fig. 2). This choice is additionally supported by positive outcomes from our prior co-registration experiments involving hematoxylin images [9]. All steps described below are performed using rigid motion transformations (translation and rotation) through automatically extracted SIFT features and global optimization algorithms [1, 8].

Prior to co-registration, all WSIs were down-sampled with the scale factor of $1/64$ and $1/16$. The down-sampling used the nearest neighbor approach in which every 64th or 16th pixel from the WSI was selected without interpolating the gray tones from the neighboring pixels.

In the first step (#1) all images down-sampled with the scale factor of $1/64$ were organized into a stack and then co-registered (Fig. 3). In this process, the first image from the stack served as the reference image to which the second image from the

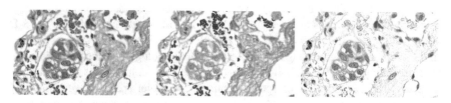

Fig. 2 Color deconvolution of a histological image (left) to eosin (center) and hematoxylin (right) stains. Image contrast is higher in the hematoxylin image than in the eosin or RGB image making the hematoxylin image a good candidate for SIFT feature extraction

stack was aligned. Subsequently, the third image was aligned to the second, the fourth to the third, and so on. The result of this co-registration of N images is a set of rigid transformation parameters: $(\alpha, x, y)_i$, $i \in \{1, \ldots, N\}$, which define the computed transformation of the ith image (angle of rotation around upper-left corner, horizontal and vertical translation, respectively). Based on these parameters, a point corresponding to the position of the centroid of an ROI on each of the down-sampled images was found. A corresponding and 4 times larger ROI is drawn around the centroid on each image in this co-registered stack. In each layer, the new ROI is parallel to the image edges to exclude interpolation errors resulting from image rotation (Fig. 3B). Coordinates of this enlarged ROI are transferred to images down-sampled with the scale factor of 1/16 that are subsequently cropped for the ROIs (Fig. 3C) that are further processed.

In the second step (#2) of the workflow, the images down-sampled with the 1/16 scale factor are co-registered (Fig. 3). Identically to the first step, for each down-sampled and co-registered image a centroid of the ROI is determined and a new ROI parallel to the image's borders is drawn. The ROI coordinates are then scaled up by the factor of 4. At this point the size of the ROI is the same as the size of the ROI marked by the user on the first WSI (Fig. 3E, compare to blue ROI denoted on Fig. 3A).

In the third step (#3), the co-registration of ROIs cropped from the original images was performed. The final registration comprised rigid transformation (translation and/or rotation) only. New pixel values yielded by the rotation were calculated using the nearest neighbor interpolation algorithm (Fig. 3E).

The rigid motion transformation approach was preferred over deformable methods. When sequential slices are co-registered pairwise using deformable methods, the deformations can accumulate across all the layers potentially resulting in poorer co-registration than with rigid motion transformation.

3.2 Stain Color-Normalization

Lack of reproducible H&E staining is a frequently encountered problem in histology laboratories. Substantial variability in stain color has been experienced in controlled environments where preanalytical factors (cutting and fixation) have been optimized for reproducible staining on consecutive days or consecutive slides. Generating large numbers of identically stained serial sections from a single tissue block for 3-D reconstruction is similarly affected [17, 19]. However, the effect of stain coloration on the accuracy of H&E image co-registration methodology has not been reported. To address this issue, we digitally transformed the H&E color spaces in our images to seven different target color spaces. Four of the target spaces were artificially generated and used previously [4]. The three remaining target color spaces were extracted from three example WSIs of lung adenocarcinoma downloaded from the publicly available repository (https://portal.gdc.cancer.gov/). Transferring the entire WSI to a new color space is a computationally expensive task. Thus, to simulate

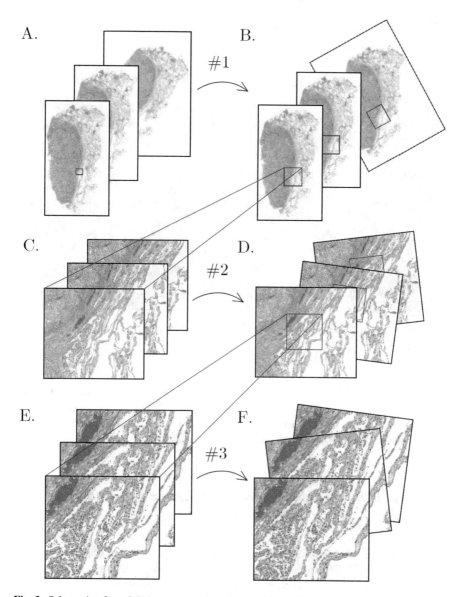

Fig. 3 Schematic of our 3-D image co-registration workflow. The co-registration was performed using downsized (steps #1 and #2) hematoxylin images deconvoluted from the original RGB images. In step #3 full resolution images were used

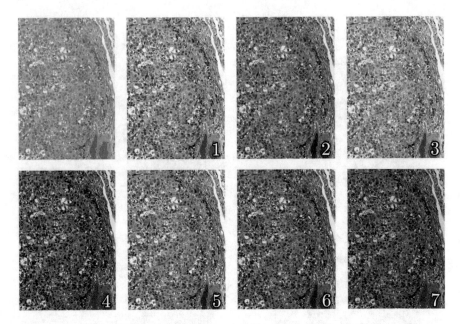

Fig. 4 Section from ROI-3 before (the most upper left) and after H&E normalization using seven color targets (1–7)

the effect of the H&E color change, we only color-transferred images of the three ROIs before step #3 of the co-registration workflow (Fig. 3F) was executed. The ROI's images were sequentially transferred to the seven predefined color spaces using Reinhard's method [16] and are included in (Fig. 4).

3.3 Evaluation of Stain Color-Normalization Effect on the Image Registration Performance

The accuracy of image co-registration can be evaluated based on image landmarks or image masks [7]. We implemented two landmark-based metrics: pair-wise target registration error (*TRE*) and accumulated target registration error (*ATRE*). The landmarks were placed by the pathologist inside or at the center of intersected nuclei or in the center of capillaries of adjacent sections. Since our regions are small, we chose to place two landmarks per section in random areas of the image. Landmark coordinates were saved to calculate *TRE* and *ATRE*.

The *TRE* was quantified for $i \in \{1, \ldots, 37\}$ pairs of sections and for each landmark point $j \in \{1, 2\}$ as follows: $TRE_{j,i} = ||x_{j,i} - x_{j,i+1}||$ that is basically the Euclidean distance between the location $x_{j,i}$ of point j on the section i and the location of the corresponding point on the following section $i + 1$. Unlike *TRE*, that is a local direct measure of co-registration accuracy, *ATRE* can quantitate the distortions accumulated through the stack by treating the displacement of each landmark j for each pair of sections i in vector form as: $X_{j,i} - X_{j,i+1}$, and by calculating the cumulative sum of the mean vectors, proceeding from sections 1 to 38. For section k, *ATRE* is defined as the Euclidean norm of the cumulative displacement vector: $ATRE_k = || \sum_{i=1}^{k} \sum_{j=1}^{2} X_{j,i} - X_{j,i+1} ||$.

Both *TRE* and *ATRE* have been well established to evaluate image co-registration locally, and they are less suited to capture global misalignments. We used the Jaccard index that involves image masks and is a measure that captures misalignments globally between sections. For $\mathcal{A}$ denoting the set of tissue pixels of section i and $\mathcal{B}$ denoting the set of tissue pixels of section $i + 1$, the Jaccard index is defined as: $J_i = |\mathcal{A} \cap \mathcal{B}| / |\mathcal{A} \cup \mathcal{B}|$, where $|\cdot|$ is the cardinality, $\cap$ is the intersection, and $\cup$ the union of $\mathcal{A}$ and $\mathcal{B}$. Prior to calculating J, each image section was co-registered with our method, then converted to a gray level image and then thresholded using a fixed cut off value. We also implemented the root mean squared error *RMSE* to evaluate the similarity of pixel intensities y on two consecutive sections i and $i + 1$ as: $RMSE = \sqrt{\frac{1}{N} \sum_{j=1}^{N} (y_{j,i} - y_{j,i+1})^2}$, where N is the number of pixels in the section. The *RMSE* was calculated using a gray scale representation of the original images. The smaller the values of *RMSE*, *TRE*, and *ATRE*, the smaller the observed error. For *Jaccard* index that measures the degree of tissue overlap, the larger the index value, the better the overlap.

3.4   3-D Visualization

Lastly, to assess the efficacy of image co-registration and to visually evaluate whether our workflow can deliver 3-D views of isolated tumor cells, the co-registered ROIs were imported to 3-D Slicer (ver. 4.10.2)—an open source platform for volumetric visualization, (https://www.slicer.org/) for 3-D rendering.

4   Results

We have developed a new workflow for 3-D tissue reconstruction and visualization and tested its co-registration accuracy by perturbing colors of H&E staining in three expert-selected ROIs. The effects were evaluated by *TRE ATRE*, *RMSE* and *Jaccard* index error measures that we calculated and compared for all ROIs and for eight color spaces (the original and seven new ones). The results summarized in Table 1 include the mean and standard deviations for normal distributed variables or median and quartile deviations (QD) for non-normal distributed variables to reflect the error dispersion.

Table 1 Values of *TRE*, *ATRE*, Jaccard index, *RMSE* for non-normalized images and color-images normalized using seven (1–7) different color spaces. Metrics from the color-normalized experiments that are statistically different from those obtained for non-normalized images are bolded

Normalization		None	1	2	3	4	5	6	7
ROI-1									
TRE	Median	8.44	8.16	7.93	8.25	8.65	8.44	7.98	8.48
	QD	5.30	4.62	5.11	4.22	4.90	4.10	4.34	4.35
ARTE	Median	41.44	40.62	**45.25**	40.90	**41.16**	**42.18**	**36.96**	**43.78**
	QD	8.26	10.01	13.28	9.6	10.70	10.10	9.97	9.57
Jaccard	Mean	0.47	**0.44**	**0.49**	**0.45**	**0.50**	**0.49**	**0.49**	**0.49**
	Std	0.04	0.02	0.02	0.02	0.02	0.02	0.02	0.02
RMSE	Mean	10.37	**10.70**	10.52	**10.59**	**10.58**	**10.64**	10.57	10.45
	Std	0.99	0.41	0.39	0.41	0.39	0.39	0.39	0.39
ROI-2									
TRE	Median	5.80	5.23	5.31	5.74	5.18	5.17	5.98	5.36
	QD	2.62	2.58	2.82	3.40	3.01	2.78	3.23	2.79
ATRE	Median	51.16	**54.62**	**47.06**	51.69	**48.65**	**44.34**	**46.44**	**49.17**
	QD	25.42	25.86	22.45	25.22	22.68	20.26	22.96	24.13
Jaccard	Mean	0.51	**0.47**	**0.52**	**0.49**	**0.53**	**0.51**	**0.52**	**0.53**
	Std	0.03	0.02	0.02	0.02	0.02	0.02	0.02	0.02
RMSE	Mean	10.26	**10.63**	10.43	10.49	10.41	**10.57**	10.44	10.28
	Std	1.13	0.41	0.39	0.40	0.41	0.39	0.40	0.41
ROI-3									
TRE	Median	5.45	6.46	6.25	5.94	6.02	5.59	5.92	6.09
	QD	4.18	3.75	3.53	3.41	3.43	3.55	3.68	3.49
ATRE	Median	60.01	**57.18**	63.74	**66.89**	**71.05**	**69.10**	**72.48**	**66.40**
	QD	27.36	26.51	30.15	30.94	32.63	32.42	32.45	30.05
Jaccard	Mean	0.47	**0.43**	**0.49**	0.46	**0.54**	0.48	**0.50**	**0.51**
	Std	0.8	0.3	0.3	0.3	0.3	0.3	0.3	0.3
RMSE	Mean	9.96	**10.60**	10.36	**10.46**	10.38	**10.50**	**10.40**	10.24
	Std	1.59	0.32	0.32	0.32	0.33	0.32	0.33	0.34

The normality of error value distributions was checked by the Shapiro-Wilk test. Since the majority of *TRE* and *ATRE* results did not meet the conditions of normality ($p > 0.05$), we applied a non-parametric Wilcoxon Rank-Sum test to compare values of *TRE* and *ATRE* and identify whether there is a statistically significant difference between the errors from non-normalized and each color-normalized set of images. No statistically significant difference was observed between *TRE* calculated for the non-normalized and color-normalized images ($p > 0.05$) in all ROIs. On the other hand, *ATRE* increased significantly ($p < 0.05$) over the baseline (non-normalized

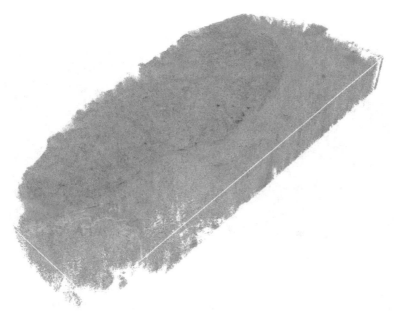

Fig. 5 3-D rendering of a WSI stack outputted in step #1 in Fig. 3

images) for nearly every color-normalization scheme. QD values of *TRE* and *ATRE* were high compared to the medians suggesting a large spread in the error values.

Distributions of the *Jaccard* index passed the test for normality for all experiments. Therefore, the comparison of error measures from non-normalized images and all the color-normalized was performed with the Student's dependent t-test for paired samples. Statistically significant difference was obtained for all color normalization schemes for ROI-1 and ROI-2 ($p < 0.05$), and for five schemes for ROI-3. The highest value of the *Jaccard* index was obtained for color normalization with H&E color scheme No. 4 (Fig. 4). Note, that *Jaccard* standard deviations from experiments with color-normalized data were often lower by two folds or more than those obtained for non-normalized images.

In most color-normalization experiments and all experiments with non-normalized images, the normality of *RMSE* distribution was confirmed by the Shapiro-Wilk test. Mean values of the *Jaccard* index *RMSE* calculated in color-normalized regions exceeded those from the non-normalized regions. Interestingly, standard deviations of *RMSE* from color-normalized images were much lower than those calculated from non-normalized images.

Lastly, the co-registered WSIs from step #1 (Fig. 5), and the ROIs after conclusion of the co-registration were imported and then volume rendered in the 3-D Slicer. The rendered volumes were clipped and zoomed in to visualize clusters of tumor cells in selected ROIs (Fig. 6). One of the clipping planes traversed perpendicularly to the WSI planes through the tumor cell clusters to reveal the internal structure of the

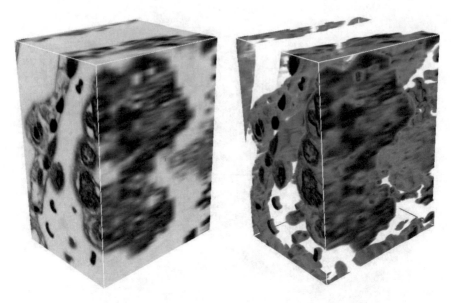

Fig. 6 3-D views of central part of ROI-1 with various opacities. The cutting plane corresponds to the first column in Fig. 7

clusters and compare the appearance of intersected clusters before and after color-normalization (Fig. 7). The voxel size of $0.39 \times 0.39 \times 3\,\mu$m was set up in the 3-D Slicer interface.

The workflow was implemented in Python 3.6.9 running on Linux Mint 19 Tara with hardware platform comprising AMD Ryzen 7 2700 (CPU), 64 GB RAM, Nvidia GeForce GTX 1070 (GPU) and an SSD drive. All image data processing routines were embedded into a single Python script that used native libraries "Register Virtual Stack Slices"—an image co-registration Java-based plugin from ImageJ [1] with default parameters (SIFT technique).

For a single ROI stack co-registration, the workflow needed about 17 min. Approximately 60% of the time was used for input/output operations (mainly reading and decompressing the WSIs). Up to 20 GB of RAM had to be available for the code.

5 Discussion

In this paper we present a new workflow dedicated to volumetric data visualization. In contrast to studies that compare accuracy of different co-registration methods to identify those that are best for general purpose 3-D visualization [5, 7], we focused on developing a workflow that can output high-quality views of isolated clusters of tumor cells—currently a focus in lung cancer pathology.

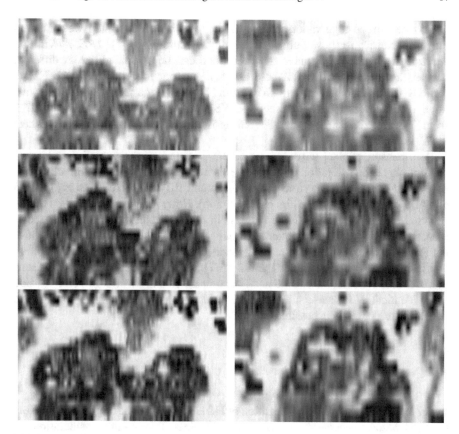

Fig. 7 Perpendicular planes of cropped volumetric images. First row: original colors; second and third rows: images after color normalization

We first compared the error values between our experiments. Due to large QD of *TRE* values, we did not observe any quantifiable effects of the color-normalization on the image co-registration. Likewise, no significant difference was observed between the mean error measure in the ROIs. In the same ROI, the *ATRE* index for color-normalized images was either a bit higher or lower than its equivalent for non-normalized images, yet without exhibiting an observable trend.

On the other hand, the normalization with the color pattern No. 4 (a relatively dark H&E hue) consistently yielded the highest *Jaccard* index (range between 0.50 and 0.53), suggesting that specimens stained darker can align better than specimens with lighter coloration: No. 1 (0.47–0.44) or non-normalized (0.51–0.47) that are also light. Interestingly, the color-normalization increased the average of *RMSE* and lowered the standard deviations of *RMSE* and *Jaccard*, thereby suggesting that the color normalization reduces hue differences and also increases tissue overlap between adjacent sections. These effects, while appearing small from the quantitative standpoint, seem to visibly improve visualization of the tumor cells (Fig. 7).

To assess the co-registration accuracy of our tool, in the second step, we compared our error metrics to those published recently. According to [7], *TRE*, *ATRE*, and *Jaccard* are invariant to image resolution and can be compared across different datasets and resolutions. With these assumptions, our highest mean *TRE* (12.06 for ROI-1) was much lower than *TRE*s from [7]: 62.17 for a set of 260 WSIs from a human prostate and 145.16 for a set of 47 WSIs from a human liver. The mean *ATRE* from [7] were: 223.89 (liver) and 577.46 (prostate) and thus higher than our highest *ATRE* of 60.55 (ROI-3).

As a measure of pixel-wise similarity, *RMSE* depends on the resolution and image content. Since the resolution of our images is much higher, we cannot directly compare *RMSE*s from our experiments (values around 10) to those reported in [7] (52.5 and 41.9 for images with the highest resolution). However, we note that the *RMSE*s reported in [7] increased with the increase in image resolution for the same specimen, suggesting that *RMSE*s obtained through our workflow are very low. The above comparisons were made using results generated with the SIFT-based co-registration approach and included in Tables 1 and 2 of [7]. To obtain quantitative comparisons that are more reliable, one would need to compare existing workflows side-by-side using identical WSI datasets. This might be feasible when stacks with serial WSIs become more publicly accessible.

6   Conclusions

In our experiments, color normalization of H&E staining did not significantly affect the SIFT-based co-registration performance of WSIs. Taking into consideration the section-to section variability of the staining, the robustness of SIFT against this variability is a desirable feature that is applicable in 3-D histopathology. Low co-registration errors of our workflow allowed us to accurately visualize clusters of tumor cells as well as the area of tumor mass in small regions. The pipeline that we developed could support the 3-D evaluation of histologically complex tumors.

Acknowledgements This work has been supported by in part by the Precision Health Grant at C-S and seed grants from the Department of Surgery at Cedars-Sinai Medical Center. The authors would like to thank Dr. Mari Mino-Kenudson from the Massachusetts General Hospital for her help in data preparation and input on the manuscript.

References

1. Arganda-Carreras, I., Sorzano, C.O.S., Marabini, R., Carazo, J.M., Ortiz-de Solorzano, C., Kybic, J.: Consistent and elastic registration of histological sections using vector-spline regularization. In: Beichel, R.R., Sonka, M. (eds.) Computer Vision Approaches to Medical Image Analysis, pp. 85–95. Springer, Berlin (2006). https://doi.org/10.1007/11889762_8

2. Falk, M., Ynnerman, A., Treanor, D., Lundström, C.: Interactive visualization of 3D histopathology in native resolution. IEEE Trans. Vis. Comput. Graph. **25**(1), 1008–1017 (2019). https://doi.org/10.1109/TVCG.2018.2864816
3. Farahani, N., Braun, A., Jutt, D., Huffman, T., Reder, N., Liu, Z., Yagi, Y., Pantanowitz, L.: Three-dimensional imaging and scanning: current and future applications for pathology. J. Pathol. Inf. **8**(1), 36 (2017). https://doi.org/10.4103/jpi.jpi_32_17
4. Gertych, A., Swiderska-Chadaj, Z., Ma, Z., Ing, N., Markiewicz, T., Cierniak, S., Salemi, H., Guzman, S., Walts, A.E., Knudsen, B.S.: Convolutional neural networks can accurately distinguish four histologic growth patterns of lung adenocarcinoma in digital slides. Sci. Rep. **9**(1) (2019). https://doi.org/10.1038/s41598-018-37638-9
5. Gibson, E., Gaed, M., Gómez, J., Moussa, M., Pautler, S., Chin, J., Crukley, C., Bauman, G., Fenster, A., Ward, A.: 3D prostate histology image reconstruction: quantifying the impact of tissue deformation and histology section location. J. Pathol. Inf. **4**(1), 31 (2013)
6. Kadota, K., Nitadori, J., Sima, C.S., Ujiie, H., Rizk, N.P., Jones, D.R., Adusumilli, P.S., Travis, W.D.: Tumor spread through air spaces is an important pattern of invasion and impacts the frequency and location of recurrences after limited resection for small stage 1 lung adenocarcinomas. J. Thoracic Oncol. **10**(5), 806–814 (2015). https://doi.org/10.1097/JTO.0000000000000486
7. Kartasalo, K., Latonen, L., Vihinen, J., Visakorpi, T., Nykter, M., Ruusuvuori, P.: Comparative analysis of tissue reconstruction algorithms for 3D histology. Bioinformatics **34**(17), 3013–3021 (2018). https://doi.org/10.1093/bioinformatics/bty210
8. Lowe, D.G.: Object recognition from local scale-invariant features. In: Proceedings of the International Conference on Computer Vision, ICCV '99, vol. 2, p. 1150. IEEE Computer Society, USA (1999)
9. Ma, Z., Shiao, S.L., Yoshida, E.J., Swartwood, S., Huang, F., Doche, M.E., Chung, A.P., Knudsen, B.S., Gertych, A.: Data integration from pathology slides for quantitative imaging of multiple cell types within the tumor immune cell infiltrate. Diagn. Pathol. **12**(1) (2017). https://doi.org/10.1186/s13000-017-0658-8
10. Magee, D., Song, Y., Gilbert, S., Roberts, N., Wijayathunga, N., Wilcox, R., Bulpitt, A., Treanor, D.: Histopathology in 3D: from three-dimensional reconstruction to multi-stain and multi-modal analysis. J. Pathol. Inf. **6**(1), 6 (2015). https://doi.org/10.4103/2153-3539.151890
11. Morales-Oyarvide, V., Mino-Kenudson, M.: Taking the measure of lung adenocarcinoma: towards a quantitative approach to tumor spread through air spaces (STAS). J. Thorac. Dis. **9**(9) (2017). https://doi.org/10.21037/jtd.2017.07.97
12. Onozato, M., Klepeis, V., Yagi, Y., Mino-Kenudson, M.: A role of three-dimensional (3D)-reconstruction in the classification of lung adenocarcinoma. Anal. Cell. Pathol. **35**(2), 79–84 (2012). https://doi.org/10.3233/ACP-2011-0030
13. Onozato, M.L., Hammond, S., Merren, M., Yagi, Y.: Evaluation of a completely automated tissue-sectioning machine for paraffin blocks. J. Clin. Pathol. **66**(2), 151–154 (2013). https://doi.org/10.1136/jclinpath-2011-200205
14. Pantanowitz, L., Valenstein, P., Evans, A., Kaplan, K., Pfeifer, J., Wilbur, D., Collins, L., Colgan, T.: Review of the current state of whole slide imaging in pathology. J. Pathol. Inf. **2**(1), 36 (2011). https://doi.org/10.4103/2153-3539.83746
15. Pichat, J., Iglesias, J.E., Yousry, T., Ourselin, S., Modat, M.: A survey of methods for 3D histology reconstruction. Med. Image Anal. **46**, 73–105 (2018). https://doi.org/10.1016/j.media.2018.02.004
16. Reinhard, E., Adhikhmin, M., Gooch, B., Shirley, P.: Color transfer between images. IEEE Comput. Grap. Appl. **21**(5), 34–41 (2001). https://doi.org/10.1109/38.946629
17. Roberts, N., Magee, D., Song, Y., Brabazon, K., Shires, M., Crellin, D., Orsi, N.M., Quirke, R., Quirke, P., Treanor, D.: Toward routine use of 3D histopathology as a research tool. Am. J. Pathol. **180**(5), 1835–1842 (2012). https://doi.org/10.1016/j.ajpath.2012.01.033
18. Ruifrok, A.C., Johnston, D.A.: Quantification of histochemical staining by color deconvolution. Anal. Quant. Cytol. Histol. **23**(4), 291–299 (2001)

19. Song, Y., Treanor, D., Bulpitt, A., Magee, D.: 3D reconstruction of multiple stained histology images. J. Pathol. Inf. **4**(2), 7 (2013). https://doi.org/10.4103/2153-3539.109864
20. Song, Y., Treanor, D., Bulpitt, A.J., Wijayathunga, N., Roberts, N., Wilcox, R., Magee, D.R.: Unsupervised content classification based nonrigid registration of differently stained histology images. IEEE Trans. Biomed. Eng. **61**(1), 96–108 (2014). https://doi.org/10.1109/TBME.2013. 2277777
21. Travis, W.D., Brambilla, E., Nicholson, A.G., Yatabe, Y., Austin, J.H., Beasley, M.B., Chirieac, L.R., Dacic, S., Duhig, E., Flieder, D.B., Geisinger, K., Hirsch, F.R., Ishikawa, Y., Kerr, K.M., Noguchi, M., Pelosi, G., Powell, C.A., Tsao, M.S., Wistuba, I.: The 2015 world health organization classification of lung tumors: impact of genetic, clinical and radiologic advances since the 2004 classification. J. Thor. Oncol. **10**(9), 1243–1260 (2015). https://doi.org/10.1097/JTO. 0000000000000630
22. Walts, A.E., Marchevsky, A.M.: Current evidence does not warrant frozen section evaluation for the presence of tumor spread through alveolar spaces. Arch. Pathol. Lab. Med. **142**(1), 59–63 (2018). https://doi.org/10.5858/arpa.2016-0635-OA
23. Warth, A.: Spread through air spaces (STAS): a comprehensive update. Transl. Lung Cancer Res. **6**(5), 501 (2017)
24. Xu, Y., Pickering, J.G., Nong, Z., Ward, A.D.: 3D morphological measurement of whole slide histological vasculature reconstructions. In: Gurcan, M.N., Madabhushi, A. (eds.) Medical Imaging 2016: Digital Pathology, vol. 9791, pp. 181–187. International Society for Optics and Photonics, SPIE (2016). https://doi.org/10.1117/12.2214871
25. Yagi, Y., Aly, R.G., Tabata, K., Barlas, A., Rekhtman, N., Eguchi, T., Montecalvo, J., Hameed, M., Manova-Todorova, K., Adusumilli, P.S., Travis, W.D.: Three-dimensional histologic, immunohistochemical and multiplex immunofluorescence analysis of dynamic vessel co-option of spread through air spaces (STAS) in lung adenocarcinoma. J. Thor. Oncol. (2019). https://doi.org/10.1016/j.jtho.2019.12.112
26. Yagi, Y., Tabata, K., Rekhtman, N., Eguchi, T., Fu, X., Montecalvo, J., Adusumilli, P., Hameed, M., Travis, W.: Three-dimensional assessment of spread through air spaces in lung adenocarcinoma: insights and implications. J. Thor. Oncol. **12**(11), S1797 (2017)

The Influence of Age on Morphometric and Textural Vertebrae Features in Lateral Cervical Spine Radiographs

Patrycja Mazur, Rafał Obuchowicz, and Adam Piórkowski

Abstract This article presents research on the relationship between age on one hand and morphometric and textural features of vertebrae in lateral cervical spine radiographs on the other. Images were collected for 93 men and 88 women as a population sample. Regions of interest were marked on each image and analyzed using the MaZda software. Statistical analysis identified features that are correlated significantly with age. The strongest correlations were found for equivalent ellipsoid diameter in the case of morphometry, and LBP, GLCM, and GRLM for textures. The influence on the results of image formats, color depth and gender is also discussed.

Keywords Texture analysis · Morphometry · LBP · GLCM · GRLM · Age · Trabecular bone

1 Introduction

Research shows that changes occur in the spine as a result of ageing. Genetic conditions, sport, lifestyle, hormonal changes, and diseases can affect the rate of these changes. Therefore, it is often the case that the condition of the spine is much worse than the patient's age would indicate.

With increasing age, there is selective loss of transversely oriented trabeculae, therefore the cervical vertebrae become wider and shorter. This leads to intervertebral disc shape changes, changes in elasticity and spinal posture, or osteopenia, which is a disease that is considered to be an early stage of osteoporosis and affects women

P. Mazur · A. Piórkowski (✉)
Department of Biocybernetics and Biomedical Engineering, AGH University of Science and Technology, A. Mickiewicza 30 Av., 30-059 Cracow, Poland
e-mail: pioro@agh.edu.pl

R. Obuchowicz
Department of Diagnostic Imaging, Jagiellonian University Medical College, Kopernika 19, 31-501 Cracow, Poland
e-mail: rafalobuchowicz@su.krakow.pl

E. Piętka et al. (eds.), *Information Technology in Biomedicine*, Advances in Intelligent Systems and Computing 1186, https://doi.org/10.1007/978-3-030-49666-1_6

more often than man. This is because bone is a tissue that is significantly influenced by hormones, which affect males and females differently [16].

Osteoporosis or osteopenia are not the only skeletal diseases. With age, people are exposed to erosion, syndesmophytes or osteophytes [1]. Another relatively common problem is spondyloarthritis [5], which may lead to structural damage [6]. Osteogenesis, which is a result of chronic inflammation, is a medical term for new bone formation. Excessive bone formation leads to changes in the shape of the spine which make it stiff.

Assessment of the age of human bones is an interesting issue for many doctors because it enables correct diagnosis or choice of appropriate treatment. One piece of research presents a scale that can be used to determine the various stages of cervical spine degeneration and its biological age [17]. A scoring system was established, as part of which MRI images are assessed. The Pearson correlation coefficient between the patient's age and the sum of values according to the proposed scale was 0.726. However, the study did not include osteoporosis, which is a relatively important factor in assessing the condition of the spine [7].

Age assessment does not only concern the spine as changes can occur in all bones. One study determined the effect of age and osteoporosis on calcaneus trabecular bone structure [4]. For this purpose, MRI images were analyzed. It was found that to differentiate the structure of a healthy person's bone trabecula from the osteoporosis of an elderly person's trabeculae, an ROI that covers the part of the calcaneus that has low density of trabeculae is best. Unfortunately, the influence of osteoporosis on bone structure was not determined. In addition, the study was carried out on a relatively small number of MRI images.

Numerous attempts to link age with bone structures have been carried out based on dental pantomograms. It is therefore worth considering age when analyzing trabecular structures in various contexts such as healing processes [2] or lytic changes resulting from disease [3].

2   Materials and Methods

The collected radiographs of the cervical spine (93 men and 88 women) were acquired from Agfa CR 25 or 35 equipment. It is worth mentioning that these X-rays were from real-life clinical diagnoses, therefore degeneration or disease may have influenced the results. The pixel spacing value for all images was 0.1×0.1 mm. Morphometric and textural analysis was performed using the qMaZda software (ver. 19.02) [12, 13]. For males, each radiograph was saved in 4 formats:

- PNG8—PNG image with a color depth of 8 bits, scaled using ImageJ software,
- CLAHE—PNG image with a color depth of 8 bits after Contrast-Limited Adaptive Histogram Equalization,
- PNG16—PNG image with a color depth of 16 bits, converted using dcm2pnm software,

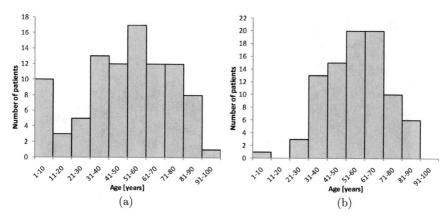

Fig. 1 Histograms of patients age—male (**a**), and female (**b**)

- DICOM—DICOM image with a color depth of 15 bits.

The analysis of all groups of male radiographs made it possible to determine the impact of the image format on the results, as is discussed in [10, 11]. The observations were described in the next stage of the work, which involved analysis of X-rays of the cervical spine of women. These images were processed only in two formats: DICOM and PNG8. The former was chosen because it presents the original color depth. The choice of the latter is justified by the conclusions from the analysis of radiographs of men.

The patients differ significantly in age (Fig. 1); however, most of them were 31–80 years old (Fig. 2).

The first step of the analysis was to define the regions of interest, namely cervical vertebral bodies. These ROIs were depicted manually (Fig. 2c, f). Due to the artifacts, not all of them were always selected. Moreover, the centers but not the edges of vertebral bodies were included in the region of interest due to the need to observe the reduction of trabeculae but not the progression of osteogenesis. Defined regions were analyzed. The obtained features described not only the texture but also the geometry and histogram of the region of interest. The statistical analysis of the results, which consisted in calculating the value of Pearson's r coefficient, made it possible to determine which of the features correlate with the patient's age. Further work will include automatic segmentation of ROI [6, 9].

2.1 X-Rays of Men's Cervical Spine

The statistical analysis made it possible to identify features that correlated significantly with the patients' age. The features were divided into two groups that were sensitive and insensitive to the image format, respectively. The first group included

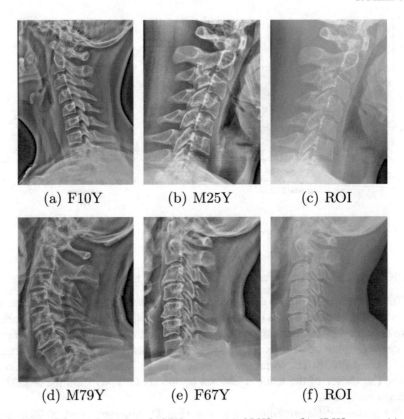

(a) F10Y   (b) M25Y   (c) ROI

(d) M79Y   (e) F67Y   (f) ROI

Fig. 2 X-ray of the cervical spine of 10 YO woman (**a**), 25 YO man (**b**), 67 YO woman (**e**), and 79 YO man (**d**) after contrast correction (CLAHE). ROI on **c** and **f**

Table 1 The 5 best Pearson correlation coefficient values for different image formats and image features (men)

Features	PNG8	CLAHE	PNG16	DICOM
YLbpCs8n15	−0.65	−0.54	−0.39	−0.12
D8HistPerc99	−0.42	−0.51	−	−
YLbpOc4n0	0.43	0.47	0.23	0.24
YD8DwtHaarS3LH	−0.40	−0.33	−0.17	−0.08
YLbpOc4n3	−0.37	−0.30	−0.33	0.04

texture features and parameters calculated on the basis of image histograms (presented in the Table 1); the second group was calculated on the basis of morphometric parameters (Table 2).

The first, third and fifth parameters from the Table 1 were calculated in the qMazda program using the Local Binary Pattern (LBP) algorithm. The designations 4n and 8n in the parameter names refer to the size of the area in which the relationships

Table 2 The 5 best Pearson correlation coefficient values for different image formats and morphometric features (men)

Morphometric features	
MorItkEquivalentEllipsoidDiameterX	0.63
MorMzS	0.59
MorMzRb	0.55
MorItkPrincipalMomentX	0.53
MorMzW6	−0.50

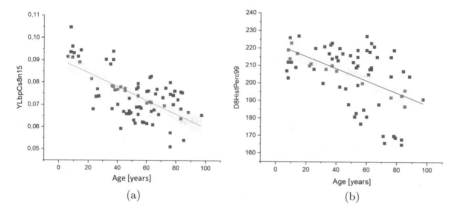

Fig. 3 Change of YLbpCs8n15 (**a**) and D8HistPerc99 (**b**) value depending on the patient's age (men)

between pixel brightness are determined. The abbreviations Oc and Cs indicate the pattern on the basis of which the parameter was calculated (Oc—over-complete, Cs—center-symmetric).

For the $YLbpOc4n0$ parameter, the highest correlation value was achieved during the analysis of images whose histogram was equalized (CLAHE). However, Pearson's r coefficient showed no correlation between a given parameter and the patient's age calculated for PNG images with a color depth of 16 bits and DICOM images.

For the $YLbpCs8n15$ parameter, the highest correlation value was obtained for PNG images with a color depth of 8 bits. However, just like in the previous case, the analysis of DICOM images and PNG images with a color depth of 16 bits produced the smallest result in the context of the correlation between the texture parameter and the patient's age. $YLbpCs8n15$ is the feature with the highest correlation, which is negative. This means that its value decreases with age (Fig. 3a).

The $D8HistPerc99$ feature results from the calculation of the histogram for the selected region of interest. It is worth noting that color depth is 16 bits for DICOM images and PNG images, therefore the correlation coefficients for a given parameter were not calculated with MaZda.

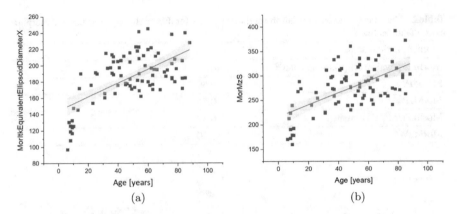

Fig. 4 Change of MorItkEquivalentEllipsoidDiameterX (**a**) and MorMzS (**b**) value depending on the patient's age (men)

The features from the Table 2 describe the shape of the ROI. They are characterized by lower sensitivity to distortions than other features. In addition, the $MorItkEquivalentEllipsoidDiameterX$ feature has the highest correlation coefficient of the all features (Fig. 4a). It can be considered for other applications [15].

One of the morphometric features is $MorMzS$, which specifies the length of the smallest rectangle which contains all points of the ROI (Fig. 4b). With age, this value increases, which may be due to the formation of syndesmophytes, which typically lengthen the ends of the cervical vertebrae.

The $MorMzRb$ feature is a Blair-Bliss coefficient that defines the ratio of the ROI surface area to the sum of the distance of subsequent pixels from its center. For the data analyzed, it correlates positively with the patient's age.

The only negative Pearson r correlation coefficient is the result of calculations for the $MorMzW6$ feature. The parameter value is the quotient of the square of the perimeter of the selected ROI and its area.

2.2 X-Rays of Women's Cervical Spine

In the case of women's cervical spine images, only two formats were analyzed: DICOM and PNG images with a color depth of 8 bits. Despite this, sensitivity of some features to the image format was observed (Table 3).

The $D8HistVariance$ parameter has the highest correlation with patient's age. This feature is based on the calculation of the histogram for the selected region of interest. Its value increases with the patient's age (Fig. 5a).

$YD5GlcmN2Correlat$ and $YD5GlcmN3Correlat$ are texture features that are calculated on the basis of the Grey-Level Co-occurrence Matrix (GLCM) algorithm. The correlation values are stable for DICOM and PNG8 formats (Fig. 5b).

Table 3 The 5 best Pearson correlation coefficient values for different image formats and image features (women)

Features	DICOM	PNG8
D8HistVariance	NAN	0.38
YD5GlcmN2Correlat	0.30	0.34
YD5GlcmN3Correlat	0.32	0.33
YD5GrlmZGLevNonUn	−0.15	−0.34
YD5GrlmNGLevNonUn	−0.14	−0.34

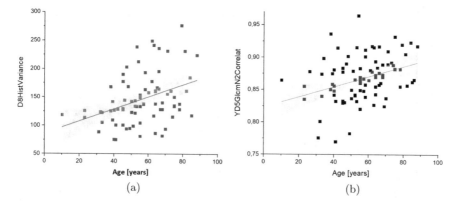

(a)   (b)

Fig. 5 Change of D8HistVariance (**a**) and YD5GlcmN2Correlat (**b**) value depending on the patient's age (women)

$YD5GrlmNGLevNonUn$ and $YD5GrlmZGLevNonUn$ are texture features that are calculated on the basis of the Grey-level Run-Length Matrix (GRLM) algorithm. Both features differ only in the direction of the algorithm. For DICOM images, Pearson's r value is so low that it cannot be considered that there is any correlation between patient age and these texture features. For PNG images with a color depth of 8 bits, this value is higher but is still very low. Such a correlation between data can be described as very weak.

Higher correlation coefficient values were obtained for features that did not show sensitivity to the image format. These were, as with the analysis of male X-rays, morphometric features. However, significant correlation values for female X-rays were obtained for completely different features than for male X-rays (Table 4).

$MorMzW8$ and $MorMzRh$ are features with a positive correlation with age (Fig. 6a). The former defines the ratio of width to length of the smallest rectangle, which contains all points located in the ROI; the latter is Haralick's ratio. $MorMzL$ is a morphometric feature that defines the width of the smallest rectangle that contains all points belonging to a region of interest. In the case of radiographs of female cervical spine X-rays, this width decreases with age. Other features which also have a negative correlation coefficient are $MorMzW7$ and $MorMzEr$. The former deter-

Table 4 The 7 best Pearson correlation coefficient values for different image formats and morphometric features (women)

Morphometric features	
MorMzW8	0.64
MorItkElongation	−0.61
MorMzRh	0.50
MorItkPrincipalMomentY	−0.49
MorMzEr	−0.47
MorMzW7	−0.44
MorMzL	−0.42

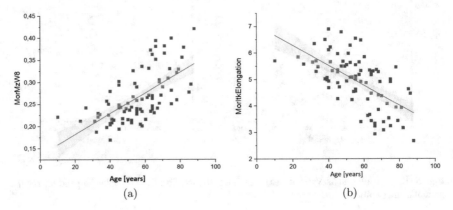

(a)   (b)

Fig. 6 Change of MorMzW8 (**a**) and MorItkElongation (**b**) value depending on the patient's age (women)

mines the ratio of the diameter of the circle describing the ROI area to the diameter of the largest circle that can be inscribed in this area. This feature describes the circularity of the object well. The latter, $MorMzEr$, determines the average distance of pixels contained in the region of interest from the center of gravity of the object.

3 Discussion

In the case of x-rays of men, texture features that correlated with age resulted from calculations based on the LBP algorithm [8]. Two methods were used: $YLbpOc4n0$ and $YLbpCs8n15$, both of which differ in terms of the size of the neighborhood. Pearson's coefficient for the former was positive and for the latter was negative. In contrast, in the case of x-ray images of the female cervical spine, the values of texture features correlating with age resulted from the use of the Grey-level Run-Length Matrix algorithm (GRLM). These parameters ($YD5GrlmNLevNonUn$ and

$YD5GrlmZLevNonUn$) obtained statistically significant values only when PNG images with a color depth of 8 bits were analyzed. It is worth noting that Pearson's r coefficients for texture features of female X-rays are lower than for texture features of male X-rays. Perhaps this shows a greater difference in female aging and the impact of osteoporosis, which mainly affects women.

Features that show changes in values depending on a patient's age are also the result of the histogram calculation. With age, the trabecular bones deteriorate, which affects the amount of X-rays absorbed during examinations.

An interesting fact is that features calculated on the basis of the LBP algorithm played a significant role in the analysis of male X-rays, but showed no significant correlation with age for female spinal images. In their case, age-dependent changes were displayed in the value of GRLM features. The features of the histogram of images with significant correlation with age were calculated for female X-rays based on variance, while for male X-rays they were based on the $Perc99$ function.

The results showed that the image format is very important for analysis in qMaZda software. PNG images with a color depth of 8 bits turned out to be the best. Contrast-Limited Adaptive Histogram Equalization (CLAHE) also had positive effects, especially for features based on the histogram. Choosing DICOM images or PNG images with a color depth of 16 bits may result in some algorithms not returning a numeric value. This shows that not only the format but also the color depth is very important for such analysis.

Pearson's R-value also reached significant values for morphometric parameters of ROI. For male X-rays, one of the shape features correlated with age is $MorMzS$, which defines the length of the smallest rectangle containing all ROI points. The width of this rectangle turned out to be important for female radiographs. The difference between the sexes is also illustrated by the $MorItkPrincipalMoment$ feature, where values for male X-rays correlated for the x axis, and for female X-rays they correlated for the y axis. As with texture features and histogram features, shape-related parameters for female X-rays also have a lower age-correlation coefficient than those obtained through the analysis of male X-rays. Further works include textural analysis of the trabecular bone for CT and MRI modalities [14].

Acknowledgements This publication was funded by AGH University of Science and Technology, Faculty of Electrical Engineering, Automatics, Computer Science and Biomedical Engineering under grant number 16.16.120.773.

References

1. Bielecka, M., Obuchowicz, R., Korkosz, M.: The shape language in application to the diagnosis of cervical vertebrae pathology. PLOS ONE **13**(10), 1–17 (2018). https://doi.org/10.1371/journal.pone.0204546
2. Borowska, M., Szarmach, J., Oczeretko, E.: Fractal texture analysis of the healing process after bone loss. Comput. Med. Imaging Graph. **46**, 191–196 (2015)

3. Chrzan, R., Jurczyszyn, A., Urbanik, A.: Whole-body low-dose computed tomography (wbldct) in assessment of patients with multiple myeloma-pilot study and standard imaging protocol suggestion. Pol. J. Radiol. **82**, 356 (2017)
4. Herlidou, S., Grebe, R., Grados, F., Leuyer, N., Fardellone, P., Meyer, M.E.: Influence of age and osteoporosis on calcaneus trabecular bone structure: a preliminary in vivo mri study by quantitative texture analysis. Magn. Reson. Imaging **22**, 237–243 (2004)
5. Korkosz, M., Gluszko, P., Marcinek, P.: Comment on bone mineral density and bone turnover markers in a group of male ankylosing spondylitis patients. JCR: J. Clin. Rheumatol. **8**(6), 359–360 (2002)
6. Nurzynska, K., Piorkowski, A., Bielecka, M., Obuchowicz, R., Taton, G., Sulicka, J., Korkosz, M.: Automatical syndesmophyte contour extraction from lateral c spine radiographs. Pol. Conf. Biocybern. Biomed. Eng. **13**(10), 164–173 (2017)
7. Palanivel, D.A., Natarajan, S., Gopalakrishnan, S., Jennane, R.: Multifractal-based lacunarity analysis of trabecular bone in radiography. Comput. Biol. Med. **116**, 103, 559 (2020)
8. Smolka, B., Nurzynska, K.: Power LBP: a novel texture operator for smiling and neutral facial display classification. Procedia Comput. Sci. **51**, 1555–1564 (2015)
9. Strzelecki, M.: Texture boundary detection using network of synchronised oscillators. Electron. Lett. **40**(8), 466–467 (2004)
10. Strzelecki, M., Kociolek, M., Materka, A.: On the influence of image features wordlength reduction on texture classification. In: International Conference on Information Technologies in Biomedicine, pp. 15–26 (2018)
11. Kociołek, M., Strzelecki, M., Obuchowicz, R.: Does image normalization and intensity resolution impact texture classification? Comput. Med. Imaging Graph. **81**, 101716 (2020)
12. Szczypiński, P.M., Klepaczko, A., Kociołek, M.: Qmazda - software tools for image analysis and pattern recognition. In: 2017 Signal Processing: Algorithms, Architectures, Arrangements, and Applications (SPA), pp. 217–221. IEEE (2017)
13. Szczypiński, P.M., Strzelecki, M., Materka, A., Klepaczko, A.: Mazda - a software package for image texture analysis. Comput. Methods Programs Biomed. **94**, 66–76 (2009)
14. Tabor, Z., Latala, Z.: 3d gray-level histomorphometry of trabecular bone-a methodological review. Image Anal. Ster. **33**(1), 1–12 (2014)
15. Tatoń, G., Rokita, E., Korkosz, M., Wróbel, A.: The ratio of anterior and posterior vertebral heights reinforces the utility of DXA in assessment of vertebrae strength. Calcif. Tissue Int. **95**(2), 112–121 (2014)
16. Twomey, L., Taylor, J.: The lumbar spine: structure, function, age changes and physiotherapy. Aust. J. Physiother. **40**, 19–30 (1994)
17. Wierzbicki, V., Pesce, A., Marrocco, L., Piccione, E., Colonnese, C., Caruso, R.: How old is your cervical spine? cervical spine biological age: a new evaluation scale. Eur. Spine J. **24**, 2763–2770 (2015)

Evaluation of Shape from Shading Surface Reconstruction Quality for Liver Phantom

Mateusz Bas and Dominik Spinczyk

Abstract The complexity and limitations of common laparoscopic procedures induce designing of solutions that allow for efficient and precise methods of guidance throughout the surgery. Using Shape from Shading methods for reconstruction of surfaces in biomedical engineering and medicine creates a whole new approach in diagnostic and therapeutic procedures. The goal of presented work is to assess the quality of phantom liver surface reconstruction from monocular laparoscopic image frames using Shape from Shading algorithm by comparing the acquired shape with ground-truth 3D model from Time-of-Flight camera using Singular Value Decomposition registration algorithm.

Keywords Surface reconstruction · Surface registration · Shape reconstruction quality · Shape from shading

1 Introduction

The development of information technology has strongly influenced the areas of medicine, resulting in the emergence of new techniques for performing surgical procedures. Modern computer components such as high-performance graphics cards enable fast image processing and rendering of accurate 3d models in real time. Such progress allows the creation of methods that support minimally invasive surgeries using augmented reality. Biomedical sciences have also been enriched with

M. Bas · D. Spinczyk (✉)
Faculty of Biomedical Engineering, Silesian University of Technology, Roosevelta 40, 41-800 Zabrze, Poland
e-mail: dominik.spinczyk@polsl.pl

M. Bas
e-mail: mateusz.bas@polsl.pl

© The Editor(s) (if applicable) and The Author(s), under exclusive license to Springer Nature Switzerland AG 2021
E. Piętka et al. (eds.), *Information Technology in Biomedicine*, Advances in Intelligent Systems and Computing 1186, https://doi.org/10.1007/978-3-030-49666-1_7

the achievements of Computer Vision, in the form of diagnostic and therapeutic support algorithms. The complexity and limitations of common laparoscopic procedures induce designing of solutions that allow for efficient and precise methods of guidance throughout the surgery.

The goal of navigation in surgery is to register the preoperative personalized anatomical model of the patient to the reference frame of patients body position during the surgery. Accomplishing of that goal means dealing with certain challenges that arise during designing of such method. These difficulties are associated with:

- positioning of the laparoscopic camera relatively to the anatomical organ,
- depth reconstruction using monocular laparoscopic images,
- registration of anatomical organ surface between different imaging modalities.

Reconstruction of anatomical models is an important aspect of surgical navigation system. This task allows to acquire the surface of the organ from the preoperative imaging in form of different representations like isosurfaces, points or splines. Prior attempts of organs surface reconstruction included using the global surface interpolation algorithm to reconstruct 3D lung model in a form of B-spline surface [16] and performing stereoscopic reconstruction of liver surface using two laparoscopic cameras in both in-vitro environment [15] and clinically [14].

The issue with surgical navigation in minimally invasive procedures is that the technique is used clinically only in neurosurgical procedures where the surgical field remains rigid [1]. Physical properties of organs and natural processes occurring in the human body introduce deformable transformations of anatomical objects making it impossible to apply a rigid preoperative model as a guide.

By extending the task of surgical navigation to other anatomical areas a problem related to non-rigid surface matching and modeling of shape deformations in real time appears. Solution to these issues can be accomplished by implementing computer vision algorithms such as Shape from Shading (SfS) algorithm [17] providing a reconstruction of 3D surface of a surface from a given monocular image. Such approach is capable of generating real-time surfaces during image-guided minimally invasive procedures allowing for tracking of organ's deformation.

The goal of presented work is to assess the quality of phantom liver surface reconstruction from monocular laparoscopic images sequence using SfS algorithm by comparison of acquired shape with ground-truth 3D model from Time-of-Flight camera using Singular Value Decomposition (SVD) registration algorithm.

2 State of the Art

Using methods for reconstruction anatomical organs' surfaces in biomedical engineering and medicine creates a whole new approach to diagnostic and therapeutic procedures.

Authors of [10] presented a method of creating a panorama visualization from multiple endoscopic images. Shape from Shading algorithm was used for reconstruction the 3D surface from each endoscopic image frame. Using Speeded-up Robust Feature (SURF) authors established the correspondences between adjacent endoscopic image frames. To recreate the surface of wider and three-dimensional view the reconstructed surfaces have been registered using Iterative Closest Point algorithm providing a registration error of less than 4mm.

In [5] surface shading model was used to recreate the surface of liver seen in the 2D laparoscopic images and register the reconstructed model with the 3D liver model acquired from a preoperative volume. Preprocessing of the input images considered filtering with a 23×23 median filter to remove high frequencies. The camera images were then divided into patches by applying watershed algorithm. A global camera pose transformation was estimated based on the assumption about Lambertian (diffusive) reflectance model of the liver's surface and pixel values in each patch. Lastly the preoperative and reconstructed model are registered based on previously calculated transformation. Authors provided a measure of the Target Visualisation Error by indication 15 visual cues like edges and corners in the images. The average TVE value of 11.3 (4.7) pixel was measured which corresponds to millimetric distances in the scene.

A Lambertian shading constraint, along with neo-Hookean elastic model, contour cues and anatomical landmarks were used to provide a method for liver's 3D model reconstruction from monocular laparoscopic images and deformable registration of the preoperative model to the laparoscopic image [9]. Authors were able to achieve a registration error of less than 1 cm for the inner liver structures. This calculates to a 4% registration error considering the liver's largest transverse diameter.

In [11] a method for reconstruction of uterus surface using Deformable-Shape-from-Motion-and-Shading algorithm is presented. The organ's 3D model is acquired based on shading of the scene and present light specularities. a A novel approach considering a case of near-lighting endoscopes used with Shape from Shading algorithm is proposed in [8].

The popularity of laparoscopic methods forces the development of image navigation in minimally invasive procedures. In response to the needs posed by laparoscopic procedures on female reproductive organs, the Uteraug system was created [7] which is used to support the procedure of myomectomy i.e. the removal of benign uterine tumors that cause pain. At present, it is the only prototype of the augmented reality system used in laparoscopy that takes into account the deformability and displacement of organs.

Even though that using 3D surface from monocular image reconstruction algorithms plays a crucial role in development of modern surgical navigation systems it remains insufficiently reviewed. The case is still an open research problem, despite existing commercial systems that do not reveal the specifications of algorithms used.

3 Materials and Methods

This section presents a description of the workbench and equipment used during the acquisition of data, a characterization of performed preprocessing and surface reconstruction and registration methods.

The problem described in the work is only an initial stage of a system implementation that could allow tracking of changes in the shape and position of organs in the laparoscopic image, updating the pre-operative model and performing image navigation in minimally invasive abdominal procedures.

3.1 Shape from Shading Algorithm

Shape recovery is a classic Computer Vision problem. The goal of methods is to obtain a three-dimensional representation of the scene based on 2D images [17]. This algorithm is an important element when tracking of organ's surface deformations is needed. Using the SfS algorithm, a 2D monocular image and shading constraints it is possible to create an indirect method of registering a three-dimensional pre-operative model.

To solve the problem of surface reconstruction from monocular laparoscopic image an approach considering Lambertian model of reflection was used. The Lambertian (diffusion) surface model assumes that the surface reflects the incident light in all directions uniformly. The brightness of such a surface is proportional to the energy of the incident light. The amount of light falling on the surface is proportional to the area seen from the location of the lighting source. The area of incidence of light is a function of the angle between the normal surface and the direction of the light source. The Lambertian surface can be modeled as:

$$I_l = A\rho \vec{N} \cdot \vec{S},$$ (1)

where A—light source intensity, ρ—surface albedo, $\vec{N} = (n_x, n_y, n_z)$—surface normal, $\vec{S} = (s_x, s_y, s_z)$—light source position.

This model is often used as a solution to the problem of recreating a 3D surface from an image, mainly due to the simplicity of implementation.

3.2 The Workbench

Workbench used for acquisition of data consisted of:

• Kyotokagaku IOUSFAN Abdominal Phantom [2]
• Olympus Laparoscope [4]

Fig. 1 Kyotokagaku
IOUSFAN abdominal
phantom

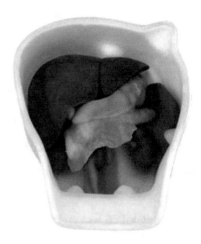

- Swissranger 4200 Time-of-Flight camera [3]

The workbench was based on the Kyotokagaku IOUSFAN phantom (Fig. 1) which is used for ultrasound imaging. The use of an open phantom was required to be able to place markers on the surface of the selected organ for measuring of surface registration quality. The Time-of-Flight camera was fixed on a tripod pointed at the phantom. Laparoscopic camera was handheld.

3.3 Proposed Method

The following method solves the registration problem of a Time-of-Flight (ToF) camera 3D surface to the surface acquired from the algorithm. In in the case of clinical use this corresponds to the reconstruction of surface from laparoscopic image frame and fitting of the three-dimensional model of the organ along with pathological tissues and key anatomical structures in the area of the operating field, segmented from magnetic resonance imaging or computed tomography.

The proposed method (Fig. 2) for assessment of surface reconstruction quality of a phantom liver using algorithm consist of following steps:

1. Calibration of laparoscopic camera
2. Acquisition of laparoscopic video sequence
3. Depth reconstruction of phantom liver surface with SfS algorithm
4. Phantom liver model acquisition with Time-of-Flight camera
5. Manual selection of markers visible in ToF camera amplitude image and laparoscopic sequence images
6. Marker-based registration of surfaces using SVD algorithm
7. Registration quality measures calculation

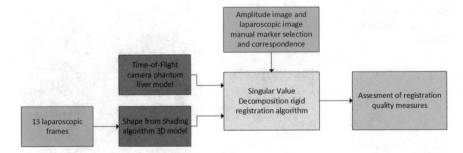

Fig. 2 Workflow of the proposed method

The algorithm was created to check the accuracy of surface reconstruction from a single image by matching to a model with known dimensions from a ToF camera.

3.4 Camera Calibration

Using the checkerboard pattern of known square size, it is possible to calibrate the camera and obtain the internal and external parameters as well as distortion correction polynomial coefficients [6]. The laparoscopic camera was calibrated using a chessboard pattern with square size of 5 mm. Obtained internal polynomial coefficients allowed for rectification of the images and removal of distortion. Internal parameters including calculated focal length values were later used as one of input parameters of SfS algorithm. The checkerboard pattern must be photographed with a camera from different angles, filling the widest possible field of view.

In the case of the pinhole camera model the equation for the projection of a point in three-dimensional space onto a two-dimensional plane of the camera transducer is as follows:

$$\begin{pmatrix} u \\ v \\ 1 \end{pmatrix} = \begin{pmatrix} f_x & \gamma & c_x \\ 0 & f_y & c_y \\ 0 & 0 & 1 \end{pmatrix} \begin{pmatrix} r_{11} & r_{12} & r_{13} & t_1 \\ r_{21} & r_{22} & r_{23} & t_2 \\ r_{31} & r_{32} & r_{33} & t_3 \end{pmatrix} \begin{pmatrix} x \\ y \\ z \\ 1 \end{pmatrix} \tag{2}$$

where u, v—projection of 3D surface point on camera sensor, f_x, f_y—focal lengths of camera lens, c_x, c_y—crossing points of optical axes and camera sensor, r, t—rotation and translation of the camera, x, y, z—coordinates of the surface point in 3D, γ—image skew value.

Fig. 3 Example
laparoscopic image of the
liver phantom

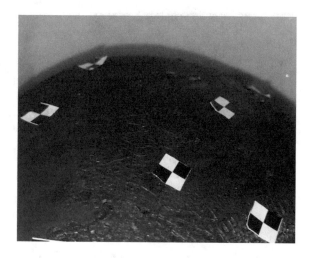

3.5 Laparoscopic Images Sequence Acquisition

The visible light images of the liver phantom have been acquired using the Olympus
Laparoscope [4]. Figure (Fig. 3) shows an example view obtained from the laparoscope. An important advantage related to the reconstruction of surface from single
laparoscopic image is that the light source of the laparoscope can be assumed as
being in the same location as the camera. This allows to introduce constraints for the
SfS algorithm in the step of performing the surface reconstruction.

Continuous acquisition of laparoscopic view was used. A set of 13 frames presenting the liver phantom was selected as input of the surface reconstruction algorithm.

3.6 Phantom Liver Model from Time-of-Flight Camera

The 3D image of the phantom was captured with the MESA Imaging SwissRanger
4000 camera [3]. The resulting depth image has a resolution of 176×144 pixels. An
amplitude (Fig. 4a) image is also provided for later marker selection and correspondence finding. The camera was placed on a tripod in such a way that the phantom in
the image was visible from above.

Acquired depth map of the phantom contained all organs of the abdomen. The 3D
surface of the phantom liver was obtained using manual segmentation of the liver in
the amplitude image. Segmented liver part of the phantom is presented in (Fig. 4b).

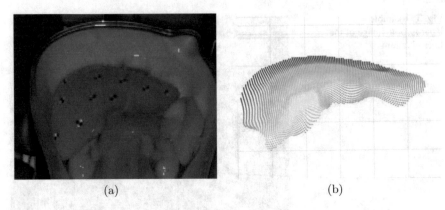

(a)   (b)

Fig. 4 **a** Time-of-Flight camera amplitude image, **b** Time-of-Flight camera output depth map

3.7 Manual Selection of Markers Visible in ToF Camera Amplitude Image and Laparoscopic Image Frames

The surface of the liver phantom has been covered with 2×2 checkerboard pattern markers which were next manually selected (Fig. 5) in the visible light camera images and the amplitude image of the ToF camera. This step provides Ground Truth correspondences between both modalities.

3.8 Marker-Based Registration of Surfaces Using SVD Algorithm

Given the correspondences between the Time-of-Flight camera liver model and reconstructed surface from the laparoscopic image in the previous step it is possible to register these point clouds using the minimization of Euclidean distance with Singular Value Decomposition algorithm [12]. Assuming the following expression as a function minimizing the distance of clouds:

$$f = \sum_{i=1}^{N} |p_i - (Rq_i + T)|^2 \tag{3}$$

where N—number of point clouds points, p_i—moving points set, q_i—fixed points set, R—rotation of the moving points set, T—translation of the moving points set, it is required to find such R and T for which the function has the smallest value. The method for finding rotation rotation variables and point cloud translation is the Singular Value Decomposition algorithm:

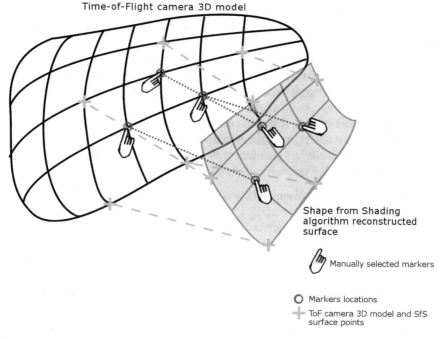

Fig. 5 Distances between ToF camera liver model and reconstructed surface points (green) and distances between reconstructed surface and ToF camera liver model markers locations (red)

$$W = PQ^T \tag{4}$$

$$SVD(W) = U\Sigma V^T \tag{5}$$

The last step of the algorithm is to calculate the R and T matrices based on the V, U and Σ matrix values:

$$R = UV^T \tag{6}$$

$$T = \mu_P - R\mu_Q \tag{7}$$

The designated R and T matrices are substituted for the variables in equation of the point clouds distance minimizing function and mean values of points locations μ_P and μ_Q are calculated. Lastly the final position of the matched cloud is computed.

3.9 Testing Scenarios and Evaluation Methods

First testing case was related to assessing the quality of reconstruction of phantom liver using SfS algorithm assuming that the light source location overlaps the laparoscopic camera position and that the imaged surface reflects light according to the Lambertian light reflection model. The SfS algorithm input image was a raw image from the laparoscopic image frame.

Second testing case assumed assessing the quality of reconstruction of phantom liver with the input image blurred with Gaussian filter. Considering Gaussian filtering a low-pass image filtration it should lead to a reduction in the number of sharp edges of the surface which as a result allows for a better rigid registration of the liver model to the reconstructed surface. It should be noted that too much image blur may cause the algorithm to not detect small changes in the image.

To evaluate the quality of phantom liver surface reconstruction with the use of SfS algorithm following geometric distance measures were used:

- M1—mean Euclidean distance between reconstructed surface and ToF camera liver model markers locations,
- M2—Hausdorff distance between reconstructed surface and ToF camera liver model markers locations,
- M3—mean Euclidean distance between ToF camera liver model and reconstructed surface points,
- M4—Hausdorff distance between ToF camera liver model and reconstructed surface points.

Assuming that we are performing only a rigid registration of the two surfaces values of all measures that are near zero indicate a perfect registration scenario. This would mean that the surface reconstructed from laparoscopic image completely matches the 3D model created with Time-of-Flight camera.

4 Results

In this section results of carried out research are presented. The fundamental case of research assumed reconstructing the liver phantom's surface and performing registration to the Time-of-Flight camera 3D model which was considered a Ground Truth for the shape of surface. Another case assumed filtering the input image with Gaussian filter. The real correspondences between the models were acquired by manually selecting markers in both modalities. Based on known positions of markers and surface points locations registration was carried out and quality measures were calculated. The reconstruction quality measured are presented in Table 1.

The overall averaged values of measures indicate that the SfS algorithm phantom liver surface reconstruction quality is unsatisfactory. With resulting distances of over 1cm the algorithm cannot be used in clinical systems for aiding minimally invasive surgeries applications. For example, such significant dislocation of reconstructed liver tumor surface in relation to its real location may mislead the surgeon and threaten the life of a patient.

The second case of testing shows that the Gaussian filtering of input image reduces the measured distances. The average value of measure M1 reduced from 1.65 to

Table 1 Results of SfS reconstructed surface and Time-of-Flight camera phantom liver model registration

	Raw input images				Blurred input images			
	M1 (cm)	M2 (cm)	M3 (cm)	M4 (cm)	M1 (cm)	M2 (cm)	M3 (cm)	M4 (cm)
1.	1.56	5.11	0.56	1.63	0.81	1.92	0.41	1.80
2.	1.89	3.73	0.22	1.11	1.53	1.99	0.26	1.03
3.	1.48	2.26	0.27	1.57	1.34	2.20	0.25	1.39
4.	1.49	2.06	0.29	1.41	1.46	2.39	0.30	1.12
5.	1.39	1.88	0.27	1.11	0.93	1.37	0.31	1.57
6.	1.87	3.35	0.29	1.33	1.09	1.33	0.36	1.83
7.	1.54	2.07	0.34	1.70	1.19	1.31	0.36	1.78
8.	1.97	2.41	0.38	1.70	1.12	1.47	0.37	1.37
9.	1.57	2.47	0.31	1.79	0.95	1.55	0.35	1.88
10.	1.57	2.24	0.35	1.76	1.01	1.55	0.32	1.74
11.	1.64	2.76	0.37	1.32	1.29	1.96	0.33	1.43
12.	1.67	2.53	0.36	1.76	1.35	1.98	0.36	1.60
13.	1.90	2.48	0.33	1.51	1.47	1.98	0.36	1.56
Average	1.65	2.72	0.33	1.52	1.20	1.77	0.33	1.55

1.52 cm (8% decrease). For the measure M2 we observed that the values decreased from 2.72 to 1.77 cm (35% decrease). Measures M3 and M4 remained at similar values. Unfortunately the values did not decrease to a degree that would make the algorithm usable clinically.

5 Discussion

Summarizing the research results, strong input image blurring gives better surface matching results. This is the due to the smoothing of the reconstructed shape. The milder surface curvatures allow for enhanced registration quality to the liver model. On the other hand using Gaussian filtering means removing high frequencies from the image which are associated with details of the the reconstructed surface. By losing information about details it is further impossible to track non-rigid deformations of the model.

The values of the presented measures state the inaccurate fitting of the liver model from the Time-of-Flight camera to the reconstructed surface. A broader literature review of the remaining surface reconstruction from single laparoscopic image methods is needed. A search for approaches indicating certain reconstruction assumptions and constraints that allow for a more accurate reproduction of the organ surface is required.

The main purpose of the work was to test the quality of reproduction of the phantom liver surface using the SfS algorithm and by registering the reconstructed model to a three-dimensional phantom model obtained using a Time-of-Flight camera assumed as a Ground Truth shape. The goal was achieved through research. On their basis, it was determined that using the proposed method it is not possible to reproduce the exact surface of the liver phantom. Therefore, it is not acceptable to use this method in clinical procedures.

Other methods of surface reconstruction from the monocular image should be taken into account as well as testing the operation of SfS algorithms on images presenting real organs should be performed due to the fact that there are significant differences in the surface light reflection models between a real human liver and the phantom presented.

Further work may include combining SfS surface reconstruction algorithm with non-rigid registration methods like presented in our previous work [13]. This approach may allow to track the deformations of organs seen in the surgical field and laparoscopic images sequence and apply the shape changes to the patient's preoperative model.

References

1. BrainLab Crainial Navigation Application. https://www.brainlab.com/surgery-products/overview-neurosurgery-products/cranial-navigation/
2. Kyotokagaku IOUSFAN specification. https://www.mice-groupe.com/materiel-de-simulation/113-abdominal-intraoperative-laparoscopic-ultrasound-phantom-iousfan.html
3. MESA Imaging SwissRanger 4000 specification. http://www.adept.net.au/cameras/Mesa/SR4000.shtml#specs
4. Olympus Laparoscope specification. https://www.olympus-europa.com/medical/rmt/media/en/Content/Content-MSD/Documents/Brochures/HD-Laparoscope_product-brochure_EN_20000101.pdf
5. Bernhardt, S., Nicolau, S.A., Bartoli, A., Agnus, V., Soler, L., Doignon, C.: Using shading to register an intraoperative ct scan to a laparoscopic image. Lecture Notes in Computer Science (including subseries Lecture Notes in Artificial Intelligence and Lecture Notes in Bioinformatics) **9515**, 35–45 (2016)
6. Burger, W.: Zhang's Camera Calibration Algorithm: In-Depth Tutorial and Implementation (2016)
7. François, T., Ement Debize, C., Calvet, L., Collins, T., Pizarro, D., Bartoli, A.: Uteraug: augmented reality in laparoscopic surgery of the uterus (February 2019), pp. 1–3 (2017)
8. Goncalves, N., Roxo, D., Barreto, J., Rodrigues, P.: Perspective shape from shading for wide-FOV near-lighting endoscopes. Neurocomputing **150**(Part A), 136–146 (2015)
9. Koo, B., Özgür, E., Le Roy, B., Buc, E., Bartoli, A.: Deformable registration of a preoperative 3D liver volume to a laparoscopy image using contour and shading cues. In: Lecture Notes in Computer Science (including subseries Lecture Notes in Artificial Intelligence and Lecture Notes in Bioinformatics), vol. 10433 LNCS, pp. 326–334. Springer (2017)
10. Kumar, A., Wang, Y.Y., Liu, K.C., Hung, W.C., Huang, S.W., Lie, W.N., Huang, C.C.: Three dimensional panorama visualization for endoscopic video. In: IFMBE Proceedings, vol. 52, pp. 39–42. Springer (2015)

11. Malti, A., Bartoli, A., Collins, T.: Template-based conformal shape-from-motion-and-shading for laparoscopy. Lecture Notes in Computer Science (including subseries Lecture Notes in Artificial Intelligence and Lecture Notes in Bioinformatics) **7330 LNCS**, 1–10 (2012)
12. Marden, S., Guivant, J.: Improving the performance of ICP for real-time applications using an approximate nearest neighbour search. In: Australasian Conference on Robotics and Automation, ACRA (2012)
13. Spinczyk, D., Bas, M.: Anisotropic non-rigid iterative closest point algorithm for respiratory motion abdominal surface matching. BioMedical Eng. OnLine **18**(1), 25 (2019)
14. Spinczyk, D., Karwan, A., Rudnicki, J., Wróblewski, T.: Stereoscopic liver surface reconstruction. Wideochirurgia I Inne Techniki Maloinwazyjne **7**(3), 181–187 (2012)
15. Spinczyk, D., Karwan, A., Zylkowski, J., Wróblewski, T.: In vitro evaluation of stereoscopic liver surface reconstruction. Wideochirurgia I Inne Techniki Maloinwazyjne **8**(1), 80–85 (2013)
16. Spinczyk, D., Pietka, E.: Automatic generation of 3D lung model. Adv. Soft Comput. **45**, 671–678 (2007)
17. Zhang, R., Tsai, P.S., Cryer, J.E., Shah, M.: Shape from shading: a survey. IEEE Trans. Pattern Anal. Mach. Intell. **21**(8), 690–706 (1999)

Pancreas and Duodenum—Automated Organ Segmentation

Piotr Zarychta

Abstract The goal of this preliminary research is to present an automated segmentation of abdominal organs: pancreas and duodenum. The paper shows the automatic extraction of pancreas and duodenum in clinical abdominal computed tomography (CT) scans. The proposed method allows building a feature vector that automates and streamlines the fuzzy connectedness (FC) method. All described steps of the presented methodology have been implemented in MATLAB and tested on clinical abdominal CT scans. The atlas based segmentation combined with the FC method gave Dice index results at the following level: 70.18–84.82% for pancreas and 68.90–88.06% for duodenum.

Keywords Atlas based segmentation · Pancreas · Duodenum · Fuzzy connectedness

1 Introduction

The pancreas is a single human organ located within the abdominal cavity. It is essentially horizontal and is situated in the retroperitoneal space. The position of pancreas corresponds to the height of the first and second lumbar vertebrae. There are three parts in the pancreas, which are: pancreas head, pancreas body and pancreas tail. The head of the pancreas is covered by the duodenum and lies near the inferior vena cava and the right kidney. The pancreas body is located in front of the lumbar vertebrae and crosses the aorta, left kidney and left adrenal gland and the superior mesenteric artery. The pancreas tail is situated in front of the left kidney and is adjacent to the spleen [1].

The pancreas performs both intra- and exocrine functions. The first of these is the secretion of hormones that are primarily involved in controlling glucose in the body.

P. Zarychta (✉)
Faculty of Biomedical Engineering, Silesian University of Technology, Roosevelta 40, Zabrze, Poland
e-mail: piotr.zarychta@polsl.pl

E. Piętka et al. (eds.), *Information Technology in Biomedicine*, Advances in Intelligent Systems and Computing 1186, https://doi.org/10.1007/978-3-030-49666-1_8

95

The exocrine function of the pancreas is in turn associated with the function of the digestive tract—this organ producing many different enzymes that are important in the digestive process (in the pancreatic juice there are also bicarbonates, which have the ability to neutralize gastric acid) [1].

The duodenum, which a is part of the digestive tract, plays an important role in the proper functioning of the entire body. The duodenum connects the stomach with the small intestine, its length is about 25–30 cm., and the shape resembles a horseshoe. Pancreatic and hepatic ducts escape into it, forming the so-called Vater's papilla. The role of the duodenum is to digest fats, carbohydrates and proteins, and it is also responsible for the absorption of nutrients [1].

The duodenum consists of four parts—top, descending, bottom and ascending. The upper part of the duodenum called the duodenal bulb is located highest, next to the gallbladder and liver. Under the upper part there is a slightly narrower descending part. In this area, the Vater's papilla (or major duodenal papilla) is located, in which the mouth of the pancreatic duct and the common bile duct are situated. Slightly higher, above the Vater's papilla, is the minor duodenal papilla, connecting to the accessory pancreatic duct. The descending part, turning, goes into the lower part, also called horizontal. This part is larger, more pleated than the previous ones, and crosses the spine. The next part, ascending, climbs upwards, forming a duodenum-jejunum fold. This fragment connects to the jejunum [1].

The incidence of pancreatic cancer is increasing worldwide. This cancer ranks fifth among the most common causes of cancer-related deaths in the United States and fourth in Japan. In Poland, nearly 3,000 new cases are reported annually. The first signs of pancreatic cancer are non-specific, making it difficult to have an early diagnosis. The incidence of pancreatic cancer increases with age. The high mortality of patients with pancreatic cancer is due to the fact that the disease is usually detected at a very advanced stage, when metastases are already present and the pancreatic tumor is inoperable [2, 3].

Radiological diagnostics plays a key role in the diagnosis of pancreatic cancer. Diagnosis of pancreatic cancer is determined by imaging and endoscopic examinations. The multi-phase computed tomography of the abdomen is usually considered to be the reference method in this case. It is currently widely used to assess the extent of a lesion detected in the pancreas, determine the severity of the disease and look for metastases of pancreatic cancer. Magnetic resonance imaging can also be helpful. The result of the histopathological examination is necessary to make the final diagnosis.

Duodenal cancer is a rare gastrointestinal tumor. And although neoplastic diseases originating from the small intestine constitute about 1–3% of all cancerous tumors, the diagnosis of the tumor is difficult (mainly due to low accessibility of the organ for examination). Imaging tests play a fundamental role in diagnostics, and especially the abdominal computed tomography.

Proper pancreas and duodenum segmentation plays a very important role in the case of cancer diagnosis. Both pancreas and duodenum have large inter-subject variability among the population (especially in position, shape and size). The CT intensity of the pancreatic region and also the duodenal region is very similar to that of their neighboring structures (abdominal organs). For these reasons the segmentation of these both organs is a considerable challenge.

In recent years, many organ segmentation methods [4] have been proposed in literature. Among them, multi-atlas segmentation schemes have been widely used for abdominal organ segmentation from CT images and from contrast-enhanced CT images [5–7]. The accuracy of segmentation of the pancreas as well as the duodenum is still significantly lower (below 73% for the Dice similarity coefficient) than in the case of other abdominal organs (i.e. the liver, heart, stomach or kidneys) for which the Dice similarity coefficients are above 90% [6–8].

The proposed automatic extraction of pancreas and duodenum in the abdominal clinical CT scans based on the atlas and a feature vector, which automates and streamlines the fuzzy connectedness method, gives quite good results: 70.18–84.82% as Dice similarity coefficient for the pancreas and 68.90–88.06% as Dice similarity coefficient for the duodenum. At this stage, the results of these preliminary researches seem to be very effective and promising.

A quite similar version of the described method has been tested on the bone structures of the knee joint. The results of segmentation based on the atlas in combination with fuzzy methods gave a Dice similarity coefficient of 85.52–89.48% (for patella, tibia and femur [9, 10].

2 Methodology

2.1 Workflow

The block diagram (Fig. 1) consists of the following steps. The first one is the preprocessing (binarization, average filtering, detecting of edges, marking the seed points—on the basis of atlas based segmentation and implementation of the morphological operations). In the next step the watershed transform was implemented and further on the basis of the convex hull algorithm, a polygon containing all separated fragments of the segmented organ was determined. In the following step, the fuzzy connectedness method with a seed point determined on the basis of atlas segmentation was implemented. The last step is the postprocessing (average filtering combined with the implementation of morphological operations). This approach in the most typical case resulted in the separation of pancreas or duodenal structures from images of the abdominal cavity of the human body.

2.2 Preprocessing

The preprocessing stage includes the following steps: binarization with upper and lower threshold, average filtering, detecting of edges, marking the seed points (on

Fig. 1 Block diagram

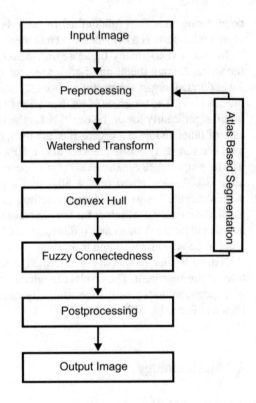

the basis of atlas based segmentation) and implementation of the morphological operations. The preprocessing in both cases (pancreas and duodenum segmentation) consisted in limiting, as much as possible, the number of image elements intended for further analysis. This effect was first obtained by binarization with the lower and upper thresholds, followed by average filtering combined with the determination of the edges of various objects present in the image of a given abdominal scan, and finally by using morphological operations. Binarization (0–300 HU) exposed the soft organs in the abdominal image. Average filtering together with the detecting of edges by means of the Canny method allowed (in the general case, neighbouring organs are separated) to be eliminated unwanted abdominal objects, leaving only those objects which include seed points. The implementation of morphological operations allowed, most often, to be broken the narrow links between adjacent structures of the internal organs of the abdominal cavity.

2.3 Watershed Transform and Convex Hull

According to MATLAB definition, the watershed transform finds *catchment basins* or *watershed ridge lines* in an image by treating it as a surface where bright pixels represent high elevations and dark pixels represent low elevations. In this work, the implementation of watershed transform allowed to obtain an image divided into areas with continuous edges, and further on the basis of the convex hull algorithm, a polygon containing all separated fragments of the segmented organ was determined (it worked well even in cases where air was present in the duodenum).

2.4 Fuzzy Cconnectedness

According to literature [11], the fuzzy connectedness approach can be defined based on the fuzzy affinity relation. In this case the generalized definition of fuzzy connectedness introduces the iterative method. The iterative method permits the FC to be determined in relation to the marked image point (seed or starting point). The seed points have been marked on the basis of the atlas based segmentation (centroids). In this paper the FC approach is not described in detail. An exhaustive description thereof can be found in [9, 12–14].

2.5 Postprocessing

The postprocessing, like the preprocessing, is based on the execution of subsequent steps, with the aim of obtaining a separate structure of the pancreas or duodenum with smoothed edges. For this purpose, it was based on average filtering combined with the implementation of morphological operations.

2.6 Atlas Based Segmentation

In practical solutions, especially in the medical field, automatic methods are desirable. Therefore, in the case of segmentation of soft structures, such as the pancreas or duodenum, it was decided to combine the atlas based segmentation method with the FC method. This allowed to avoid user's interaction in marking the seed points, which were obtained on the basis of the mean feature vector. In order to calculate the average feature vector for the teaching group the following steps were taken:

– extraction of pancreas and duodenum structures by an expert—usually requiring a lot of work (many volumes have to be analysed) to be done by an expert (radiologist). This step is time-consuming, but nonetheless necessary in order to build a large elementary atlas;

- feature vector finding for each scan in the volume (Fig. 2b)—in this work, the following features have been calculated: centroid, skeleton and area of the extracted structures as well as the area of the entire abdominal cavity;
- normalization of scans within the volume (Fig. 2c)—this is a very important step, due to the different number of scans in each volume;
- division of the normalized scans (features) into 11 sets (Fig. 2c)—this step has been implemented in order to adapt all the scans (features) to their most faithful representation in the atlas segmentation. Such division is the result of preliminary studies taking into account the layer thickness in CT examinations and a compromise between the acceptable effectiveness of the segmentation method (FC) and the time required to determine the features within the individual volume;

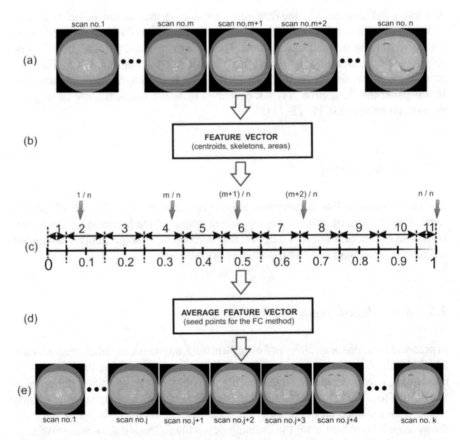

Fig. 2 Atlas based segmentation **a** teaching group, **b** feature vector **c** determining diagram of the average feature vector, **d** average feature vector and **e** testing group

- averaging features within each of the 11 sets (Fig. 2d)—this step has allowed to obtain average features within each of the 11 sets;
- initialization of the FC method by the determined sets of averaged features (by the sets of averaged features determined earlier) (Fig. 2e).

3 Discussion and Results

3.1 Materials

The methodology has been tested on 20 clinical CT studies of the abdominal cavity. The CT data have been acquired for females and males of different ages [15].

3.2 Experiments and Evaluation

The obtained dataset of clinical scans has been divided into two groups. These were the teaching and the testing group. The teaching group consisted of 10 clinical CT studies of abdominal cavity. Based on this group, the average feature vector (centroid, skeleton and area of the extracted structures, as well as the area of the entire abdominal cavity) have been determined. The rest of the obtained clinical dataset constituted the testing group. On the basis of the scans of the teaching group, the normalized values of x and y coordinates for centroid were obtained, due to the size of the scans (due to different size of the scans). These coordinates were used in the next step as seed points in the implemented FC method.

The extracted structures of the pancreas and duodenum together with the outline marked by an expert have been shown in (Figs. 3 and 4), respectively.

The proposed methodology of using atlas based segmentation combined with FC method applied to pancreas structures and duodenum structures produced results (average value for testing group) at the level of 77.293% and 76.906% for the Dice index, respectively, in the analysis of clinical CT studies of the abdominal cavity.

The obtained values of the Dice index for the analyzed CT series (testing group) have been collected in Table 1 (atlas based segmentation combined with FC method).

Table 1 Values of Dice index for the analyzed CT series for pancreas and duodenum

Set	1	2	3	4	5	6	7	8	9	10
Pancreas	75.08	70.18	84.82	75.46	75.75	78.58	77.01	75.50	80.09	80.47
Duodenum	88.06	68.90	76.61	75.36	80.94	76.24	75.08	73.22	79.57	75.08

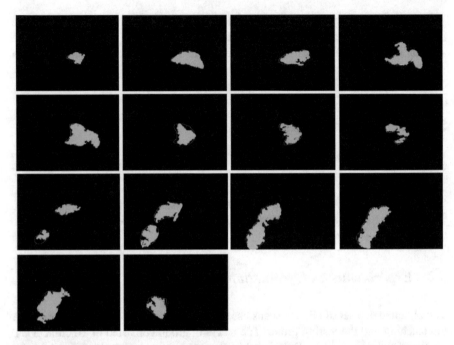

Fig. 3 Extracted pancreas structures for the case no. 13

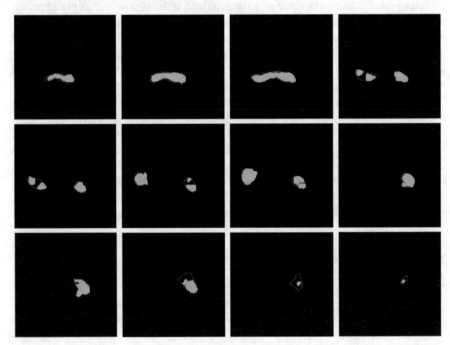

Fig. 4 Extracted duodenum structures for the case no. 13

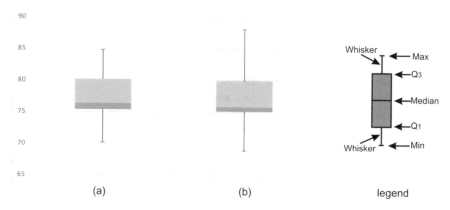

Fig. 5 Discrepancy in the obtained values of Dice index **a** pancreas and **b** duodenum

The discrepancy in the obtained values of the Dice index between atlas based segmentation combined with FC method for pancreas and duodenum has been shown on the box-and-whisker plot (Fig. 5).

This paper presents a multistep image processing method that in the author's opinion, seems to be a ready product. Therefore, such a multistep processing of images requires many decisions to be made about parameters characterising the performance of the corresponding algorithms. According to the block diagram shown in the Fig. 1, in the stage of preprocessing, binarization was first carried out with an upper and lower threshold. In the most typical case, these thresholds were set at 0 and 150 HU for the pancreas, and 30 and 120 HU for the duodenum, respectively. The next step was based on averaging filtration, in which has been used a square matrix 3×3, with the detecting of edges by means of the Canny method. In the last step of preprocessing based on the morphological operations, first erosion was performed for the entire scan, then a separate area of the scan containing the object overlapping the seed point (pixel) was left, and in the last step after filling the holes in this object, a dilatation operation was performed with the same structural element as in the case of erosion. In the general case, the implementation of preprocessing allows the seperation of the neighbouring organs, elimination of unwanted abdominal objects, leaving only those objects that contain seed point.

Usually, the preprocessing stage is insufficient to extract the desired anatomical structures. Therefore, in the next step, the watershed transformation and the fuzzy connectedness approach were implemented. In the FC approach has been implemented a 5×5 neighborhood window within the region, containing pancreas or duodenum structures with the surrounding tissues. This way permits the most typical cases of under-segmentation to be eliminated without much impact on the overall analysis time.

For the FC method, the input parameters are as follows: seed points—coordinates according to previously determined centroids for the pancreas and duodenum, respectively, intensity—corresponds to seed points, and standard deviation—is 22 for the pancreas and 19 for the duodenum.

In cases where air was present in segmented structures, it was necessary to implement a convex hull algorithm. In this way, a polygon containing all separated fragments of the segmented organ was determined.

Post-processing is based on the following steps to obtain a separate segmented structure (pancreas or duodenum) with smoothed edges. At this stage, it is always the same sequence, i.e. averaging filtration, erosion, filling holes in a separate object, and dilatation operation with the same structural element.

The parameters described above maximize the quality of the obtained results, and the presented method was tested on abdominal CT scans described in detail in [15].

4 Conclusions

Automatic segmentation of pancreas and duodenum is a difficult task for practical implementation. The inaccuracy and uncertainty of biomedical data, as well as a whole range of additional factors, such as individual differences in the structure of both organs and the presence of air within the segmented organs (especially in duodenum), are important here. For this reason, it was decided to combine the information flowing from the atlas based segmentation with the FC algorithm, which resulted in obtaining results convergent with experts' outlines. At this stage, the described automated methodology dedicated to the pancreas and duodenum extraction based on atlas segmentation seems to be very effective and promising.

References

1. Bochenek, A., Reicher, M.: The human anatomy. Wydawnictwo Lekarskie PZWL, Warsaw (1990)
2. Goslinski, J.: Pancreatic cancer—first symptoms, Oncological portal (2019)
3. Ito, M., Makino, N., Ueno, Y.: Glucose intolerance and the risk of pancreatic cancer. Transl. Gastrointest. Cancer 2(4), 223–229 (2013)
4. Summers, R.: Progress in fully automated abdominal CT interpretation. Am. J. Roentgenol. 207(1), 67–79 (2016)
5. Iglesias, J., Sabuncu, M.: Multi-atlas segmentation of biomedical images: a survey. Med. Image Anal. 24(1), 205–219 (2015)
6. Karasawa, K., Oda, M., Kitasaka, T., Misawa, K., Fujiwara, M., Chu, C., Zheng, G., Rueckert, D., Mori, K.: Multi-atlas pancreas segmentation: atlas selection based on vessel structure. Med. Image Anal. 39, 18–28 (2017)
7. Wolz, R., Chu, C., Misawa, K., Fujiwara, M., Mori, K., Rueckert, D.: Automated abdominal multi-organ segmentation with subject-specific atlas generation. IEEE Trans. Med. Imaging 32(9), 1723–1730 (2013)
8. Roth, H., Lu, L., Lay, N., Harrison, A., Farag, A., Sohn, A., Summers, R.: Spatial aggregation of holistically-nested convolutional neural networks for automated pancreas localization and segmentation. Med. Image Anal. 45, 94–107 (2018)

 9. Zarychta, P.: A new approach to knee joint arthroplasty. Comput. Med. Imaging Graph. **65**, 32–45 (2018)
10. Zarychta, P.: Patella—atlas based segmentation. In: Pietka, E., Badura, P., Kawa, J., Wieclawek, W., (eds.) Information Technologies in Medicine, Advances in Intelligent Systems and Computing, vol. 1011, pp. 314–322 (2019)
11. Udupa, J., Samarasekera, S.: Fuzzy connectedness and object definition: theory, algorithms, and applications. Graph. Models Image Process. **58**, 246–261 (1996)
12. Zarychta, P.: ACL and PCL of the knee joint in the computer diagnostics. In: Napieralski A., (ed.) 21st International Conference Mixed Design of Integrated Circuits and Systems MIXDES, pp. 489–492 (2014)
13. Zarychta, P., Zarychta-Bargiela, A.: Anterior and posterior cruciate ligament-extraction and 3D visualization. In: Pietka E., Kawa J., (eds). Information Technologies in Biomedicine, Advances in Intelligent and Soft Computing, vol. 69. Springer, Berlin, pp. 115–122 (2010)
14. Zarychta P.: Automatic registration of the medical images T1- and T2-weighted MR knee images. In: Napieralski A., (ed.) International Conference Mixed Design of Integrated Circuits and Systems MIXDES, pp. 741–745 (2006)
15. Spinczyk, D., Zysk, A., Sperka, P., Stronczek, M., Pycinski, B., Juszczyk, J., Biesok, M., Rudzki, M., Wieclawek, W., Zarychta, P., Woloshuk, A., Zylkowski, J., Rosiak, G., Konecki, D., Mielczarek, K., Rowinski, O., Pietka, E.: Supporting diagnostics and therapy planning for percutaneous ablation of liver and abdominal tumors and preclinical evaluation. Comput. Med. Imaging Graph. **78**, 101664 (2019)

Evaluation of the Effect of a PCL/nanoSiO$_2$ Implant on Bone Tissue Regeneration Using X-ray Micro-Computed Tomography

Magdalena Jędzierowska, Marcin Binkowski, Robert Koprowski, and Zygmunt Wróbel

Abstract This paper evaluates the regeneration process of large bone defects filled with a highly porous (nano) composite implant. A polycaprolactone—based scaffold modified with nanometric silica was introduced into bone defects created in the distal femoral epiphyses of rabbits. The bone tissue regeneration process was evaluated 1, 2, 3 and 6 months after implantation. Empty bone defects served as a control. The osseointegration process was evaluated using the parameters of cancellous bone microstructure. 16 bone tissue samples were imaged using X-ray micro-computed tomography (XMT). There were 1000 2D images in each measurement, which in total gave 16000 2D images. In the end, in this work 200 2D images were picked for detailed analysis. The studies have shown that the PCL/nanoSiO$_2$ composite implant supports successfully the initial phase of bone regeneration. In each of the reference periods, a greater volume of new bone tissue was observed for the implanted samples.

Keywords X-ray micro-computed tomography (XMT) · Bone regeneration · Scaffold · Polycaprolactone (pcl) · Silica (sio$_2$)

M. Jędzierowska (✉) · R. Koprowski · Z. Wróbel
Faculty of Science and Technology, Institute of Biomedical Engineering,
University of Silesia in Katowice, ul. Będzińska 39, Sosnowiec 41-200, Poland
e-mail: magdalena.jedzierowska@us.edu.pl

R. Koprowski
e-mail: robert.koprowski@us.edu.pl

Z. Wróbel
e-mail: zygmunt.wrobel@us.edu.pl

M. Binkowski
X-ray Microtomography Lab, Department of Computer Biomedical Systems,
Faculty of Computer and Materials Science, Institute of Computer Science,
University of Silesia, Sosnowiec 41-200, Poland
e-mail: binkowski.marcin@gmail.com

© The Editor(s) (if applicable) and The Author(s), under exclusive license
to Springer Nature Switzerland AG 2021
E. Piętka et al. (eds.), *Information Technology in Biomedicine*, Advances in Intelligent
Systems and Computing 1186, https://doi.org/10.1007/978-3-030-49666-1_9

1 Introduction

Bone and cartilage tissue damage in people is one of the biggest problems of modern medicine, which boosts the development of biomaterials market. This is related to the fact that regeneration of large bone defects usually necessitates a scaffold which supports bone structure reconstruction. In practice, autogenous bone grafts are considered the gold standard. However, their use also entails side effects [12]. An alternative for doctors is tissue engineering that allows to apply the principles of biology and engineering in order to enable the creation of functional substitutes which can be applied to the damaged tissue [11]. Placing an implant in the bone is associated with the creation of an interface where a living tissue is combined with a biomaterial, which is of great importance to the success of implant treatment in humans. This phenomenon was observed for the first time in 1950 by Professor Branemark and called osseointegration. It is now widely recognized that the implant is integrated into the bone tissue when there is no motion in direct contact, so that the implant may function properly under normal loads [10].

Implants acting as bone scaffolds are usually made from biodegradable, porous materials, which during the regeneration process are a kind of "mechanical" support for the damaged bone tissue [1]. Meeting the requirements of an ideal implant is a big challenge for tissue engineering today. A promising solution seems to be polymer composite materials, which, thanks to their combined structure and a wide range of doping possibilities are one of the most widely studied materials for regenerative medicine [15, 26]. With the increase of requirements for the implant itself, there is a growing need for new alternative test methods or supplementary methods to the existing ones. X-ray micro-computed tomography (XMT) fulfils this need. It is increasingly used to study scaffold architecture and the process of bone tissue regeneration [8, 11, 27, 28]. XMT offers non-destructive and non-invasive testing, allowing for imaging of, inter alia, three-dimensional scaffolds of implants and bone tissue microstructure [3, 9]. In addition, it allows for the quantitative study of trabecular bone, its mechanical properties and remodelling processes [17].

Besides the commonly used histology and SEM, more and more scientists have been using XMT. Shim et al studied in vivo the possibility of restoring new bone tissue in the skull defects in rabbits using polymer scaffolds [19]. The new bone formation was studied by means of X-ray micro-computed tomography, histology and histometric analysis. The significance of hybrid scaffolds in regenerative medicine was also stressed by Shao et al, who evaluated, inter alia, a hybrid scaffold: medical-grade PCL (mPCL) seeded with bone marrow stem cells (BMSC), implanted into the bone defects of the medial condyle of the femur of New Zealand rabbits [18]. 3 months after implantation the volume of the newly formed bone was significantly higher for the samples from mPCL than for control samples (empty bone defects), whereas after a period of six months, the levels of the new bone tissue for both bones with implants and the reference were very similar. It is worth remembering that the studies of bone implant suitability in animal models are just a stage preceding the key clinical trials, which verify the implant suitability in humans.

The literature shows that the range of biomaterials for use in regenerative medicine is very rich. One such biomaterial is polycaprolactone (PCL)—a bioresorbable polymer exhibiting good biocompatibility [29], used in cartilage and bone regeneration [30]. Although PCL is not an osteoinductive material, it may be modified with, for example, growth factors or other molecules in order to enhance its osteoinductive potential [4, 5, 16, 22].

The purpose of this article is to assess the regeneration of bone defects filled with a new highly porous (nano)composite material: polycaprolactone (PCL) modified with nanometric silica (SiO_2). The undertaken in vivo studies are intended to confirm the suitability of the implant for clinical applications in humans with bone defects. The stimulating effect of the PCL/nanoSiO$_2$ implant on bone cells should accelerate the process of regeneration of damage caused by resection of cysts or neoplastic bone defects. Previously conducted in vitro studies proved that the material is biocompatible and bioactive, characterized by good mechanical and physicochemical parameters (the results are in the process of publishing). The effect of the implant was studied on a rabbit model 1, 2, 3 and 6 months after implantation. X-ray micro-computed tomography was used for imaging bone tissue samples. Empty bone defects served as a control.

2   Materials and Methods

2.1   Scaffold Preparation for Implantation

The implants came from the Department of Biomaterials, Faculty of Materials Science and Ceramics, AGH University of Science and Technology in Krakow. The material from which the implant was formed was obtained by phase inversion and lyophilisation of a mixture of polycaprolactone (60 kDa, Sigma-Aldrich) with nanometric silica (of average particle size of 5–10 nm, Sigma-Aldrich). The final material contained a 5% weight share of SiO_2. The material had an average pore size ranging from 50 to 300 μm. The average porosity of the implant was $52 \pm 4.2\%$. By using the nanometric silica as a bioactive filler, the material gained osteoconductive properties [21]. Three-dimensional scaffolds were formed from the PCL/nano-SiO$_2$ composite in a cylindrical shape. The cylinders had an average length of 12 mm and an average diameter of 3 mm. The ready implants were subjected to low-temperature sterilization (40 °C) using hydrogen peroxide plasma.

2.2   Implantation Procedure

All tests were carried out with the approval of the ethics committee, approval number: 959/2012. 8 male New Zealand rabbits aged from 5 to 7 months and weighing 2–

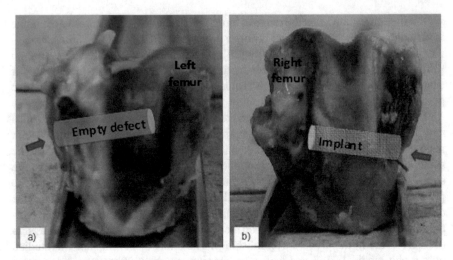

Fig. 1 Distal femoral heads with schematically designated places of drilling bone tunnels (red arrow). **a** The left base of the distal femoral head together with the marked empty bone defect—a control sample. **b** The right base of the distal femoral head together with the marked implanted biomaterial: PCL/nanoSiO$_2$

2.5 kg were subjected to testing. Properly formed and sterile implants were implanted into the distal femoral heads. Bone tunnels were drilled in the distal femoral epiphyses laterally and distally. The created defects were cleaned, so as to remove any bone particles resulting from drilling the tunnel. Finally, implants were saturated in the blood of the animal, and then their diameter was re-measured (mean diameter of the implant after saturation was 4.5 mm). The bone tunnels were filled with saturated implants (right distal femoral epiphyses) or left empty (left distal femoral epiphyses), so as to constitute control samples (see Fig. 1). After a period of 1, 2, 3 and 6 months the rabbits were euthanized (two for each control period). Then the whole knees were cut out surgically, the femoral heads were dissected, and then they were purified from the residue of the muscle tissue and tendons in 96% ethanol. In the end, 16 samples were obtained—8 with bone defects filled with PCL/nanoSiO$_2$ implants and 8 control samples.

2.3 Imaging and Visualization of the Test Samples by Means of XMT

The samples were then scanned using the XMT v|tome|x s (GE Sensing & Inspection Technologies, Phoenix|xray, Wunstorf, Germany). The test samples were placed on a rotating table in the scanner chamber. There were 1000 2D images in each measurement, which in total gave 16000 2D images for analysis. Image reconstruction was performed in the software provided by the scanner manufacturer (Datos 2.0).

The analysed samples were reconstructed in an 8bit format. Threedimensional visualization of the samples was done in Drishti ver. 2.3.3.

2.4 Determination of Histomorphometric Parameters for the Acquired Images

Histomorphometric parameters describing the bone tissue were calculated by means of the CT Analyser ver.1.13.2.1 (CTAn) (Skyscan, Belgium). The analysis was carried out for specific regions of interest, selected according to the procedure described below.

Images were selected for the analysis of bone microarchitecture from a collection of cross-sections obtained by XMT scanning. The samples were placed perpendicular to the axis of the drilled tunnel, and then, knowing the length of the created defects, two points were selected—in the $\frac{1}{4}$ and $\frac{3}{4}$ of the length of the tunnel. Starting from each of the selected locations, 10 subsequent cross-sections were marked (into the tunnel) (see Fig. 2).

Then, for the designated cross-sections, a cylindrical region (volume) of interest (VOI) was selected, which was subject to further analysis. The selected VOI included:

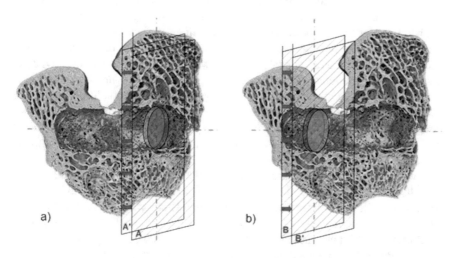

Fig. 2 Three-dimensional visualization of the cross-sections of the right base of the femoral head along the axis of symmetry of the bone tunnel with marked locations of image selection for the analysis of bone microarchitecture. **a** The first set of images for analysis was designated from the plane A (located in the $\frac{1}{4}$ of the length of the bone tunnel) to the plane A', so that the thickness of the selected area amounted to 0.16 mm, which corresponds to 10 cross-sections. **b** The second set of images for analysis was determined from the plane B (located in the $\frac{3}{4}$ of the length of the bone tunnel) to the plane B', so that the thickness of the selected area amounted to 0.16 mm, which corresponds to 10 cross-sections. Visualization was performed using the program Drishti

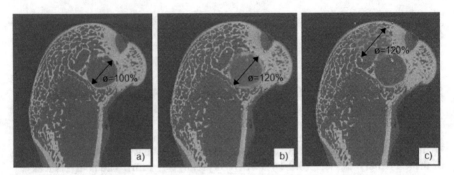

Fig. 3 Images of the cross-sections of the right base of the femoral head from the program CTAn. Images designated by the plane A (see Fig. 2) for the sample 3 months after implantation. **a** Cross-section before selecting a region of interest (ROI) with the marked size of the implant. **b** Cross-section with the ROI (marked in colour) containing the implant and the surrounding bone tissue. **c** Cross-section with the marked reference area covering the unchanged cancellous bone of the greatest density and the same diameter as the ROI containing the implant

the implant/defect (100%) together with the surrounding cancellous bone (20%) (Fig. 3b). The selected volume corresponded to the most significant area in bone tissue regeneration, where both the body's response to the implant and the implant behaviour within the body can be observed [14]. It is worth noting that intra-individual factors may result in a different structure of cancellous bone in test animals.

Therefore, for each of the cross-sections, additional regions of interest (reference) were selected, covering the unchanged cancellous bone with the greatest density (according to the operator's visual judgment) with a diameter equal to the VOI comprising the implant/defect (Fig. 3c). The VOI selection procedure was carried out manually with the greatest precision, always by the same operator. Since the regions of interest were identified on the basis of the visibility of the drilled tunnel, such identification was not possible for the samples after 6 months, when the process of bone reconstruction was almost complete and it was impossible to find the implantation site. In addition, in two control samples (both after 2 months after surgery) the bone tunnels were drilled incorrectly, and the bone defects were created in the medullary canals. To sum up, the samples after 6 months and the two control samples two months after the surgery were excluded from histomorphometric studies. In the end, 10 samples were analysed—6 with implants (two per each time period) and 4 controls (two for 1 and 3 months), which in total gave 200 2D images for analysis.

Then, automatic segmentation of bone tissue was performed in the CTAn for the selected images. Binarization thresholds were selected individually for each sample, always by the same operator.

Finally, the following parameters were calculated for all the selected areas: bone volume to total volume (BV/TV), trabecular number (Tb.N), trabecular thickness (Tb.Th), connectivity, structural model index (SMI) and trabecular separation (Tb.Sp).

3 Results

The presented results of histomorphometric analysis illustrate the sought parameters for individual volumes of interest with respect to the corresponding reference areas (unchanged areas of cancellous bone) and thus are expressed as percentages (Table 1). All the results are given as the mean.

For the femoral heads of right knees (tunnels filled with PCL/nanoSiO$_2$ implant), bone volume to total volume (BV/TV) increased from 49.58% in the first month to 55.17% in the second month and 68.71% in the third month. In the case of the reference samples, in which the drilled bone tunnel was left to self-heal, BV/TV after one month was 23.16%, and after 3 months 67.84%. BV/TV values are shown in Fig. 4. The number of bone tissue trabeculae within the studied area also increased, both for the implanted samples and the reference ones (see Fig. 5). Tb.N for the implanted bones increased from 48.55% in the first month to 54.27% in the second month, finally in the third month reaching a value of 63.96%. The number of bone tissue trabeculae also increased for the areas with an empty tunnel, from 28.26% in the first month to 68.22% in the third month. Structural model index (SMI) decreased with time, both for the group with the implant and the reference one (see Fig. 6). In the case of the tunnels filled with the implant, SMI after one month was 184.82%, after 2 months 126.04%, and after 3 months 75.93%. For the reference samples, it decreased from 222.51% after one month to 115.96% after three months. According to the literature [2, 20], a decline in the value of SMI indicates a change in the bone structure from "rood-like structure" towards "plate-like structure". There was also a slight decrease in trabecular separation. Tb.Sp in the implanted samples decreased from 107.69% after one month to 101.79 after 2 months and 74.83% after three months. For the empty bone tunnels, Tb.Sp was 109.43% after 1 month, and after 3 months it decreased to 105.54%.

Table 1 Percentages of bone microarchitecture parameters determined using CTAn

Month	BV/TV (%)		Tb.N (%)		Tb.Th (%)	
	Implant	Reference	Implant	Reference	Implant	Reference
1	49.58	23.16	48.55	28.26	100	94.74
2	55.17	–	54.27	–	102.02	–
3	68.71	67.84	63.96	68.22	79.4	100
Month	Connectivity (%)		SMI (%)		Tb.Sp (%)	
	Implant	Reference	Implant	Reference	Implant	Reference
1	60.92	36.52	184.82	222.51	107.69	109.43
2	43.86	–	126.04	–	101.79	–
3	45.41	62.52	75.93	115.96	74.83	105.54

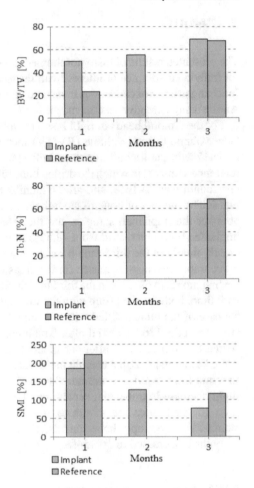

Fig. 4 Bone volume to total volume (BV/TV) in [%] of the samples after 1, 2 and 3 months, determined using the program CTAn

Fig. 5 The number of bone tissue trabeculae in [%] of the samples after 1, 2 and 3 months, determined using the program CTAn

Fig. 6 SMI in [%] of the samples after 1, 2 and 3 months, determined using CTAn

4 Discussion

The studies have demonstrated that the PCL/nanoSiO$_2$ (nano)composite implant may accelerate bone regeneration within the bone defect of the distal femoral head in New Zealand rabbits. Thus, it appears advisable to continue the research on the implant in relation to bone defects in humans. Furthermore, it has been shown that the applied method of X-ray micro-computed tomography (XMT) is suitable for assessing the process of osseointegration, thanks to the possibilities of threedimensional presentation of data and determination of the parameters of bone tissue microstructure.

Based on a review of literature it can be said that most of the research groups used histology as a major method for assessing reconstruction and remodelling of bone tissue, using X-ray micro-tomography only as a complementary test, although the results of XMT in every case correlated with histology [18, 19, 25]. The correctness of XMT measurements and the ability to replace histological tests with X-ray micro-tomography in quantitative analysis of bone tissue was previously confirmed [24]. When studying the regeneration of bone defects of the tibia and femur in sheep, implanted with a PLA/TCP biocomposite, Van der Pol et al used only the parameter of bone volume to total volume (BV/TV) and the possibility of 3D visualization, from among a wide range of data that XMT can provide, to evaluate osseointegration [13]. Based on the above, in this publication, we decided to present these and other parameters of bone tissue microstructure to emphasize their significance and effectiveness in assessing cancellous bone remodelling.

On the basis of the basic histomorphometric parameter which is bone volume to total volume (BV/TV), it has been shown that the bone tissue volume increased between the first and third month after implantation. The biggest difference between the implanted and reference samples occurred in the first month when the increase in BV/TV for PCL/nanoSiO$_2$ was on average 26% higher than for the references. This value decreased significantly in the third month, when, according to data from CTAn, an increase in the bone volume was almost identical. On this basis, it can be concluded that the implant successfully supports the initial phase of bone regeneration, accelerating it. This is also confirmed by the number of bone tissue trabeculae (Tb.N), whose number after 1 month was almost twice higher for the implanted sample. However, in the third month, Tb.N was slightly higher for the reference. Similar observations are presented in paper [18], wherein after 6 months bone remodelling was at the same level for both the bone with a tested scaffold and for the control sample. According to the literature [23], osteoporotic cancellous bone changed its structure from "plate-like" to "rood-like", so there was an increase in SMI. For the test samples of cancellous bone, this index decreased with time, so it can be assumed that the process of bone remodelling was correct and therefore the bone structure was strengthened. 6 months after implantation, the bone defect was completely invisible for both the implanted as well as the reference sample. After this time, bone tissue regeneration was complete.

It should be also pointed out that many authors in their studies showed that biomaterials containing SiO$_2$ are able to increase the expression of genes involved in bone regeneration and stimulate cell proliferation [5, 6, 29]. Furthermore, the introduction of nanoparticles increases the roughness of the biomaterial structure, which also supports the aforementioned cell proliferation [7].

5   Summary

In conclusion, the study demonstrated that for the used animal model the femurs of New Zealand rabbits, the polymerceramic composite with a polycaprolactone matrix and nanometric silica (SiO$_2$) as a modifying phase is safe and may help in the reconstruction of large bone defects. Moreover, it may accelerate the regeneration of damaged tissue. Promising results indicate the largest, approx. 26% increase in bone volume one month after implantation compared to the reference (BV/TV after

1 month for the defect filled with the implant: 49.58%, 23.16% for the defect left to selfregenerate). In addition, the method of X-ray micro-computed tomography is a modern and effective method suitable for assessing the osseointegration process.

Acknowledgements The authors thank Dr inż. Ewa Stodolak-Zych from AGH University of Science and Technology in Krakow, Faculty of Materials Science and Ceramics, Department of Biomaterials, for providing materials for research and valuable consultations.

References

1. Bose, S. et al.: Recent advances in bone tissue engineering scaffolds. Trends Biotechnol. 30, 10, 546–54 (2012). https://doi.org/10.1016/j.tibtech.2012.07.005
2. Boyd, S.K.: Micro Computed Tomography. In: Sensen, C.W., B.H., (eds.) Advanced Imaging in Biology and Medicine Technology, Software Environments, Applications, pp. 3–25. Springer, Berlin (2009)
3. Cancedda, R. et al.: Bulk and interface investigations of scaffolds and tissue–engineered bones by X–ray microtomography and X–ray microdiffraction. Biomaterials 28(15), 2505–24 (2007). https://doi.org/10.1016/j.biomaterials.2007.01.022
4. Dang, W. et al.: A bifunctional scaffold with CuFeSe 2 nanocrystals for tumor therapy and bone reconstruction. Biomaterials 160(92–106) (2018). https://doi.org/10.1016/j.biomaterials.2017.11.020
5. Dziadek, M. et al.: Biodegradable ceramic-polymer composites for biomedical applications: a review. Mater. Sci. Eng. C. (2016). https://doi.org/10.1016/j.msec.2016.10.014
6. Feng, J. et al.: Stimulating effect of silica-containing nanospheres on proliferation of osteoblast-like cells. J. Mater. Sci. Mater. Med. 18(11), 2167–72 (2007). https://doi.org/10.1007/s10856--007-3229-9
7. Gentile, F. et al.: Cells preferentially grow on rough substrates. Biomaterials 31 (28), 7205–12 (2010). https://doi.org/10.1016/j.biomaterials.2010.06.016
8. Guldberg, R.E. et al.: 3D imaging of tissue integration with porous biomaterials. Biomaterials 29(28), 3757–61 (2008). https://doi.org/10.1016/j.biomaterials.2008.06.018
9. Ho, S.T., Hutmacher, D.W.: A comparison of micro CT with other techniques used in the characterization of scaffolds. Biomaterials 27(8), 1362–76 (2006). https://doi.org/10.1016/j.biomaterials.2005.08.035
10. Khan, S.N. et al.: Osseointegration and more–a review of literature. Indian J. Dent. 3(2), 72–76 (2012). https://doi.org/10.1016/j.ijd.2012.03.012
11. van Lenthe, G.H. et al.: Nondestructive micro-computed tomography for biological imaging and quantification of scaffold-bone interaction in vivo. Biomaterials 28(15), 2479–90 (2007). https://doi.org/10.1016/j.biomaterials.2007.01.017
12. Lohmann, P. et al.: Bone regeneration induced by a 3D architectured hydrogel in a rat critical-size calvarial defect. Biomaterials 113, 158–169 (2016). https://doi.org/10.1016/j.biomaterials.2016.10.039
13. van der Pol, U. et al.: Augmentation of bone defect healing using a new biocomposite scaffold: an in vivo study in sheep. Acta Biomater. 6(9), 3755–62 (2010). https://doi.org/10.1016/j.actbio.2010.03.028
14. Puleo, D.: a, Nanci, a: Understanding and controlling the bone-implant interface. Biomaterials. 20(23–24), 2311–21 (1999)
15. Rezwan, K. et al.: Biodegradable and bioactive porous polymer/inorganic composite scaffolds for bone tissue engineering. Biomaterials 27(18), 3413–31 (2006). https://doi.org/10.1016/j.biomaterials.2006.01.039

16. Roosa, S.M.M. et al.: The pore size of polycaprolactone scaffolds has limited influence on bone regeneration in an in vivo model. J. Biomed. Mater. Res. A. **92**(1), 359–68 (2010). https://doi. org/10.1002/jbm.a.32381
17. Rüegsegger, P., et al.: A microtomographic system for the nondestructive evaluation of bone architecture. Calcif. Tissue Int. **58**(1), 24–9 (1996)
18. Shao, X.X. et al.: Evaluation of a hybrid scaffold/cell construct in repair of high-load-bearing osteochondral defects in rabbits. Biomaterials **27**(7), 1071–80 (2006). https://doi.org/10.1016/ j.biomaterials.2005.07.040
19. Shim, J.-H. et al.: Stimulation of healing within a rabbit calvarial defect by a PCL/PLGA scaffold blended with TCP using solid freeform fabrication technology. J. Mater. Sci. Mater. Med. **23**(12), 2993–3002 (2012). https://doi.org/10.1007/s10856-012-4761-9
20. Stauber, M., Müller, R.: Volumetric spatial decomposition of trabecular bone into rods and plates–a new method for local bone morphometry. Bone **38**(4), 475–84 (2006). https://doi.org/ 10.1016/j.bone.2005.09.019
21. Stodolak-Zych, E. et al.: Effect of silica nanoparticle characteristics on the bioactivity of nanocomposites based on bioresorbable polymer. In: Zviad, K. (ed.) Second International Conference for Students and Young Scientists on Materials Processing Science, pp. 59–65 (2012)
22. Stodolak-Zych, E. et al.: Osteoconductive nanocomposite materials for bone regeneration. Mater. Sci. Forum. **730–732**(November 2012), 38–43 (2012). https://doi.org/10.4028/www. scientific.net/MSF.730-732.38
23. Teo, J.C.M. et al.: Correlation of cancellous bone microarchitectural parameters from microCT to CT number and bone mechanical properties. Mater. Sci. Eng. C. **27**(2), 333–339 (2007). https://doi.org/10.1016/j.msec.2006.05.003
24. Thomsen, J.S. et al.: Stereological measures of trabecular bone structure: comparison of 3D micro computed tomography with 2D histological sections in human proximal tibial bone biopsies. J. Microsc. **218**(Pt 2), 171–9 (2005). https://doi.org/10.1111/j.1365-2818.2005.01469.x
25. Walsh, W.R. et al.: β-TCP bone graft substitutes in a bilateral rabbit tibial defect model. Biomaterials **29**(3), 266–271 (2008). https://doi.org/10.1016/j.biomaterials.2007.09.035
26. Wang, X., et al.: Enhanced bone regeneration using an insulin- loaded nano-hydroxyapatite/collagen/PLGA composite scaffold. Int. J. Nanomed. **13**, 117–127 (2018)
27. Wang, Y. et al.: Micro-CT in drug delivery. Eur. J. Pharm. Biopharm. **74**(1), 41–9 (2010). https://doi.org/10.1016/j.ejpb.2009.05.008
28. Westhauser, F. et al.: Micro-computed-tomography-guided analysis of in vitro structural modifications in two types of 45S5 bioactive glass based scaffolds. Materials (Basel). **10**(12) (2017). https://doi.org/10.3390/ma10121341
29. Wiecheć, A., et al.: The study of human osteoblast-like MG 63 cells proliferation on resorbable polymer-based nanocomposites modified with ceramic and carbon nanoparticles. ACTA Phys. Pol. A. **121**(2), 546–550 (2012)
30. Williams, J.M. et al.: Bone tissue engineering using polycaprolactone scaffolds fabricated via selective laser sintering. Biomaterials. **26**(23), 4817–27 (2005). https://doi.org/10.1016/j. biomaterials.2004.11.057

Sound and Motion in Physiotherapy and Physioprevention

Effect of Various Types of Metro-Rhythmic Stimulations on the Variability of Gait Frequency

Robert Michnik, Katarzyna Nowakowska-Lipiec, Anna Mańka,
Sandra Niedzwiedź, Patrycja Twardawa, Patrycja Romaniszyn,
Bruce Turner, Aneta Danecka, and Andrzej W. Mitas

Abstract The research discussed in the article involved the assessment of the effect of various types of metro-rhythmic stimulations and the manner of their application on the variability of gait frequency in a group of persons without locomotor function disorders. Tests of gait were attended by 22 adults in two equal groups: group 1—persons, who were not informed how to behave after hearing sounds, group 2—persons clearly instructed before the test to walk in the rhythm of music (stimulation). The tests of locomotor functions were performed using a Zebris FDM-S

R. Michnik (✉) · K. Nowakowska-Lipiec · A. Danecka
Department of Biomechanics, Silesian University of Technology,
40 Roosevelta Street, 41-800 Zabrze, Poland
e-mail: Robert.Michnik@polsl.pl

K. Nowakowska-Lipiec
e-mail: Katarzyna.Nowakowska-Lipiec@polsl.pl

A. Danecka
e-mail: Aneta.Danecka@polsl.pl

A. Mańka · P. Twardawa · P. Romaniszyn · A. W. Mitas
Department of Informatics and Medical Devices, Silesian University
of Technology, 40 Roosevelta Street, 41-800 Zabrze, Poland
e-mail: Anna.Manka@polsl.pl

P. Twardawa
e-mail: PatrTwa708@student.polsl.pl

P. Romaniszyn
e-mail: Patrycja.Romaniszyn@polsl.pl

A. W. Mitas
e-mail: Andrzej.Mitas@polsl.pl

S. Niedzwiedź
Student' Scientific Circle "Biokreatywni" Department of Biomechanics,
Silesian University of Technology, 40 Roosevelta Street, 41-800 Zabrze, Poland
e-mail: SandNie863@student.polsl.pl

B. Turner
dBs Music, HE Facility, 17 St Thomas Street, Bristol, UK
e-mail: Bruce.Turner@dbsmusic.co.uk

E. Piętka et al. (eds.), *Information Technology in Biomedicine*, Advances in Intelligent
Systems and Computing 1186, https://doi.org/10.1007/978-3-030-49666-1_10

treadmill. The analysis involved changes in gait frequency during the gait accompanied by various types of sound stimulations (arrhythmic stimulus, rhythmic stimulus at a rate corresponding to gait frequency at a preferable speed, rhythmic stimulus presented at a rate corresponding to gait frequency increased by 10%, rhythmic stimulus presented at a rate of the double gait frequency). It was demonstrated that acoustic stimuli heard during gait can affect its frequency. The frequency of gait was mostly influenced by rhythmic stimuli, the rate of which varied from the frequency of steps at a preferable pace. The short-term sound-based stimulation was also affected by the fact whether a examined person had been informed on how to react to stimulation.

Keywords Gait · Gait frequency · Rhythmic auditory stimulation · Treadmill

1 Introduction

"Rhythmic Auditory Stimulation (RAS) is a tool supporting rehabilitation of movements that are naturally rhythmic. Auditory cueing is mainly used to improve or restore lost body movement function. The purpose of introducing RAS into therapy is to provide a stimulus facilitating the maintenance of correct movement patterns and rhythmic cues during movement" [20]. Performing a activity characterized by repetitive movements which is cued by auditory stimuli is called sensorimotor synchronization (SMS) [13]. The mechanism of entraining the body to external rhythms applies to the entire human body, which extends the use of metrorhythmic stimuli to different groups of patients and types of therapy [19]. RAS is not limited to gait therapy but can be successfully used to entrain whole body movements, including arm and hand movement since rhythmic stimulations work well with any therapy based on physical activity. Many studies on RAS indicate its use for patients with limited or impaired mobility is desirable, mainly for patients with stroke, traumatic brain injury or Parkinson's disease. There are no restrictions on the age of patients since RAS can be used both for children and adults [7, 12, 19, 20].

Auditory cueing used in SMS can have various forms, starting from the metronome and ending with music containing more complex elements which allow participants to more accurately synchronise their movements [21]. In some rehabilitation programs instead of artificial sounds like metronome or simple music sounds, footstep sounds, referred to as ecological RAS, are used. Another option is the use of bilateral stimuli [6]. In any case RAS cues should be adjusted to the parameters of the subject's movement [13]. Typically, tempo of stimuli is equal or slightly different than patient's cadence, depending on the methodology and patient characteristics [20]. Due to music characteristics and greater accumulation of information in it, the musical stimulus has a stronger impact on gait than a metronome. Additional information such as melody, harmony and rhythm between the main beats allows to optimize the movement path based on those additional information [21].

The analyzed parameters and chosen method of conducting therapy depend on the study group and the aim of rehabilitation. The treadmill is often used because of the ability to control the gait speed of the subject and a simple way to match the stimulus tempo to the gait tempo. An alternative to these are studies in an open field.Measures include gait symmetry, gait ability, balance ability, lower extremity function analysis and gait variability. It is important to evaluate gait variability as it can change in two ways—synchronization to the rhythm may reduce the temporal variability but at the same time it can have a damaging effect on the body, adversely increasing gait variability [21].

Each RAS therapy should be adapted to the needs of the patient and his disability to achieve improvement of specific movement parameters, as close as possible to the values obtained for people without movement disorders [3, 8]. Type of used stimuli and its characteristics can lead to different effects on movement [21]. Music type, especially temporal patterns, can change the walking speed and stride length [7]. Bilateral rhytmic auditory stimulation can lead to increased improvement of gait symmetry and ability and various gait test like the Timed Up and Go test, Berg Balance Scale, and Fugl-Meyer Assessment in stroke patients [6].

Reported findings of RAS for movement rehabilitation are promising [13]. Studies on various patient groups show that the use of rhythmic stimuli affects the mechanism of movement, especially step cadence, stride length, and helps maintain correct posture and symmetric muscle activation patterns [20]. The effects of introduction RAS into therapy have been most widely investigated in stroke and Parkinson's patients due to the characteristics of the symptoms they experience. In the group of Parkinson's disease patients, RAS can be used to work on gait pattern [7, 20]. Parkinson patients can walk longer after RAS session [7]. Stroke patients can benefit from RAS as it may improve gait parameters like gait symmetry, pattern and velocity, cadence, stride length, muscle activation, and range of limb movement [4, 20]. Treadmill walking with cued footfall improve gait coordination [13]. Metrorhythmic stimuli are also used for healthy people, mainly to improve sport performance. It is possible to cue rhythmic movement in a way that the tempo of this movement fits the tempo of the stimulus even in cases where the movement is clearly marked [13]. A similar experiment to ours was carried out by Styns et al [17]. The study revealed that subjects walk faster to music than to metronome. The subjects are able to synchronize their walk to various stimuli, but they did it most effectively when the tempo of the stimuli was close to 120 BPM [17]. Wittwer et al. [21] determined the effect of rhythmic music and metronome stimuli on gait parameters in healthy older adults. Mean spatio-temporal variability was low at baseline and did not change with both stimuli and participants walked faster to music than metronome. Study findings suggest stimuli type and its frequency should be considered when evaluating effects of RAS on gait.

Synchronization of physical activity to external metrorhythmic stimuli can affect trajectory of movement, time of its occurence and can help learn complex movements [13]. It is still unknown why some patient groups are cued in more effective way than others. Undetermined information also applies to the stimuli used: what the stimulus effectiveness depends on, how different RAS affect gait entrainment and how rhythmic representations are established [13].

The research work aimed to assess the effect of various types of metro-rhythmic stimulations and the manner of their application on the variability of gait frequency in a group of persons without locomotor function disorders.

2 Material and Method

The research-related tests involved 22 adults without locomotor systems disorders and locomotor dysfunction. All participants agreed to participate in the tests.

The examined subjects were divided into two groups, each of which consisted of 11 members:

- Group 1 (age: 23.1 ± 1.6 years, weight: 66.1 ± 22.4 kg, body height:171.9 ± 11.6 cm) was composed of persons who were not instructed before the test that during gait with metro-rhythmic stimulation they should try to adjust their gait frequency to the sounds they heard,
- Group 2 (age: 26.3 ± 7.2 years, weight: 65.9 ± 9.1 kg, body height: 170.3 ± 8.3 cm) included persons clearly instructed before the test that they should walk in the rhythm of music (metro–rhythmic stimulation).

The assessment of locomotor functions was performed during gait on a ZEBRIS FDM-T treadmill (ZebrisMedical GmbH, Isny, Germany).

At the first stage, each examined person individually adjusted their preferable gait velocity when walking on the treadmill (vp). The examined subjects started walking at a relatively low speed. Afterwards, the operator increased the velocity of gait by 0.1 km/h until a given examined person stated that they were walking at their preferable speed. Afterwards, the then-current speed was increased by 1.5 km/h and, next, decreased repeatedly by 0.1 km/h to return to the speed regarded as preferable. After each change of speed, the operator asked whether the then-present speed of gait was preferable. In the case of uncertainty, the procedure was repeated.

Once the preferable speed had been adjusted, each examined person walked on the treadmill at the aforesaid speed in order to get accustomed to it.

The next phase involved a 60-s long recording of the gait (GP) in relation to the preferable speed (vp). The results of the above-presented procedure were used to identify the average frequency of gait in relation to the preferable speed.

The subsequent stage included the recording of gait during metro-rhythmic stimulation. The speed adjusted on the treadmill corresponded to the preferable speed of gait (vp). Before each presentation of a stimulus, the examined person walked for 30 s in accordance with their own rhythm of steps and no sound was played then. Gait with the sound stimulus lasted 90 s. The tests were performed in relation to four types of stimulation:

- GA (arrhythmic stimulus played at a rate of 120 BPM, time 4/4, ambient style)— because of the lack of accents in the stimulus and gradual transition between individual tones, changes in tempo could not be sensed by the listeners in respect of the effect on audio-motor synchronisation (connected with the performance of movements synchronised with the timing of accentuated moments in, e.g. a music piece fragment)—the stimulus was played at the tempo consistent with the composer's intention. In the above-presented case, music was supposed to provide relaxation, assumedly leading to the symmetrisation and "tranquilising" of gait;

- GR (rhythmic stimulus played at a rate corresponding to the frequency of gait and determined during tests of preferable speed, time 4/4, motivating music)— rhythmed periodic stimulus with accents in strong parts of the bar (quarter notes in the 1st and 3rd measure) and an 8-bar phrase. Additional non-accentuated rhythmic units were at regular intervals in the weak parts of the bar (quarter notes in the 2nd and 4th measure). The composition included synthesized sounds; the 8-bar phrase was followed by a single or double striking of the plate idiophone (high hat) of natural sound. Selected fragments of the stimulus, in the bars preceding the beginning of a new phrase, were preceded by dotted notes (dotted eighth note and sixteenth note). The stimulation was of a motivating nature, characteristic of music played during sports training (e.g. aerobics);
- GR110 (rhythmic stimulus as above, played at a rate corresponding to gait frequency increased by 10%; the tempo was determined during the tests of gait at a preferable speed);
- GR200 (rhythmic stimulus as above, played at a rate corresponding to doubled gait frequency; the tempo was determined during the tests of gait at a preferable speed).

The assessment involved the susceptibility of healthy examined subjects to metro-rhythmic stimuli. Detailed analysis was concerned with the variability of gait frequency.

The average gait frequency as well as the standard deviation for gait at a preferable speed and gait accompanied by various types of metro-rhythmic stimulation were determined for each examined person. The cadence variation coefficient was determined for each examined subject in relation to each successive test.

The research also involved the identification of the difference between pre-set frequency (obtained on the basis of the tests involving the preferable speed) and the frequency determined in relation to the tests involving various types of simulation. Percentage differences in the cadence variation coefficient were determined for all subsequent tests. Gait frequency, its deviation and coefficients of frequency variability were determined for 45 s long intervals:

- in relation to gait not accompanied by metro-rhythmic stimulation: from the 15th to the 60th s of recorded gait,
- in relation to gait accompanied by metro-rhythmic stimulation: from the 60th to the 105t s, i.e. the analysis covered the fragment starting 30 s after the playing of the sound stimulus.

The analysis of results was performed with reference to two groups (Group 1, Group 2). It was necessary to verify if the above-named quantitative variables differed as regards the participants who were not informed about how to behave after hearing sound stimuli and those who, before the test, were clearly instructed to walk in the rhythm of music after hearing metro-rhythmic stimulation.

3 Results

Tables 1 and 2 present the distribution of gait frequency results and its standard deviation in relation to gait not accompanied by any sounds and that accompanied by various types of metro-rhythmic stimulation.

The obtained values of gait frequency and their standard deviations related to each examined person were used to determine the coefficient of cadence variation for the tests of gait not accompanied by sounds and that accompanied by metro-rhythmic stimulation. The average values and the standard deviation of the cadence variation coefficient in relation to subsequent tests of gait are presented in Fig. 1.

The results obtained in the tests were subjected to statistical analysis. The normality of the distribution of obtained gait frequency values, the standard deviation of frequency and the cadence variation coefficient in relation to both groups were verified using the Shapiro-Wilk test. The statistical analysis, i.e. the Mann-Whitney Utest for independent samples, revealed a statistically relevant difference in gait

Table 1 Gait frequency results concerning the test without sounds and the test with metro-rhythmic stimulation

		Group 1					Group 2				
		Mean	Std	Median	Min	Max	Mean	Std	Median	Min	Max
Cadance[step/min]	GP	107.36	4.54	108	98	113	107.64	5.16	109	98	114
	GA	105.64	4.99	106	98	112	105.82	5.19	107	96	111
	GR	105.82	5.62	107	95	113	108.18	4.49	109	100	114
	GR110	104.82	4.75	106	98	111	114.45	5.11	114	108	124
	GR200	104.55	5.65	107	94	111	109.18	9.59	108	96	134

Table 2 Results of gait frequency standard deviation concerning the test without sounds and the test with metro-rhythmic stimulation

		Group 1					Group 2				
		Mean	Std	Median	Min	Max	Mean	Std	Median	Min	Max
Std of cadance [step/min]	GP	1.55	1.18	1.55	1.36	1.27	1.36	1.27	1.64	2.27	2.18
	GA	0.82	0.40	0.52	0.50	0.47	0.67	0.65	0.92	1.49	0.75
	GR	1.00	1.00	2.00	1.00	1.00	1.00	1.00	1.00	2.00	2.00
	GR110	1.00	1.00	1.00	1.00	1.00	1.00	1.00	1.00	1.00	1.00
	GR200	3.00	2.00	2.00	2.00	2.00	3.00	3.00	4.00	6.00	3.00

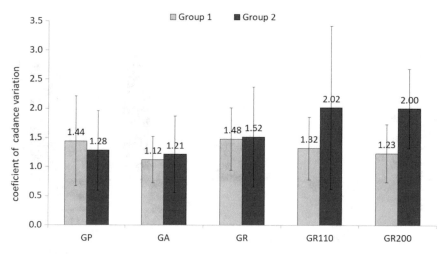

Fig. 1 Cadence variation coefficient concerning the test without sounds and the test with metro-rhythmic stimulation

frequency only in relation to the test with stimulation GR110 (p = 0.0008) (for Group 1 and Group 2). The values of gait frequency standard deviation (p = 0.006) and the values of cadence variation coefficient (p = 0.039) differed between the above-named groups only in relation to the test of gait with stimulation GR200. The remaining tests of gait did not reveal statistically relevant differences of analysed variables between Group 1 and 2. Figure 2 presents percentage differences in relation to the cadence variation coefficient between the tests involving metro-rhythmic stimulation and those without simulation. The highest percentage differences of the cadence variation coefficient were observed in relation to the test with simulation GR110 and that with simulation GR200. As regards the tests of gait accompanied by rhythmic stimulation, the aforesaid differences were significantly higher in Group 2, i.e. participants clearly instructed before the tests to walk in the rhythm of music when hearing sounds.

4 Discussion

The overview of information concerning previous research on the rhythmical sound stimulation revealed the effect of acoustic sounds on the time-spatial parameters of gait in patients suffering from various neurological disorders [1, 2, 5, 6, 9, 11, 22, 23]. Changes were also observed in healthy persons [10, 14, 18, 21]. In previous research-related tests, the frequency of sound signal playing was determined on the basis of individual preferences and changed within the range of 22.5% of the participant's primary gait frequency. The time-scale calculus related to the assessment of sound effect varied in individual publications. The parameters were compared on

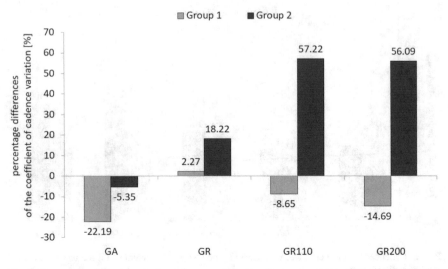

Fig. 2 Percentage differences in the cadence variation coefficient in relation to the test with metro-rhythmic stimulation and the test without stimulation

the same day or within several weeks, during which patients underwent a rhythmic stimulation-based treatment.

The reference publications stated that the use of sounds usually positively affected the gait frequency in the tests where the rhythm of the sound was equal to or higher than the preferable cadence [2, 5, 6, 9, 11, 15, 16, 21, 23].

The analysis of the results obtained in the research work revealed that acoustic stimuli heard during gait can affect its frequency.

When analysing the values of the standard deviations from gait frequency (Table 2), it was noticed that, in both groups, the average values of deviations in relation to gait with an arrhythmic model were nearly by twice lower than those related to gait not accompanied by stimulation. In addition, the deviations for gait with stimulus GR and GR110 were lower as well. The foregoing leads to the conclusion that the rhythmic stimulus at the rate corresponding to gait frequency determined during the tests of gait with the preferable speed and the rhythmic stimulus at the rate corresponding to gait frequency increased by 10% did not impede walking. The tests involving the use of stimulus GR200 revealed significantly high standard deviations of gait frequency in comparison with those obtained for gait without stimulation and with the preferable speed, particularly in relation to Group 2. This can indicate that examined subjects could not adjust to stimulation of the above-named rate. The analyses presented above lead to the conclusion that hearing sound stimuli during gait at a rate slightly (10%) faster than preferable gait frequency did not impede walking. In addition, among persons who had been clearly instructed (Group 2) to walk in the rhythm with them, the stimuli led to an increase in gait frequency (Table 1).

The lowest gait frequency variability was observed in relation to GA, i.e. gait with the arrhythmic stimulus, where music had a relaxation role, indirectly leading to the symmetrisation and "tranquilising" of gait (Fig. 1). The highest variability was observed in relation to gait with variously timed stimuli (GR110, GR200) in Group 2, i.e., the participants tried to adjust their gait frequency to sounds. In Group 1, i.e. the participants not instructed on how to react to stimulation, the variability of gait frequency did not change significantly in relation to the gait not accompanied by sound stimulation. In relation to the tests of gait accompanied by stimulation GP, GA and GR, it was observed that differences in the values of the cadence variation coefficient between Group 1 and Group 2 were small. However, the difference between the groups was significantly higher in relation to the tests with sound stimulation GR110 and GR200, i.e. the tests of gait accompanied by rhythmic stimulation at a rate different from the frequency of gait performed with preferable speed. The values of the cadence variation coefficient in relation to Group 1 in the tests involving GR110 and GR200 were similar to those obtained in the remaining tests. The cadence variation coefficient in Group 2 was significantly higher in relation to the tests with GR110 and GR200, which could indicate that the persons who were clearly instructed before the test to walk in the rhythm of music tried to abide by the instruction.

The foregoing was also confirmed by percentage differences of the cadence variation coefficient between the test involving metro-rhythmic stimulation and that without the stimulation (Fig. 2). In relation to the tests with stimulation GR110 and GR200 in Group 2, the above-named values amounted to 57% and 56% respectively, whereas in relation to Group 1, they did not exceed 15%. Because of the fact that the tempo of metro-rhythmic stimulation did not correspond to gait in relation to the pre-set preferable speed of gait on the treadmill, the results of the tests with sounds GR110 and GR200 were characterised by significantly higher gait frequency variability.

The above-presented analyses indicate that gait parameters will be most modified by rhythmic stimuli having a tempo different from the frequency of gait determined when identifying gait with preferable speed. The aforesaid information is important because of the fact that until today the research-related stimulation has been primarily performed using the metronome [9, 14–16, 18, 21–23]. It is possible to come across publications concerning tests where stimuli were natural sound signals such as steps [9], clasping, clicking, gunshots etc. [5]. The vast overview of publications on the issue revealed the lack of works involving tests where participants were stimulated by composed pieces of music, including arrhythmic stimuli and rhythmic musical pieces of motivating nature, typical of music used in sports training.

The research also revealed that during the first and short-term use of sound stimuli, the frequency of gait will also be affected by the fact whether a given examined person was informed on how to react to metro-rhythmic stimulation. Until today, there has been no research concerning the above-presented issue.

The above-presented results of the research work can be regarded as reliable, yet it is undoubtedly possible to indicate certain limitations of the tests and analyses. Primarily, in order for statistical analysis to provide reliable results, the tests should have involved a larger number of participants in equinumerous groups. In addition, it would be recommendable to perform long-term tests, where participants would be subjected to the long-term effect of metro-rhythmic stimulation during gait and, next, would be subjected to the aforesaid test after a certain period of time. Similar tests should also be performed during unforced gait on the treadmill. Particularly interesting could be the extension of tests by including other types of metro-rhythmic stimulation. Tests could also be extended by including the analysis of the variability of other time-spatial parameters of gait as a result of rhythmic auditory stimulation, e.g. the time of a gait cycle, the length of a step etc. As future plans, it would be worth checking how the above stimuli affect the gait of people with dysfunctions, e.g. after a stroke or with Parkinson's disease. Nonetheless, the above-presented research work represents significant substantive value as it presents the effect of various types of metro-rhythmic stimulation and the manner of their application on gait frequency variability in a group of persons without locomotor system dysfunctions. The research concerning the above-presented issue has not been performed until today.

5 Conclusions

The analysis of the results obtained in the above-presented tests enabled the formulation of the following conclusions:

- acoustic stimuli heard during gait can affect gait frequency,
- arrhythmic stimuli, related to music tasked with relaxation, indirectly "tranquilise" the speed of gait,
- hearing sound stimuli during slightly faster gait (by 10%) than the preferable gait frequency does not impede walking,
- gait frequency is most modified by rhythmic stimuli, the tempo of which differs from gait with preferable speed,
- during the first short-time sound stimulation, gait frequency was affected by whether a given examined person had been informed how to react to stimuli.

References

1. Arias, P., Cudeiro, J.: Effect of rhythmic auditory stimulation on gait in parkinsonian patients with and without freezing of gait. PLoS One 5(3), e9675 (2010)
2. Conklyn, D., Stough, D., Novak, E., Paczak, S., Chemali, K., Bethoux, F.: A home-based walking program using rhythmic auditory stimulation improves gait performance in patients with multiple sclerosis: a pilot study. Neurorehabil. Neural Repair 24(9), 835–842 (2010)
3. Jochymczyk-Woźniak, K., Nowakowska, K., Michnik, R., Gzik, M., Kowalczykowski, D.: Three-dimensional adults gait pattern - reference data for healthy adults aged between 20 and 24. In: Innovation in biomedical engineering Gzik, M., Tkacz, E., Paszenda, Z., Piętka, E. (Eds.) Advances in Intelligent System and Computing, vol. 925 2194–5357, 169–176. Springer International Publishing, Cham (2019)
4. Kim, J., Jung, M., Yoo, E., Park, J., Kim, S., Lee, J.: Effects of rhythmic auditory stimulation during hemiplegic arm reaching in individuals with stroke: an exploratory study. Hong Kong J. Occup. Therapy 24(2), 64–71 (2014)

5. Ko, B.W., Lee, H.Y., Song, W.K.: Rhythmic auditory stimulation using a portable smart device: short-term effects on gait in chronic hemiplegic stroke patients. J. Phys. Ther. Sci. **28**(5), 1538–1543 (2016)
6. Lee, S., Lee, K., Song, Ch.: Gait training with bilateral rhythmic auditory stimulation in stroke patients: a randomized controlled trial. Brain Sci. **8**(9), 164 (2018)
7. Leman, M., Moelants, D., Varewyck, M., Styns, F., van Noorden, L., Martens, J.-P.: Activating and relaxing music entrains the speed of beat synchronized walking. PLoS One **8**(7), e67932 (2013)
8. Michnik, R., Nowakowska, K., Jurkojć, J., Jochymczyk-Woźniak, K., Kopyta, I.: Motor functions assessment method based on energy changes in gait cycle. Acta Bioeng. Biomech. **19**(4), 63–75 (2017)
9. Murgia, M., Pili, R., Corona, F., Sors, F., Agostini, T.A., Bernardis, P., Casula, C., Cossu, G., Guicciardi, M., Pau, M.: The use of footstep sounds as rhythmic auditory stimulation for gait rehabilitation in Parkinson's disease: a randomized controlled trial. Front Neurol. **9**, 348 (2018)
10. Roerdink, M., Bank, P.J.M., Lieke, C., Peper, E., Bee, P.J.: Walking to the beat of different drums: practical implications for the use ofacoustic rhythms in gait rehabilitation. Gait Post. **33**, 690–694 (2011)
11. Roerdink, M., Lamoth, C.J.C., Kwakkel, G., van Wieringen, P.C.W., Beek, P.J.: Gait coordination after stroke: benefits of acoustically paced treadmill walking. Phys. Ther. **87**(8), 1009–1022 (2007)
12. Romaniszyn, P., Kania, D., Nowakowska, K., Sobkowiak, M., Turner, B., Myśliwiec, A., Michnik, R., Mitas, A.: RAS in the Aspect of Symmetrization of Lower Limb Loads. (in:) Information Technologies in Medicine 7th International Conference, ITIB 2019, Kamień Śląski, Poland, June 18-20, 2019., Pietka E., Badura P., Kawa J., Wieclawek W. (eds.), Cham: Springer, Advances in Intelligent System and Computing, vol. 1011, 436–447 (2019)
13. Schaefer, R.S.: Auditory rhythmic cueing in movement rehabilitation: findings and possible mechanisms. Philos. Trans. R Soc. Lond. B Biol. Sci. **369**(1658), 20130402 (2014)
14. Schreiber, C., Remacle, A., Chantraine, F., Kolanowski, E., Moissenet, F.: Influence of a rhythmic auditory stimulation on asymptomatic gait. Gait Post. **50**, 17–22 (2016)
15. Shahraki, M., Sohrabi, M., Torbati, H.T., Nikkhah, K., NaeimiKia, M.: Effect of rhythmic auditory stimulation on gait kinematic parameters of patients with multiple sclerosis. J. Med. Life **10**, 33–37 (2017)
16. Shin, Y.K., Chong, H.J., Kim, S.J., Cho, S.R.: Effect of Rhythmic Auditory Stimulation on Hemiplegic Gait Patterns. Yonsei Med. J. **56**(6), 1703–1713 (2015)
17. Styns, F., van Noorden, L., Moelants, D., Leman, M.: Walking on music. Hum. Mov. Sci. **26**, 769–785 (2007)
18. Terrier, P., Dériaz, O.: Persistent and anti-persistent pattern in stride-to-stride variability of treadmill walking: influence of rhythmic auditory cueing. Hum. Mov. Sci. **31**, 1585–1597 (2012)
19. Thaut, M.H., McIntosh, G.C., Hoemberg, V.: Neurobiological foundations of neurologic music therapy: rhythmic entrainment and the motor system. Front. Psychol. **5**, 1185 (2014)
20. Thaut, M.H., Hoemberg, V. (eds.): Handbook of Neurologic Music Therapy (2014). ISBN: 9780198792611
21. Wittwer, J.E., Webster, K.E., Hill, K.: Music and metronome cues produce different effects on gait spatiotemporal measures but not gait variability in healthy older adults. Gait Post. **37**(2), 219–22 (2013)
22. Wright, R.L., Bevins, J.W., Pratt, D., Sackley, C.M., Wing, A.M.: Metronome cueing of walking reduces gait variability after a cerebellar stroke. Front. Neurol. **7**, 84 (2016)
23. Yoon, S.K., Kan, S.H.: Effects of inclined treadmill walking training with rhythmic auditory stimulation on balanceand gait in stroke patients. J. Phys. Ther. Sci. **28**(12), 3367–3370 (2016)

Cross-Modal Music-Emotion Retrieval Using DeepCCA

Naoki Takashima, Frédéric Li, Marcin Grzegorzek, and Kimiaki Shirahama

Abstract Music-emotion retrieval is important for treatments of mood disorders and depression based on music. Although existing approaches only investigate one-way retrieval from music to emotions, an approach from emotion to music might be needed for proper application of music-based therapies. This can be achieved by sensor-based music retrieval which firstly recognises a specific emotion based on physiological data acquired by wearable sensors and then identifies music suitable for that emotion. In this paper, we propose *Cross-modal Music-emotion Retrieval* (CMR) as the first step to achieve retrieval of music based on sensor data. Our approach uses *Deep Canonical Correlation Analysis* (DeepCCA) which projects music samples and their associated emotion sequences into a common space using deep neural networks, and maximises the correlation between projected music samples and emotion sequences using CCA. Our experiments show the superiority of our approach for CMR compared to one-way retrieval.

Keywords Music emotion retrieval · Machine learning · Cross-modal retrieval

N. Takashima (✉) · K. Shirahama
Department of Informatics, Kindai University 3-4-1 Kowakae, Higashiosaka City, Osaka
577-8502, Japan
e-mail: takashima.naoki@kindai.ac.jp

K. Shirahama
e-mail: shirahama@info.kindai.ac.jp

F. Li · M. Grzegorzek
Institute of Medical Informatics, Lübeck University, Ratzeburger Allee 160, 23538 Lübeck,
Germany
e-mail: li@imi.uni-luebeck.de

M. Grzegorzek
e-mail: grzegorzek@imi.uni-luebeck.de

133

E. Piętka et al. (eds.), *Information Technology in Biomedicine*, Advances in Intelligent
Systems and Computing 1186, https://doi.org/10.1007/978-3-030-49666-1_11

1 Introduction

Emotion recognition is an important topic for affective computing with potential applications in medicine. The literature has shown that music-based therapies using emotion recognition could be effectively used for treatments of mood disorders and depression [15, 18].

To use such therapies, it is needed to automatically link music to emotions. Most of existing solutions for this are based on *one-way retrieval* approaches which take one music excerpt as input and return a list of emotions associated to this input. Such methods have been mostly developed by streaming services like Spotify,[1] Amazon Music,[2] etc. But, those services mainly perform retrieval based on external factors like venue categories, visual scenes and users' listening histories [20]. For this reason, the development of an automatic Music-Emotion Retrieval (MER) system which detects emotions of users and identifies music corresponding to these emotions has attracted the attention of the machine learning research community [22].

The aforementioned one-way music to emotion retrieval approaches have one limitation: they link a music sample to a 'general' emotions roughly perceived by groups of users such as happiness, anger or sadness. This makes it difficult to take into account 'perceptual variation' which refers to the differences in emotional perceptions of a music sample between different users. Perceptual variation for instance often depends on whether users know a song. If a user knows a specific song, they might feel some emotions based on their past experiences with it. If they do not know it, they can express emotions from a more neutral state. To address perceptual variation, we need to consider the opposite retrieval way from emotion to music by assembling different emotions perceived for the same music. In other words, this associates different emotions to the same music and enables us to take into account different perceptions of the same music by different users. Moreover, the opposite retrieval way from emotion to music can take as input a 'specific' (nuanced) emotion of a user like cheerfulness, madness and disappointment, and retrieve music samples that match this specific emotion. We therefore propose a *bidirectional retrieval* approach which can not only retrieve general emotions based on the analysis of music samples evoking similar emotions, but also identify music samples associated to more nuanced specific emotions.

In addition, we aim at incorporating sensor-based emotion recognition into a bidirectional MER system. To link sensor data to music, we need to develop and combine the following two systems. Firstly, a bidirectional MER system that takes a specific emotion as input and finds music samples suitable for the emotion. Secondly, an emotion recognition system based on physiological sensor data such as blood pressure, heart rate and skin conductance. Using the output of the emotion recognition component as input of the bidirectional MER system, music can be retrieved based on specific emotions recognised from the sensor data.

---

[1] https://www.spotify.com.

[2] https://music.amazon.com.

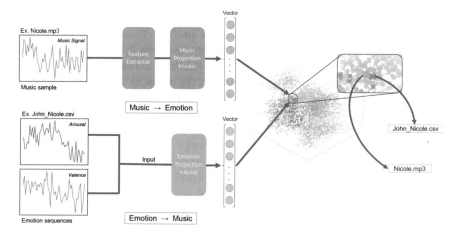

Fig. 1 An overview of our CMR approach

In this paper, we propose *Cross-modal Music-emotion Retrieval* (CMR) to obtain the first component of the aforementioned sensor-based MER system. Existing MER approaches only conduct retrieval that uses a music sample as a query to find a general emotion perceived by multiple users for this music sample. CMR can additionally achieve retrieval of music samples using a specific emotion as a query. To consider both general and specific emotions, we use the Circumplex model of emotions which is popular in the field of affective computing [12, 13]. It decomposes emotions along two axes following Russell's circumplex model of emotions: arousal (level of stimulation) and valence (level of pleasantness) [22].

Figure 1 shows an overview of our bidirectional CMR approach which associates music samples with their associated two-dimensional emotion sequences representing arousal and valence values over time. In Fig. 1, acoustic features are extracted from a music sample "Nicole.mp3" and then fed into a music projection model to obtain a projection vector. On the other hand, it is assumed that the two-dimensional emotion sequence "John_Nicole.csv" is obtained from the subject John when listening to Nicole.mp3. This emotion sequence is input into an emotion projection model that transforms it into a vector of the same dimensionality as the music vector. In other words, the music sample and the emotion sequence are projected into a common space. In this space, associated music samples and emotions are projected close to each other. This kind of similarity relation in the common space is the core of our bidirectional CMR approach. In Fig. 1, an example of retrieval from music to emotion shows that emotion sequences similar to John_Nicole.csv are retrieved using Nicole.mp3 as a query. In contrast, giving John_Nicole.csv as a query would lead to the retrieval of several associated music samples, including Nicole.mp3. This way our CMR approach can accomplish bidirectional retrieval between music and emotion.

Instead of using the common Euclidean distance as similarity measure, our CMR approach employs *Deep Canonical Correlation Analysis* (DeepCCA) [2] which performs the projection to maximise the correlation between relevant music samples and emotion sequences in the common space. This is based on our assumption that while the degree of perceiving emotions differs from user to user, each user relates emotions to music in a relatively correlated way. More concretely, two subjects might be more or less emotionally affected by a song. But, in such a situation, it is assumed that both of the subjects react in the same "emotional direction" when listening to the same specific song (e.g., they are more or less happy when listening a "happy" song, sad when listening a "sad" song, and so on). Furthermore, DeepCCA has shown that it can be successfully used for bidirectional retrieval between image and text data [2]. In our work, DeepCCA is adapted to the MER context and allows us to take into account perceptual variation of emotions. The experimental results show that our CMR approach using DeepCCA yields retrieval performances approximately twice better than baseline MER approaches.

This paper is organised as follows: Sect. 2 reviews the literature of conceptualisation approaches for emotions and music retrieval systems. Section 3 describes details of our CMR approach based on DeepCCA, and Sect. 4 reports the experimental results showing the effectiveness of our CMR approach through the comparison with baseline approaches. Finally, Sect. 5 presents the conclusion and our future work.

2 Related Work

The conceptualisation of human emotions is studied in the field of psychology. This section presents the two main conceptualisation approaches, reviews the literature on music retrieval systems and shows the differences between them and ours.

2.1 Emotion Conceptualisation

Existing approaches to conceptualise emotions can be divided into 'categorical' and 'dimensional'. Categorical approaches refer to the idea of classifying human emotions in discrete categories. Ekman's model is the most famous categorical approach [5]. An essential idea of this model is the concept of *basic emotions* which defines and lists universal primary emotions (e.g. happiness, sadness, anger, fear disgust and surprise) from which all the other secondary emotions can be derived [5, 14]. Another famous categorical approach is Hevner's adjective list [8] which divides affective terms into eight clusters and arranges them in a circle, as shown in Fig. 2. The adjectives within each cluster are similar, while opposing clusters contain emotions with opposing meanings [22]. One of the main drawbacks of categorical approaches

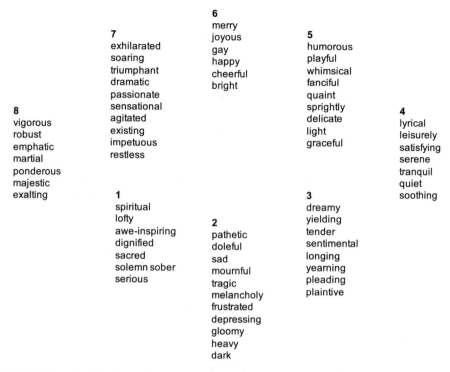

Fig. 2 Hevner's adjective list of eight emotion clusters [8]

is that it is difficult to express the richness and diversity of emotions using a limited number of categories only.

Dimensional approaches define emotions using several characteristic axes such as valence (positive vs negative), arousal (level of energy) and potency (powerful vs powerless) [16]. According to this, an emotional state can be defined as a point in the emotional space structured by the characteristic axes. In particular, arousal and valence are more popular than the others because they have shown to be the most efficient representation of emotions. Russel was the first to propose the Circumplex model which is a two dimensional model measuring levels of valence and arousal, as illustrated in Fig. 3. The Circumplex model is the most common model used by existing MER approaches [4], because the continuity of the emotional space allows a more fine-grained modelisation of emotions than categorical approaches.

2.2 Music Retrieval System

Existing MER approaches such as [10, 17, 23] focus on music retrieval based on emotions. Acoustic hand-crafted features are traditionally extracted from music samples,

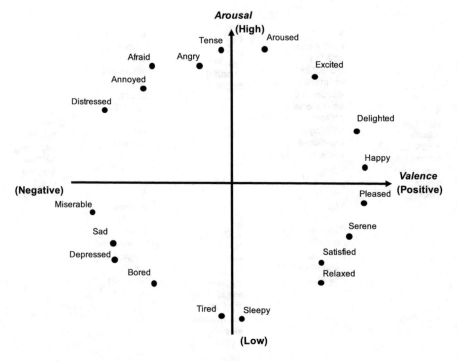

Fig. 3 Russel's Circumplex model of emotions [16]

such as Mel-Frequency Cepstrum Coefficients (MFCC) which represent vocal tract characteristics and Fundamental tone (F0) indicating the lowest frequency sound. Those features are high-dimensional and can adversely impact the retrieval speed of real-time MER systems [17] proposed a method to reduce the dimensionality of acoustic features while preserving retrieval performances. This approach is evaluated by a retrieval accuracy using K-nearest neighbor [10] proposed a mood-based music retrieval system that classifies music into four moods including happiness, anger, sadness and fear by analyzing acoustic features of tempo (fast/slow) and articulation (staccato/legato). Music Retrieval in the Emotion Plane [23] is an emotion-based music retrieval platform. It represents a music sample depending on arousal and valence ratings, and their relevance is measured by Euclidean distance.

Additionally, some existing works investigate cross-modal approaches using different modalities and report excellent performances. For example, [19] proposed a personalised video soundtrack recommendation system. The system detects mood-tags in movie scenes and venue categories, and recommends soundtracks that match the detected mood-tags as well as user's listening history [24] proposed a cross-modal audio-lyrics retrieval system that maximises the correlation between relevant music samples and lyrics in a common space using DeepCCA.

Most of existing MER approaches like [10, 17, 23] are one-way retrieval, so they cannot take perceptual variation into account. Compared to them, our approach based on bidirectional retrieval can consider perceptual variation. In addition, while one-way retrieval only exploits links from music to emotion, our bidirectional retrieval additionally uses links from emotion to music. In other words, our method analyses a larger amount of data than previous ones, which leads to building an improved retrieval model. Finally, different from the existing cross-modal approach between music and mood-tags [19] and the one between music and lyrics [24], we propose the first cross-modal approach between music and emotions.

3 Cross-Modal Music-Emotion Retrieval

Figure 4 shows a network architecture of our CMR approach using DeepCCA. We use VGGish[3] developed by Google to extract acoustic features from a music sample. VGGish is similar to the VGG model used in image recognition, and involves a Convolutional Neural Network (CNN) trained on the benchmark dataset Audioset [6] to classify music samples for the Acoustic Event Detection (AED) classification task [7]. VGGish firstly calculates MFCC features and feeds them into the CNN which outputs a 128-dimensional feature vector f_m. f_m is then given as an input of our music projection model, as shown in Fig. 4(a). Also, the emotion sequence associated to the music sample is simplified into a two-dimensional vector f_e by averaging arousal and valence values over time. Subsequently, f_e is fed into an emotion projection model, as depicted in Fig. 4(b). Both music and emotion projection models are trained so that the correlation between their outputs-respectively $\hat{f}_m$ and $\hat{f}_e$-is maximised in the common space using a 'Canonical Correlation Analysis' (CCA). The music projection model (a), the emotion projection model (b), and CCA layer for DeepCCA (c) in Fig. 4 are described below.

3.1 Encoding of Music Samples

The music projection model in Fig. 4(a) is a Multi-Layer Perceptron (MLP) model consisting of five layers. By following the standard recommendation, each layer is subdivided into Fully Connected (FC), Batch Normalisation (BN), softplus and dropout layers. A FC layer consists of multiple units that perform the following non-linear transformation on the input vector x to produce an output vector Y representing a higher-level feature:

$$Y = \sigma(wx + b) \tag{1}$$

where w is the weight matrix for the linear transform, b is the bias, and σ is an activation function. In our studies, we chose the softplus function defined by $\sigma(x) = \log(1 + e^x)$.

---

[3] https://github.com/tensorflow/models/tree/master/research/audioset.

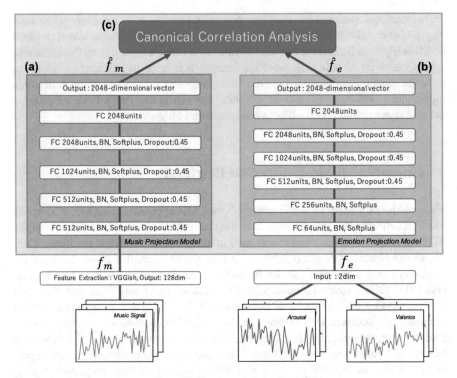

Fig. 4 A network architecture of our CMR approach using DeepCCA

In addition, a BN layer normalises the distribution of unit outputs from the previous layer [9]. A dropout layer drops outputs from several units at a certain rate [21]. These BN and dropout layers are used to prevent the model from over-fitting, which refers to excessively learning on training data thus losing generalisation capacity on test data.

3.2 Encoding of Emotion Values

Our emotion projection model is also a MLP model, and consists of six layers, as shown in Fig. 4(b). As in Sect. 3.1, each layer is subdivided into FC, BN, softplus and dropout layers. The emotion projection model input consists in a two-dimensional vector that represent the averaged arousal and valence values associated to a music sample.

3.3 Learning a Common Space

The CCA layer in Fig. 4(c) is based on DeepCCA [2, 24]. It trains the music and emotion projection models to maximise the correlation between associated music samples and emotion sequences in a common space. Specifically, both outputs from the music projection model ($\hat{f}_m$) and the emotion projection model ($\hat{f}_e$) are 2048-dimensional vectors. In the training phrase of the CCA layer, weights and biases of the music and emotion projection models are optimised so as to maximise the correlation between $\hat{f}_m$ and $\hat{f}_e$.

The objective function for the CCA layer training can be mathematically formulated as:

$$\left(W_m^*, W_e^*, \theta_m^*, \theta_e^* \right) = \underset{(W_m, W_e, \theta_m, \theta_e)}{\mathrm{argmax}} \ \mathrm{corr} \left(W_m^T \hat{f}_m, W_e^T \hat{f}_e \right) \tag{2}$$

where W_m and W_e are 2048×2048 transformation matrices of the linear projection weights in the canonical correlation. Additionally, $W_m^T \hat{f}_m$ and $W_e^T \hat{f}_e$ are called canonical components, and expressed by inner products of the transformation matrices W_m and W_e and the output vectors $\hat{f}_m$ and $\hat{f}_e$ with the projection models. W_m and W_e are trained and updated to maximise the correlation between the canonical components. Moreover, $\theta_m = (w_m, b_m)$ and $\theta_e = (w_e, b_e)$ are parameters that include the weight matrices w for linear transform and the biases b of projection MLP models. The CCA layer training aims at examining numerous sets of W_m, W_e, θ_m and θ_e, and finding the optimal one (W_m^*, W_e^*, θ_m^*, θ_e^*) which maximises the right hand of Eq. (2).

The authors of [2] showed that the optimisation problem given by Eq. (2) can be reformulated as:

$$\left(W_m^*, W_e^*, \theta_m^*, \theta_e^* \right) = \underset{(W_m, W_e, \theta_m, \theta_e)}{\mathrm{argmax}} \ \mathrm{tr} \left(W_m^T C_{me} W_e \right)$$

$$\text{Subject to} : W_m^T C_{mm} W_m = W_e^T C_{ee} W_e = I \tag{3}$$

where I is the identity matrix, C_{me} is the cross-covariance matrix of $\hat{f}_m$ and $\ddot{f}_e$, and C_{mm} and C_{ee} are the covariance matrices of $\hat{f}_m$ and $\hat{f}_e$, respectively. The optimal parameters θ_m^*, θ_e^*, W_m^* and W_e^* are obtained by solving the maximisation problem under constraints given by Eq. (3) using a gradient descent approach. For this purpose, we use Adam optimiser that automatically fine-tunes the learning rate during the training phase (the initial learning rate is set to 1^{-5}) [11].

4 Experimental Results

This section compares our CMR approach with existing approaches and demonstrates its effectiveness. In particular, we firstly describe the dataset used to train the model, and the evaluation measure. Then, an overall evaluation of our CMR approach and a discussion about the effectiveness of DeepCCA are reported.

4.1 Experimental Setting

4.1.1 Dataset

We use *Media Eval Database for Emotional Analysis in Music* (DEAM) dataset [1] to train music and emotion projection models, and evaluate the performance of our CMR approach. DEAM dataset contains 1802 free audio source signals and their corresponding arousal and valence emotion sequences which are annotated every 0.5 s. Music samples and their corresponding emotion sequences are then split to form a training and evaluation datasets of 1441 and 361 elements, respectively.

4.1.2 Evaluation Measure

We use *Mean Reciprocal Rank* (MRR) to measure the retrieval performance of our CMR approach. MRR is written as:

$$\text{MRR} = \frac{1}{|Q|} \sum_{i=1}^{|Q|} \frac{1}{r_i} \qquad (4)$$

where Q is the number of the queries and r_i corresponds to the rank of the most relevant sample for the ith query. For retrieval from emotion to music, r_i is computed as follows: A test emotion is used as a query. The correlations between its projection using the emotion projection model (f_e) and projections of all test music samples using the music projection model (f_ms) are computed. Test music samples are then ranked in decreasing order of correlations, and r_i is determined by picking the rank of the music sample associated with the query emotion. Finally, a MRR score is calculated as the average of inverses of r_i for all the Q test music samples. The higher a MRR score is, the better the retrieval performance is. A MRR score for retrieval from music to emotion is computed similarly. In addition, we provide the average of r_i to intuitively show at which position the music sample (or emotion) relevant to the query is ranked on average.

4.2   Overall Evaluation of Our CMR Approach

Most of existing MER models are one-way while our model is bidirectional. In addition, most one-way models calculate the relevance score of a music sample (or emotion) to a query as their Euclidean distance, and rank emotions (or music samples) in the test set based on such scores. Compared to this, our model computes relevance scores of music samples (or emotions) to a query as their correlations. To validate our choices to use the bidirectional model and correlations, we compare our model to the four models shown in Table 1. First, we build two regression models, *Reg-M2E* and *Reg-E2M*, which use a 128-dimensional acoustic vector f_m and a two-dimensional emotion vector f_e for a music sample, as shown in Fig. 1. Reg-M2E uses f_m to predict f'_e that should be close to f_e. Similarly, f'_m which a prediction of f_m is computed based on f_e by Reg-E2M. Both of Reg-M2E and Reg-E2M have the same network architecture consisting of four layers subdivided into FC, BN, softplus and dropout layers, and built using the training dataset.

Given a test music sample as a query, Baseline1 and Baseline2 in the second row of Table 1 first use Reg-M2E to predict its emotion vector f'_e. Then, retrieval from music to emotion (M2E) is performed by Baseline1 which computes a relevance score as the Euclidean distance between f'_e and f_e of each of test emotions. Similarly, the correlation between f'_e and f_e is used in M2E by Baseline2. In contrast, Baseline1 and Baseline2 in the bottom row of Table 1 begin with predicting an acoustic feature f'_m using Reg-E2M. Baseline1 carries out retrieval from emotion to music (E2M) by computing a relevance score as the Euclidean distance between f'_m and f_m of each of test music samples, and Baseline2 performs E2M based on the correlation between f'_m and f_m.

Table 1 shows the comparative results between the above-mentioned baseline models and our CMR model for M2E and E2M. The comparison between Baseline1 and Baseline2 shows that the retrieval performance of the latter is better than the one of the former in both M2E and E2M. This indicates the effectiveness of using correlations instead of Euclidean distances. Furthermore, the superior performance of our CMR model over Baseline2 demonstrates the effectiveness of the bidirectional retrieval between music and emotion taking into account perceptual variation of emotions.

Table 1 Comparison between baseline one-way models and our bidirectional CMR model for retrieval from music to emotion (M2E) and retrieval from emotion to music (E2M). In each cell, the number on the left and the one on the right indicate the MRR score and average rank (given out of 361 test samples), respectively

	Baseline1 (Euclidean)	Baseline2 (Correlation)	CMR
M2E	0.00435/272	0.03240/126	**0.06084/77**
E2M	0.01540/195	0.03311/131	**0.06150/79**

5 Conclusion and Future Work

In this paper, we introduced *Cross-modal Music-emotion Retrieval* (CMR) which is the first step to implement a sensor-based *Music-Emotion Retrieval* (MER) system. CMR can achieve bidirectional retrieval using *Deep Canonical Correlation Analysis* (DeepCCA) which learns a projection to maximise the correlation between the projected vectors of music samples and those of the associated emotion sequences in a common space. Furthermore, our bidirectional approach can consider the 'perceptual variation' of a music sample by different subjects, because it can associate different emotions to the same music. The experimental results show the effectiveness of using the bidirectional approach and correlations based on DeepCCA.

In our future work, we will consider projection models able to take the time dimension into account, which is not the case of the MLPs we used in this paper. In particular, models based on Gated Recurrent Units (GRUs) [3]—which are a specific variant of Recurrent Neural Networks—will be investigated. In addition, since our CMR approach is the first step to achieve the sensor-based MER system, we will investigate the bidirectional retrieval between sensor data and emotions using a similar cross-modal approach presented in this paper. After projecting the sensor data, emotion sequences and music samples into a common space, we will investigate whether it is possible to retrieve music based on specific emotions recognised from sensor data.

References

1. Aljanaki, A., Yang, Y.H., Soleymani, M.: Developing a benchmark for emotional analysis of music. PloS One **12**(3), e0173,392 (2017)
2. Andrew, G., Arora, R., Bilmes, J., Livescu, K.: Deep canonical correlation analysis. In: Proceedings of the 30th International Conference on Machine Learning (ICML 2013), pp. 1247–1255 (2013)
3. Chung, J., Gulcehre, C., Cho, K., Bengio, Y.: Empirical evaluation of gated recurrent neural networks on sequence modeling. In: Proceedings of NIPS 2014 Deep Learning and Representation Learning Workshop (2014)
4. Dufour, I., Tzanetakis, G.: Using circular models to improve music emotion recognition. IEEE Trans. Affect. Comput. (2018)
5. Ekman, P.E., Davidson, R.J.: The Nature of Emotion: Fundamental Questions. Oxford University Press (1994)
6. Gemmeke, J.F., Ellis, D.P.W., Freedman, D., Jansen, A., Lawrence, W., Moore, R.C., Plakal, M., Ritter, M.: Audio set: an ontology and human-labeled dataset for audio events. In: Proceedings of the 2017 IEEE International Conference on Acoustics, Speech and Signal Processing (ICASSP 2017), pp. 776–780 (2017)
7. Hershey, S., Chaudhuri, S., Ellis, D.P.W., Gemmeke, J.F., Jansen, A., Moore, C., Plakal, M., Platt, D., Saurous, R.A., Seybold, B., Slaney, M., Weiss, R., Wilson, K.: CNN architectures for large-scale audio classification. In: Proceedings of the 2017 IEEE International Conference on Acoustics, Speech and Signal Processing (ICASSP 2017), pp. 131–135 (2017)
8. Hevner, K.: Experimental studies of the elements of expression in music. Am. J. Psychol. **48**(2), 246–268 (1936)

9. Ioffe, S., Szegedy, C.: Batch normalization: accelerating deep network training by reducing internal covariate shift. In: Proceedings of the 32nd International Conference on International Conference on Machine Learning (ICML 2015), pp. 448–456 (2015)
10. Kim, J., Lee, S., Kim, S., Yoo, W.Y.: Music mood classification model based on arousal-valence values. In: Proceedings of the 13th International Conference on Advanced Communication Technology (ICACT 2011), pp. 292–295 (2011)
11. Kingma, D.P., Ba, J.: Adam: a method for stochastic optimization. In: Proceedings of the 3rd International Conference on Learning Representations (ICLR 2015) (2015)
12. Picard, R.W.: Affective Computing. MIT Press (2000)
13. Picard, R.W.: Affective computing: challenges. Int. J. Hum. Comput. Stud. **59**(1–2), 55–64 (2003)
14. Picard, R.W., Vyzas, E., Healey, J.: Toward machine emotional intelligence: analysis of affective physiological state. IEEE Trans. Pattern Anal. Mach. Intell. **23**(10), 1175–1191 (2001)
15. Raglio, A., Attardo, L., Gontero, G., Rollino, S., Groppo, E., Granieri, E.: Effects of music and music therapy on mood in neurological patients. World J. Psychiatry **5**(1), 68 (2015)
16. Russell, J.A.: A circumplex model of affect. J. Pers. Soc. Psychol. **39**(6), 1161–1178 (1980)
17. Ruxanda, M.M., Chua, B.Y., Nanopoulos, A., Jensen, C.S.: Emotion-based music retrieval on a well-reduced audio feature space. In: Proceedings of the 2009 IEEE International Conference on Acoustics, Speech and Signal Processing (ICASSP 2009), pp. 181–184 (2009)
18. Sakka, L.S., Juslin, P.N.: Emotion regulation with music in depressed and non-depressed individuals: goals, strategies, and mechanisms. Music Sci. **1**, 1–12 (2018)
19. Shah, R.R., Yu, Y., Zimmermann, R.: Advisor: personalized video soundtrack recommendation by late fusion with heuristic rankings. In: Proceedings of the 22nd ACM International Conference on Multimedia (MM 2014), pp. 607–616 (2014)
20. Slaney, M.: Semantic-audio retrieval. In: Proceedings of the 2002 IEEE International Conference on Acoustics, Speech, and Signal Processing (ICASSP 2002), pp. 4108–4111 (2002)
21. Srivastava, N., Hinton, G., Krizhevsky, A., Sutskever, I., Salakhutdinov, R.: Dropout: a simple way to prevent neural networks from overfitting. J. Mach. Learn. Res. **15**(1), 1929–1958 (2014)
22. Yang, Y.H., Chen, H.H.: Machine recognition of music emotion: a review. ACM Trans. Intell. Syst. Technol. **3**(3) (2012). Article No. 40
23. Yang, Y.H., Lin, Y.C., Cheng, H.T., Chen, H.H.: Mr. Emo: music retrieval in the emotion plane. In: Proceedings of the 16th ACM International Conference on Multimedia (MM 2008), pp. 1003–1004 (2008)
24. Yu, Y., Tang, S., Raposo, F., Chen, L.: Deep cross-modal correlation learning for audio and lyrics in music retrieval. ACM Trans. Multimed. Comput. Commun. Appl. **15**(1), 20:1–20:16 (2019)

Computer-Based Analysis of Spontaneous Infant Activity: A Pilot Study

Iwona Doroniewicz, Daniel Ledwoń, Monika N. Bugdol,
Katarzyna Kieszczyńska, Alicja Affanasowicz, Małgorzata Matyja,
Dariusz Badura, Andrzej W. Mitas, and Andrzej Myśliwiec

Abstract The development of computer-aided infants diagnosis systems is currently popular field of research. Video recordings provide the opportunity to develop a non-invasive, objective and reproducible tool for assessing the quality of infant movements. The aim of this pilot study is attempt to numerically describe selected movement parameters of the normal activity of 10 infants. The whole group was assessed at fidgety movements by four experts. Infant limbs movement features were based on kinematic parameters like velocity and acceleration. Basic information about movement location was described as mean value. Novel parameters characterised movement range based on ellipses described on limbs trajectories have been proposed.

Keywords Computer-based video analysis · Feature extraction · Physiotherapy · Developmental neurodiagnostics

I. Doroniewicz
Department of Physiotherapy in Movement System and Developmental Age Diseases,
Academy of Physical Education in Katowice, Katowice, Poland
e-mail: i.doroniewicz@awf.katowice.pl

D. Ledwoń (✉) · M. N. Bugdol · A. W. Mitas
Faculty of Biomedical Engineering, Silesian University of Technology, Zabrze, Poland
e-mail: daniel.ledwon@polsl.pl

M. N. Bugdol
e-mail: monika.bugdol@polsl.pl

A. W. Mitas
e-mail: andrzej.mitas@polsl.pl

K. Kieszczyńska · A. Affanasowicz · M. Matyja · A. Myśliwiec
Institute of Physiotheraphy and Health Science, Academy
of Physical Education in Katowice, Katowice, Poland
e-mail: kieszczynskakasia@gmail.com

D. Badura
Katowice Institute of Information Technologies, Katowice, Poland
e-mail: drhbad@gmail.com

E. Piętka et al. (eds.), *Information Technology in Biomedicine*, Advances in Intelligent
Systems and Computing 1186, https://doi.org/10.1007/978-3-030-49666-1_12

1 Introduction

The current state of knowledge indicates that it is impossible to develop a comprehensive, objective and accessible measurement method that can be used in the process of early diagnosis of a child [9]. The available diagnostic methods can be divided into subjective and objective. The former are used to evaluate, among other things, the body posture and psychomotor skills of a child (TIMP—Test of Infant Motor Performance) [19, 22], developmental disorders of a small child (Dubowitz Score) [10], neonatal behaviour (NBAS—Neonatal Behavioral Assessment Scale) [5, 28], positioning reactions (Vojta's neurokinesiological diagnostics) [16], or infant motor skills before and following the therapy (AIMS) [2]. The literature review by Ciuraj et al. 2019 showed that these methods are characterized by the effectiveness expressed by reliability falling within the range of 0.76–0.98. The highest rating is given to the reliability of the Prechtl's Method on the Qualitative Assessment of General Movements [9]. The effectiveness of this method is emphasized by the fact that it is the most reliable method of prediction of cerebral palsy. This has been confirmed by numerous studies carried out by the method's creator himself, his followers [7, 8, 26], and by independent authors [29]. In the light of objective holistic methods such as Podo Baby [15], growth charts, morphogram or biological age assessment, which represent only a small percentage of all diagnostic capabilities, the Prechtl's method provides a starting point for deeper analysis.

Image analysis provides the opportunity to develop a simple, non-invasive and, most importantly, reproducible tool for assessing the quality of infant movements. Some studies in the literature have used video recordings. Part of the publications focus mainly on the assessment of movements to predict potential cerebral palsy and the development of various visual models for the assessment of movement [1, 17]. The comparison of computer-based analysis of general movement using magnetic sensors tracking the movement of the child's upper and lower limbs was made by the team of Philippi et al. According to the authors, the kinematic analysis of a child's movements allows for prediction of the development of cerebral palsy in children to a greater extent than the clinical evaluation [25]. Other studies emphasized the assessment of limb movements, including analyses of the kinematic properties of movements, which are: frequency, repeatability of sequences, and coordination of joints and limbs. At the same time, qualitative assessment of global spontaneous movements and lower limb movements was made based on video recordings [31].

The authors of this study focused on extracting the features of normal spontaneous activity. The proposed analysis is one of the first stages in the development of the system for the assessment of the course and quality of movement in infants. Therefore, the authors of this study decided to divide the research into several stages and start the work by the characterization of the parameters of normal movement. The aim of this study is attempt to numerically describe selected movement parameters of the normal activity of infants between 8 and 14 weeks of age.

2 Materials and Methods

The study was approved by the Biomedical Research Ethics Committee (No 5/2018) and in accordance with the Declaration of Helsinki. All patients and their parents/guardians gave written informed consent to participate in the study.

Personal data and the images of patients were collected and processed in a database that complies with the personal data protection regulations. The equipment used in the tests did not pose any threat of radiation or other energy that could in any way affect the safety of the child under observation.

2.1 Test Procedure

The recording lasted 20 min and was made using a portable video recording system in the patient's home. The stand consisted of a lying place that met the standards of hygiene and safety. The surface was soft, washable, with side stops. The stand frame was stable, with dimensions of $1 \times 1 \times 1$ m, equipped with place for mounting video camera. Spatial resolution of the camera was 1920×1080 px with frame rate 60 fps. The platform was placed on a stable and adequately illuminated ground. The position of the child during the examination was free, lying on his or her back, without any distractions. The child did not cry during the recording. The tests were always performed at the same time of the day, after sleeping and feeding.

In this pilot study we selected 10 videos clearly defined by four independent experts who were diagnosticians with experience in the Prechtl's general movement assessment of fidgety movements (continual FMs, score: ++). The movements were defined as frequent, interspersed with very short 1–2 s pauses. The movements involved the whole body, particularly the neck, shoulder, wrists, hips and ankles. Depending on the actual body posture, especially the head position, FMs was allowed to occur asymmetrically [11, 12]. Then, in each of the ten recordings, 3 min sections were selected, which were again evaluated by the same experts as the so-called golden standard of fidgety movements [12].

2.2 Research Population

The video recordings included infants in the age range of 8–14 weeks (mean: 10.6 ± 2.0) who met the inclusion criteria: they were born full-term (38–41 Hbd), by physiological delivery, from a single pregnancy, with positive perinatal history and without worrying symptoms. Mean body mass on the day of birth was 3445.0 ± 295.9 g and mean body length 55.1 ± 1.6 cm. All assessed infants received the Apgar score of 10.

2.3   Video Processing

Collected videos were subjected to undistortion procedure to reduce the impact of camera lens characteristic. Transformation map was computed based on series of images with checkerboard pattern and then applied to every video frame in OpenCV library [4]. Next, each video was manually cropped to region of interests containing the observed infant. Characteristic points of the infant's body were detected by human pose estimation algorithm implemented in OpenPose software [6]. This approach was previously used and evaluated in case of infant pose in Marchi et al. and McCay et al. works [20, 21]. As a result, locations of 25 characteristic points corresponding to joints positions, trunk and face elements were received. Due to low confidence value for some points location and observed high frequency noise, it was necessary to apply preprocessing steps for each point trajectory. First, the unconfident points (confidence value lower than 0.2) were replaced by the previous location. It reduced the large changes of location between frames caused by short-time unconfident detections, mostly when detected point has been covered. Second, the Savitzky–Golay filter (second order polynomial, 9 coefficients) were used to reduce noise.

This work focused on limbs movement analysis, therefore the impact of the whole body movement during the observation was reduced. Key points locations from each frame were shifted on the basis of the movement of the neck—this point was the new center of the coordinate system [20]. Next, changes of trunk position were removed by rotation of key points by angle between video y-axis and line crossing the neck and the point between hips. After these operations the infant's trunk was in the similar position on each frame of the video.

2.4   Features Extraction

This paper focuses on the analysis of spontaneous movements of the child's limbs. For this purpose, a set of features that can be automatically determined based on the obtained point trajectories indicating the temporal positions of wrists and ankles was determined. The selection of the features was based on a literature review on automatic analysis of spontaneous movements in computer-aided diagnostics. An additional criterion during the selection was the possibility of obtained values interpretation by experts involved in the diagnosis of children. The finally selected set of features consisted of kinematic values such as total distance travelled (trajectory length), instantaneous velocity and acceleration, for which distributions, means and standard deviations were compared [18, 20]. Due to location errors, outliers removal was carried out before the analysis. A parameter often used by other researchers dealing with this problem is the location of the mean position, both for the general movement of the child and for the movements of individual limbs. In this case, both the variability of the mean position [1, 30] and the variability of the position of the limb over time relative to the locally determined mean from a longer period of time are examined [27]. The mean position indicates the location of the high density of movements, which can provide important diagnostic information. Due to the different positions of the child in the camera coordinate system, the means in the x and y axes obtained for the 3 min analysis were normalized successively with respect to the mean obtained for shoulder width (distance between the left and right shoulder points) and the mean length of the torso (distance between the neck point and the hip point). Another feature beyond the global location of movement in relation to the child's body that can provide important diagnostic insights is the area in which the movement of a single limb is performed. The area determined by the point's trajectory in the assumed time interval is described by the parameters of the ellipse described by the set of points in the image space. Outliers were removed in order to eliminate the effect of single movements extending the area of the high density of movements. This procedure involved determining the distance from the mean for each time point. Then, for each limb analysed, the threshold was determined as the sum of the values of the third quartile and twice the interquartile range. Trajectory points exceeding the threshold were removed from further analysis. The remaining points were subjected to the procedure of removing the adjacent points in order to eliminate the effect of density of movements in an area on the resulting ellipse. For each trajectory point, points in an area with a radius of 5 pixels were removed. The parameters of the ellipse were determined based on the eigenvectors and eigenvalues of the covariance matrix of both coordinates. The following features were identified from the areas determined in this manner: ellipse areas normalized in relation to the product of infant's shoulder width and body length describing the relative area in which limb movement was observed, normalized values of the length of the major and minor axes and the aspect ratio of the ellipse, being the quotient of both these values (Fig. 1).

3   Results

The landmarks detection method was evaluated by comparing resulting positions of wrists and ankles with points selected manually for each second of analyzed fragments. The 99.68% of detected positions were closer than 40 pixels to manually marked points (distance approximately corresponds width of the wrist).

The mean values of speed (Fig. 2) obtained in most cases do not differ significantly between the corresponding right and left limbs. Referring the mean speed of the upper limbs to the value obtained by the lower limbs yields different observations for individual patients. Higher means were obtained for lower limbs in subjects with numbers 9, 2 and 4, whereas for upper limbs, they were observed in subjects 15 and 16. For the other test subjects, the speed distributions obtained by individual limbs were similar. The mode value obtained for speed was similar for all patients. This means that the most frequently recorded movement speed was similar for all patients. The differences in the means were directly related to the degree of asymmetry in the distribution of the analysed variable, which in turn resulted from instantaneous rapid

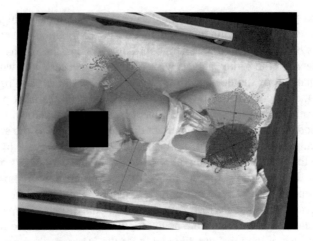

Fig. 1 Locations of individual trajectory points from an example of a 3 min part of the recording with marked values of individual parameters. The means computed for the movement of individual limbs are marked with black dots. The ellipses described on the obtained trajectories are presented in colours corresponding to those of the trajectory, but with higher transparency. The position of the major and minor axes is marked as darker lines

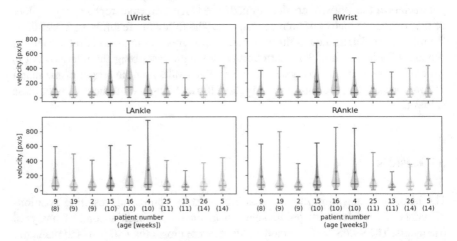

Fig. 2 Violin plots of the distributions of the instantaneous speed achieved by individual test subjects in the 3 min sections used for the analysis. For each distribution, the mean speed (dotted marker) and modes (horizontal line) were also marked. Each of the four graphs presents the distributions of the speed of a single limb for each subject (x axis). The distributions are presented in the order of the child age in weeks. Each subject was assigned one colour

changes in the movement speed. The number of movement stops had a direct effect on the mode, from which it can be concluded that there were relatively few such stops. Moderate mean movement speed with the accompanying high variation and a low number of stops is evidence of the presence of fidgety movements.

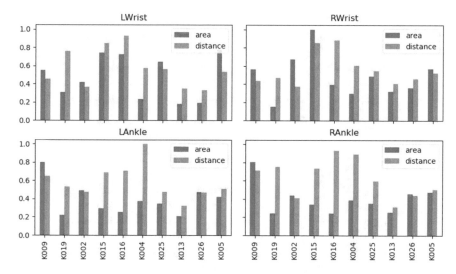

Fig. 3 Area and distance values normalized to the maximum values obtained inside the group for both parameters independently

No correlation was observed between the total length of the movement path and the area where the movement was performed (Fig. 3). The total distance travelled by point trajectory in a specific time corresponds to an appropriately scaled mean speed. Therefore, the observations concerning symmetry and comparison of lower and upper limbs in both analyses are identical. For the area of the movement of the lower limbs, similar values for the right and left sides can be observed for each subject. This symmetry is much less noticeable for the upper limbs. The difference is almost twofold in the case of patient No. 16, with very similar values of the trajectory followed by both wrists. No link was observed between the movement area for the upper and lower limbs. In some cases (e.g. 15 and 16), the greater range of wrist mobility was not reflected by the area determined for the ankles.

Figure 4 shows centroids of movement of individual limbs. The results indicate the high symmetry between the left and right sides. The movement of both ankles and wrists occurred at a similar distance from the child's long axis. It can be observed that the child No. 5 was making wrist movements in front of the trunk, while the other subjects kept their arms spread to the sides.

In the majority of the examined children, the aspect ratio had values not greater than 1.6. (Fig. 5). It can be observed that the movements of the ankles were characterized by a more circular shape than the movements of the respective wrists.

Due to the small group of respondents, the results were not analysed in relation to the age of the infants.

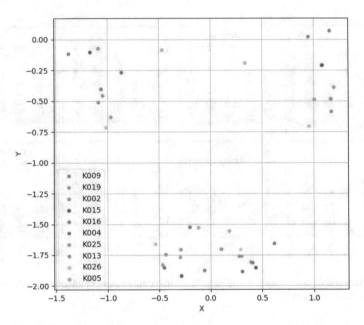

Fig. 4 Mean location from 3 min of movement. Horizontal coordinate (X) normalized to shoulder width, vertical coordinate (Y) normalized to torso length. Point (0,0) indicates the location of the neck of the subject

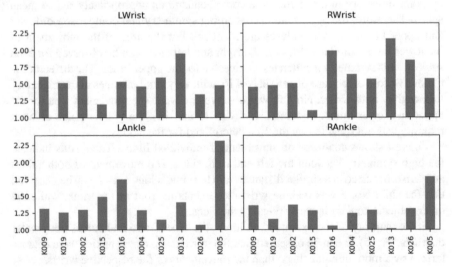

Fig. 5 The values of the ellipse shape coefficient (the quotient of the length of the long and short axes) obtained for the ellipse described on the trajectories of each limb for each subject

4 Discussion

Diagnostics in the area of potential disorders of spontaneous movements of infants is not easy, especially for young diagnosticians without experience. The observation used by a specialist to make an assessment is only seemingly an intuitive process. In fact, it involves processing of an enormous amount of information, collected from gradually acquired knowledge, skills and experience. It is clear that the more knowledge, experience and skills a diagnostician has, the more appropriate the assessment will be. In the process of assessing general movements and spontaneous activity of infants, Professor Prechtl, author of Prechtl's Method on the Qualitative Assessment of General Movements, which is a recognized method of prediction of cerebral palsy, refers to the "catalogues of normal images" [14]. It is a kind of a "computer disk" on which files with pictures of child's normal movements are stored. When assessing an infant, the diagnostician subconsciously uses the algorithms available in his or her catalogues. Creating such a catalogue requires diagnosticians to constantly improve and gain experience. The proposed algorithm is useful in the evaluation of such movements as it represents an introduction to the system for the assessment of the course and quality of movement in infants. It should be stressed, however, that the authors' aim was not to replace human with computer diagnosis or an algorithm. The paper only attempted to systematize or to specify the features of normal spontaneous movements of the child during the period of fidgety movements.

No correlation was observed between the total length of the movement path and the area where the movement was performed. Based on the authors' experience, it was assumed that with the growth of the child's central nervous system, both distance and area values would decrease. The older the infant, the less the fidgety movements are noticeable. The hypothesis should be verified on a larger group of subjects, and the age range should be increased as fidgety movements may still be observed at 22 weeks of age, and the study group included those aged up to 14 weeks.

The literature related to the description of qualitative characteristics related to speed distribution contains the definition of normal fidgety movements. These are average velocity movements, with variable acceleration in all directions [13]. In terms of quantitative research, several studies can be found in the literature. Ohgi, S. ct al. 2008 presented a comparative analysis of spontaneous upper limb movements in preterm infants with brain damage and premature infants without such damage. The results of the analysis showed that spontaneous movements of preterm infants show a non-linear and chaotic character. The movements of infants with brain damages were characterized by increased disorganization compared to the movements of children without such problems [24].

In this study an attempt was made to characterize the kinematic features of normal spontaneous movements of infants. Standard deviations make the group slightly differentiated, which can be expected due to the multiple variants and variability in the normal development of each healthy infant. Furthermore, no differences were found in the study between the right and left side of the body. Therefore, the results confirm the qualitative assessment of general fidgety movements, described as moderate with variable acceleration. Similar findings were presented by Ohgi et al. 2007 from Japan [23]. A variety of speed values were obtained, which may be indicative of the multiple variants and variability of movements. These features determine the correct psychomotor development, which is individually variable and occurs in variants. According to the neurodevelopmental concept, there are no patterns of normal development, and a healthy child, even in reflex behaviour, demonstrates the variability of responses [3]. The mode value obtained for speed was similar for all patients. This means that the most frequently recorded movement speed was similar for all patients, corresponding to the characteristics of normal fidgety movements. Analysis of the distribution of the instantaneous accelerations reveals that it is close to normal, and there are also slight intragroup differences. These are values that are assessed by diagnosticians as the "broad norm" in terms of differentiation of movement accelerations and decelerations. During the activity, children mostly present a uniform movement, but the added and correct feature is the occasional spontaneous activity consisting of short dynamic movements of the upper and lower limbs in different directions. Such dynamics is often observed and characteristic during the activity of spontaneous movements in the fidgety period.

The position of mean value of all trajectory points was developed, allowing for obtaining information on the quality of spontaneous movements. Data on the movements of upper and lower limbs in relation to the axis of the child's body and the position of the shoulders were collected. From the neurodevelopmental point of view, these are important data since they refer to the fundamental law of motor activity i.e. the principle of proximal-distal development. According to this principle, the better the infant controls the proximal parts of the body (shoulders, hips), the better he or she controls distal points (upper limbs, lower limbs). The near-zero centroid value obtained in the study may suggest "mature" movements of the upper and lower limbs, performed close to the body. In practice this means better stabilization of the torso and thus better control of the distal points such as upper and lower limbs. The study identified the most frequent position of the analysed point during the 3 min video. Therefore, the values of the selected feature may reflect the degree of maturity of spontaneous movements generated by the central nervous system. However, this model should be verified on a larger group of respondents.

It can be observed that the movements of the ankles were characterized by a more circular shape than the movements of the respective wrists. This is a natural phenomenon in early childhood, resulting from the physiological ranges of motion in the hip and knee joints. The lower limbs in infants show a lot of rotational movements in the period studied. With mobile stabilization of the torso and the ability to rotate externally, the feet can be controlled in front of the body against gravity. Consequently, the child performs the circular movements in supination, abduction and flexion of the hip and knee joints.

5 Conclusions

The results of an attempt to describe physiologicaly normative spontaneous infants limbs movement based on video recordings has been presented. The research group consisted of 10 infants in the age between 8 and 14 weeks. Inclusion criteria have been strictly followed and four experts with experience in the Prechtl's method defined whole group of fidgety movements (continual FMs, score: ++). Homogeneous testing conditions were ensured in the context of the infant's condition and video recording system. Characteristic points were extracted from the recordings and then the variability of limbs position in the field of image was analysed. A number of frequently used coefficients, such as trajectory length, average speed and acceleration and their standard deviations, as well as a description of the position of the centroid, have provided basic information on the movements of the child's limbs. The novel assessment was obtained by author's analysis of the coefficients determined for ellipses, described on the motion trajectory of the limb characteristic points. The results obtained concerning speed and acceleration confirm the presence of fidgety movements, which allows to count on the correctness of the procedure also for the other presented parameters.

Further works on the analysis of described movement parameters will include verification of repeatability for received values both during other 3 min fragments of the same recordings and between independent videos from the same infant. Next studies should concern also features extracted in frequency domain. These analyses should be carried out for the remaining points of the infant's body, which will allow more detailed description showing the relationships between the movements of individual body segments.

References

1. Adde, L., Helbostad, J.L., Jensenius, A.R., Taraldsen, G., Grunewaldt, K.H., Støen, R.: Early prediction of cerebral palsy by computer-based video analysis of general movements: a feasibility study. Dev. Med. Child Neurol. **52**(8), 773–778 (2010)
2. Almeida, K.M., Dutra, M.V.P., Mello, R.R.d., Reis, A.B.R., Martins, P.S.: Concurrent validity and reliability of the alberta infant motor scale in premature infants. J. Pediatr. **84**(5), 442–448 (2008)
3. Bobath, K.: A Neurophysiological Basis for the Treatment of Cerebral Palsy. Cambridge University Press, Cambridge (1991)
4. Bradski, G.: The OpenCV Library. Dr. Dobb's J. Softw. Tools (2000)
5. Brazelton, T.B., Nugent, J.K.: Neonatal Behavioral Assessment Scale, vol. 137. Cambridge University Press, Cambridge (1995)
6. Cao, Z., Simon, T., Wei, S.E., Sheikh, Y.: Realtime multi-person 2d pose estimation using part affinity fields. In: CVPR (2017)
7. Cioni, G., Ferrari, F., Einspieler, C., Paolicelli, P.B., Barbani, T., Prechtl, H.F.: Comparison between observation of spontaneous movements and neurologic examination in preterm infants. J. Pediatr. **130**(5), 704–711 (1997)

8. Cioni, G., Prechtl, H.F., Ferrari, F., Paolicelli, P.B., Einspieler, C., Roversi, M.F.: Which better predicts later outcome in fullterm infants: quality of general movements or neurological examination? Early Hum. Dev. **50**(1), 71–85 (1997)

9. Ciuraj, M., Kieszczyńska, K., Doroniewicz, I., Lipowicz, A.: Subjective and objective assessment of developmental dysfunction in children aged 0–3 years-comparative study. In: International Conference on Information Technologies in Biomedicine, pp. 382–391. Springer (2019)

10. Dubowitz, L., Ricciw, D., Mercuri, E.: The dubowitz neurological examination of the full-term newborn. Mental Retard. Dev. Disabil. Res. Rev. **11**(1), 52–60 (2005)

11. Einspieler, C., Peharz, R., Marschik, P.B.: Fidgety movements-tiny in appearance, but huge in impact. J. Pediatr. **92**(3), S64–S70 (2016)

12. Einspieler, C., Prechtl, H.F.: Prechtl's assessment of general movements: a diagnostic tool for the functional assessment of the young nervous system. Mental Retard. Dev. Disabil. Res. Rev. **11**(1), 61–67 (2005)

13. Einspieler, C., Prechtl, H.F., Ferrari, F., Cioni, G., Bos, A.F.: The qualitative assessment of general movements in preterm, term and young infants-review of the methodology. Early Hum. Dev. **50**(1), 47–60 (1997)

14. Ferrari, F., Einspieler, C., Prechtl, H., Bos, A., Cioni, G.: Prechtl's Method on the Qualitative Assessment of General Movements in Preterm, Term and Young Infants. Mac Keith Press (2004)

15. Gajewska, E.: Narzędzia diagnostyczne do oceny wczesnego rozwoju motorycznego stosowane w fizjoterapii dziecięcej. Neurologia Dziecięca **20**(40), 53–59 (2011)

16. Gajewska, E., Sobieska, M., Samborski, W.: Correlates between munich functional development diagnostics and postural reactivity findings based on seven provovoked postural reactions modus vojta during the first period of child's life. Ann. Acad. Med. Stetinensis **52**, 67–70 (2006)

17. Ihlen, E.A., Støen, R., Boswell, L., de Regnier, R.A., Fjørtoft, T., Gaebler-Spira, D., Labori, C., Loennecken, M.C., Msall, M.E., Möinichen, U.I., et al.: Machine learning of infant spontaneous movements for the early prediction of cerebral palsy: a multi-site cohort study. J. Clin. Med. **9**(1), 5 (2020)

18. Kanemaru, N., Watanabe, H., Kihara, H., Nakano, H., Nakamura, T., Nakano, J., Taga, G., Konishi, Y.: Jerky spontaneous movements at term age in preterm infants who later developed cerebral palsy. Early Hum. Dev. **90**(8), 387–392 (2014)

19. Kolobe, T.H., Bulanda, M., Susman, L.: Predicting motor outcome at preschool age for infants tested at 7, 30, 60, and 90 days after term age using the test of infant motor performance. Phys. Ther. **84**(12), 1144–1156 (2004)

20. Marchi, V., Hakala, A., Knight, A., D'Acunto, F., Scattoni, M.L., Guzzetta, A., Vanhatalo, S.: Automated pose estimation captures key aspects of General Movements at eight to 17 weeks from conventional videos. Acta Paediatr. Int. J. Paediatr. 1–8 (2019)

21. McCay, K.D., Ho, E.S.L., Marcroft, C., Embleton, N.D.: Establishing Pose Based Features Using Histograms for the Detection of Abnormal Infant Movements pp. 5469–5472 (2019). 1https://doi.org/10.1109/embc.2019.8857680

22. Nuysink, J., van Haastert, I.C., Eijsermans, M.J., Koopman-Esseboom, C., Helders, P.J., de Vries, L.S., van der Net, J.: Prediction of gross motor development and independent walking in infants born very preterm using the test of infant motor performance and the alberta infant motor scale. Early Hum. Dev. **89**(9), 693–697 (2013)

23. Ohgi, S., Morita, S., Loo, K.K., Mizuike, C.: A dynamical systems analysis of spontaneous movements in newborn infants. J. Motor Behav. **39**(3), 203–214 (2007)

24. Ohgi, S., Morita, S., Loo, K.K., Mizuike, C.: Time series analysis of spontaneous upper-extremity movements of premature infants with brain injuries. Phys. Ther. **88**(9), 1022–1033 (2008)

25. Philippi, H., Karch, D., Kang, K.S., Wochner, K., Pietz, J., Dickhaus, H., Hadders-Algra, M.: Computer-based analysis of general movements reveals stereotypies predicting cerebral palsy. Dev. Med. Child Neurol. **56**(10), 960–967 (2014)

26. Prechtl, H.F.: General movement assessment as a method of developmental neurology: new paradigms and their consequences the 1999 ronnie mackeith lecture. Dev. Med. Child Neurol. **43**(12), 836–842 (2001)

27. Rahmati, H., Aamo, O.M., Stavdahl, O., Dragon, R., Adde, L.: Video-based early cerebral palsy prediction using motion segmentation. In: 2014 36th Annual International Conference of the IEEE Engineering in Medicine and Biology Society, EMBC 2014 pp. 3779–3783 (2014)
28. Stewart, P., Reihman, J., Lonky, E., Darvill, T., Pagano, J.: Prenatal pcb exposure and neonatal behavioral assessment scale (nbas) performance. Neurotoxicol. Teratol. **22**(1), 21–29 (2000)
29. Støen, R., Boswell, L., De Regnier, R.A., Fjørtoft, T., Gaebler-Spira, D., Ihlen, E., Labori, C., Loennecken, M., Msall, M., Möinichen, U.I., et al.: The predictive accuracy of the general movement assessment for cerebral palsy: a prospective, observational study of high-risk infants in a clinical follow-up setting. J. Clin. Med. **8**(11), 1790 (2019)
30. Støen, R., Songstad, N.T., Silberg, I.E., Fjørtoft, T., Jensenius, A.R., Adde, L.: Computer-based video analysis identifies infants with absence of fidgety movements. Pediatr. Res. **82**(4), 665 (2017)
31. Van Der Heide, J.C., Paolicelli, P.B., Boldrini, A., Cioni, G.: Kinematic and qualitative analysis of lower-extremity movements in preterm infants with brain lesions. Phys. Ther. **79**(6), 546–557 (1999)

Behavioral and Physiological Profile Analysis While Exercising—Case Study

Patrycja Romaniszyn, Damian Kania, Monika N. Bugdol, Anita Pollak, and Andrzej W. Mitas

Abstract The essence of determining the patient's behavioural and physiological profile during therapy is an extremely important element of the overall rehabilitation process. It should therefore examine how and why external physiological responses to stimuli occur. The article presents a detailed study of one specific case. A qualitative approach was adopted to analyze the problem because of the desire to understand the situation of participation in therapy in its uniqueness. The State-Trait Anxiety Inventory, the Verbal Fluency Test, the Digit Symbol Test, thermograms and Electrodermal Activity signal used for this purpose. The effect of the study was to formulate plans and hypotheses for further research, this time in a quantitative approach.

Keywords Behavioral and physiological profile · Electrodermal Activity · Physiotherapy · Stress · Anxiety · Thermovision

P. Romaniszyn (✉) · M. N. Bugdol · A. W. Mitas
Faculty of Biomedical Engineering, Silesian University of Technology,
Roosevelta 40, 41-800 Zabrze, Poland
e-mail: patrycja.romaniszyn@polsl.pl

M. N. Bugdol
e-mail: monika.bugdol@polsl.pl

A. W. Mitas
e-mail: andrzej.mitas@polsl.pl

D. Kania
Faculty of Physiotherapy, The Jerzy Kukuczka Academy of Physical Education
in Katowice, Mikołowska 72b, 40-065 Katowice, Poland
e-mail: d.kania@awf.katowice.pl

A. Pollak
Institute of Psychology, University of Silesia in Katowice,
Bankowa 12, 40-007 Katowice, Poland
e-mail: anita.pollak@us.edu.pl

E. Piętka et al. (eds.), *Information Technology in Biomedicine*, Advances in Intelligent
Systems and Computing 1186, https://doi.org/10.1007/978-3-030-49666-1_13

1   Introduction

The essence of determining the patient's behavioural and physiological profile during therapy is an extremely important element of the overall rehabilitation process. It is worth mentioning that the main role of rehabilitation is a combination of physiological (movement) and psychological spheres—readiness for cooperation [1]. On the other hand, the rehabilitation itself is the sum of medical effects on the patient whose key goal is to restore the maximum possible functional efficiency [2].

To the best of our knowledge there is no direct definition of a behavioural and physiological profile. However behaviorism is a direction in psychology that is studied in humans and animals, as well as the analysis of the influence of environmental factors on the subsequent consequences [3]. Physiology, on the other hand, is the science of life functions and processes taking place in living organisms [4]. The 1904 Nobel Prize winner, Ivan Pavlov, also studied this profile in animals, analyzing their unconditional reflexes, but did not write about it directly.

The behavioural-physiological profile should therefore examine how and why external physiological responses to stimuli occur. In the context of therapy, on the basis of the patient's mental state and changes in their physical condition, the analysis of this profile will allow to assess the degree of involvement in the therapy process.

2   Materials and Methods

The entire presented protocol is part of the Disc4Spine project, which aims to develop a system of Dynamic Individual Stimulation and Control For Spine and Posture Interactive Rehabilitation.

2.1   Research Group

The article presents a detailed study of one specific case. A qualitative approach was adopted to obtain the most comprehensive description of participation in therapy. We are interested in both the values of variables and the relationships between them. We proceed to research without preliminary hypotheses, intending to investigate the phenomenon in its real context thoroughly [5]. A student (male, 20 years old) of the J. Kukuczka Academy of Physical Education in Katowice was examined. Before the measurements the participant was informed about the aim of the study and gave written consent to it. For the purpose of the experiment—observation of the patient while performing exercises in the device—it was necessary to ensure visibility of the relevant parts of the back muscles. Therefore the participant was informed about the need to put on a sporting outfit and to unveil the upper part of the trunk. Before the measurements were conducted, the examined person was asked to remove the

T-shirt and not to touch the back areas, due to the importance of getting the body accustomed to the ambient temperature (for about 15 min).

2.2   Equipment

Specialized equipment was used for data acquisition. Empatica E4 was employed to collect biomedical signals (electrodermal activity, EDA), which is a medical-grade wearable device that offers real-time physiological data acquisition. To perform the Verbal Fluency Test (VFT), a proprietary Android mobile application was used, which allowed to count the number of spoken words. A thermal imaging camera was used to acquire thermal images from the patient's back—FLIR A300 with 320×240 pixel resolution and accuracy $\pm 2\,°C$. The emissivity factor was set to 0.95. The distance between the patient and the camera was 2 m. The EDA signal was recorded continuously during the whole examination. The psychological tests and the Digit Symbol Test (DST) were carried out in a traditional way using paper and a pen.

2.3   Data Aquisition

The study was conducted at the Jerzy Kukuczka Academy of Physical Education in Katowice, in a specially assigned room to ensure the participant peace and intimacy. During the tests, only investigators conducting the research were present in the room.

The protocol of the whole study consisted of several steps. First, the examined person was asked to complete psychological tests. The proposed set contained a number of methods relating to the current feeling, mood and attitudes towards one's own health situation. Each tool was accompanied by precise instructions, and during their performance comfortable conditions were provided—silence and isolation from a third party. At the beginning of the survey, the respondent was asked to complete the *State-Trait Anxiety Inventory* questionnaire (STAI) [6, 7], which allowed to measurement of two forms of anxiety. Firstly, situational conditioned anxiety, characterizing the current emotional state of an individual (feelings, fears and tensions), secondly understood as a relatively constant personality trait. The tool consists of two parts, each of 20 statements. The items were evaluated on a 4-degree scale. The higher score in questionnaire may shows the higher level of anxiety.

The test procedure is designed to familiarize the participant with the equipment used in the test. At this stage of the test, the Empatica E4 sensor (after completing in the anxiety test) was also placed on the left wrist of the patient and monitored his condition during subsequent tests and exercises. Probably the most important parameter obtained from this wristband was the Electrodermal Activity signal (EDA). EDA is reflecting the neural measure of the effect on permeability of the sweat gland, observed as changes in skin resistance under the influence of low current intensity or as differences in electrical potential between different points on the skin surface [8].

For the E4, according to the technical documentation, the current is about 100 uA [9]. The Empatica E4 device allows the EDA signal to be recorded at a 4 Hz sampling rate.

Next, the assessment of cognitive performance was carried out using Verbal Fluency Tests (VFT) [10]. VFT is designed to test the semantic (categorical) or alphabetic (phonetic) verbal liquidity. Its correct execution depends on the smooth operation of execution functions and operating memory, as well as on lexical resources in long-term memory [11]. It is useful in the examination of both healthy and sick people. The test allows to check the semantic (categorical) or alphanumeric (phonetic) verbal liquidity. In this experiment VFT in letter version, lasting 60 s, was used. The letter for which words had to be pronounced, was selected each time in a random way (excluding X, Y and all Polish diacritical letters). In the whole protocol this test was performed twice—before and after exercising. The counting of spoken words and the time remaining until the end of the test as well as the continuous presentation of the leading letter were performed using a mobile application implemented by the author. During the whole test, it was checked whether the spoken words are not repeated and whether there are no names, surnames or proper names among them.

Then, to check the visuo-cognitive abilities (which include the ability to learn, maintain concentration despite distractions, plan future, solve tasks, evaluate and make choices), the examined person was asked to complete the Digit Symbol Test [12]. For this purpose, the participant was given a sheet of paper with two rows of fields at the top, with fixed number-symbol pairs. In the first line there were consecutive numbers from 1 to 9, and in the second, lower line, the corresponding symbols assigned to the numbers. The task was to draw as many symbols as possible corresponding to other, randomly given numbers from the range 1–9, within 60 s.

After performing the above tests, the next step was to carry out physiotherapy exercises in the prototype of the device, being a component of the Dynamic Individual Stimulation and Control For Spine and Posture Interactive Rehabilitation, under the supervision of a specialist. The examined person was asked to make a movement sequence, during which a series of back pictures was taken with a thermovision camera (Fig. 1). Before starting, the participant was safely positioned in the device and thoroughly instructed on how to correctly perform consecutive movements. The first exercise was to make anterior and posterior pelvic tilts for 60 s, at the frequency of one sequence (front/rear) per second. The aim was to activate the back muscles located within the lumbar section of the spine.

After leaving the device, in order to check the sensations that accompanied the participant during the test (anger, relaxation, etc.), the examined person was asked to complete the JAWS questionnaire (Job related Affective Well-Being Scale) [13].

In the presented study, the short 12-item version was used. The scale allows to determine the strength of feelings felt at a given moment resulting in performing a specific action. The respondent indicates from a list of 12 feelings (six of which are positive, and the remaining six negative), how often he experiences them. He indicates the answer on a 5-point scale (from 1—never to 5—very often). It is possible to create four categories of emotions, by sign (positive and negative) and stimulation (high and low activation level). Several results are obtained—the total overall result, the

Fig. 1 A thermal image of the patient's back during exercising

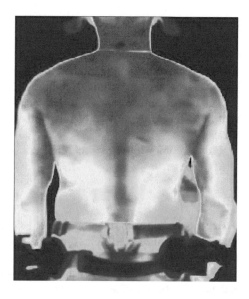

sum for positive emotions and the sum for negative emotions, as well as the sums in individual subscales: eustress—positive emotions with a high level of arousal, pleasure emotions with a low level of arousal, distress—negative emotions with a high level of arousal, unpleasant emotions with a low level of arousal.

The last two elements of the research protocol were the re-performances of the VFT, but using a different letter than previously, and a DST, in which only the number-symbol pairs were changed.

At the very end, the monitoring of the patient's condition was stopped, by removing the E4.

2.4 Data Analysis

2.4.1 Verbal Fluency Tests

The application used to count the VFT result generated a file in .csv format. The file contained: the chosen letter, the time of pronouncement of particular words and their total number, which was the most important result, because it was a proof of the verbal—letter fluency.

2.4.2 Digit Symbol Test

The results were analysed manually, checking that the test was performed correctly. Below there is the result of the DST, filled by the examined person. However, the difficulty is that the fields must be completed one after the other in the order given.

2.4.3 Thermal Image Analysis

For proper temperature analysis only 4 photos were used—before the start of the exercises, at the beginning, at the middle and at the end of exercising. The patient's body was divided into 4 areas—right/left top and right/left bottom.

The movement sequence was designed to activate the lumbar section of the back muscles, so for the purpose of this work the analysis focused mainly on the lower areas.

First, in order to extract the patient's body from the picture, thresholding was used:

$$T = \begin{cases} 0, \ T < 29.5 \\ 1, \ T \geq 29.5 \end{cases}$$

Then, mophorological opening with a 10×10 structural element was performed to remove the disturbances (holes created in the body image). In the next step, all objects with less than the maximum area were removed from the image.

Next, the patient's body was divided into 4 areas (Fig. 2b). For this purpose the key points had to be detected. First the edges were determined with a Sobel operator. On the basis of them the positions of armholes—left (AL)/right (AR)—were determined, computed as the points below which the minimum difference between successive edge points in a given row (separate for the left and right side of the image). Vertical upward lines from the AL and AR points were used to determine the position of the acromones left (ACL) and right (AR) respectively. This line allowed to remove the arms from the image, while the horizontal connection of the ACL and ACR points allowed to remove from the image the patient's neck (Fig. 2a). The level at which the neck line was computed was determined by that point of the acromine, which was higher (in case they were located asymmetrically). Both of this areas were not relevant for further analysis (separated by a dashed line in Fig. 2a).

The proposed algorithm, in accordance with the indicated points, has divided the back into 4 regions of interest (ROI) on basis of the centre of the defined body area.

In the last step, for each of the 4 photos the mode temperature within each ROI was calculated.

2.4.4 Signal Processing and Analysis

Throughout the entire study protocol, the E4 enabled markers to be placed (start of a stage) in the following order: 1st VFT, 1st DST, exercise, JAWS—psychological test, 2nd VFT, 2nd DST.

In the subsequent analysis, this facilitated the division of the signal into appropriate time segments, depending on the activity.

The initial processing of the EDA signal was Z-Score normalization, which is based on the mean and standard deviation (std)

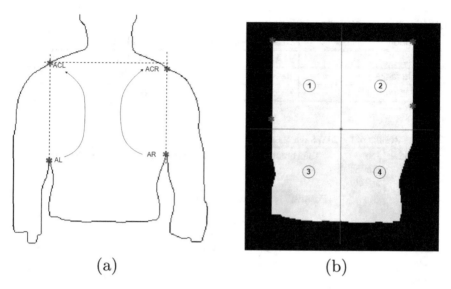

(a)   (b)

Fig. 2 a Significant points and on that basis **b** 4 ROIs of the patient's back with marked points

$$V' = \frac{V - mean}{std}.$$

To filter the signal, a wavelet transform with decomposition level set to 10 and the *MinMax Estimation* method for defrosting was used. This method used a fixed threshold chosen to yield minimax performance for mean square error against an ideal procedure.

The first feature determined from the EDA signal was the value of the galvanic skin response (GSR) and its amplitude. For this purpose, Matlab toolbox distributed under the free GNU GPL license for Electrodermal Activity (EDA) processing and analysis—EDA-master—was used. The following algorithm input parameters have been set to determine GSR: value of GSR (0.2—infinity), GSR slope (0.1—infinity), GSR risetime (0.1—infinity). Next, statistical features were determined to describe the signal in appropriate time intervals, i.e. mean signal value, standard deviation, number of GSRs per minute, number of all GSRs and their amplitudes.

3   Results

3.1   *Psychological Evaluation*

The table below (Table 1) shows the results of the STAI questionnaire.
Table 2 presents the results of the JAWS questionnaire.

Table 1 Results of the STAI questionnaire

Description	Total state—anxiety	Total trait—anxiety
Variable	STAI-X1	STAI -X2
Possible range	20–80	20–80
Actual range	53	49

Table 2 Results of the JAWS questionnaire

Description	Job related affect	Total emotions		High pleasure		Low pleasure	
		Positive	Negative	Arousal			
				High	Low	High	Low
Variable	JAWS			HPHA	HPLA	LPHA	LPLA
Possible range	12–60	6–30	6–30	3–18	3–18	3–18	3–18
Actual range	44	55	21	15	10	10	9

Table 3 Results of the VFTs performed before and after exercising

	Letter of words	Number	Average time between the words (s)
Before	U	9	6.17
After	R	17	3.57

3.2 Verbal Fluency Tests

Table 3 shows the results of the Verbal Fluency Test performed before and after the exercises. The letter to which the test person was supposed to pronounce the word, the number of words and the time between successive answers are presented.

3.3 Digit Symbol Test

The table below (Table 4) shows the results of the DST performed before and after the exercises. The test results was analyzed in terms of both the total number of completed fields (*Summary filled*) and the number of correctly matched number-symbol pairs (*Correct*).

Table 4 Results of the DSTs before and after exercising

	Correct	Summarily filled
Before	38	38
After	47	48

Table 5 Mode back temperature in different ROI areas during exercising

	1	2	3	4
Before	33.93	33.83	31.94	32.15
Beginning	33.88	33.75	31.90	32.04
During	34.27	33.82	32.06	32.08
End	33.91	33.84	31.95	32.16

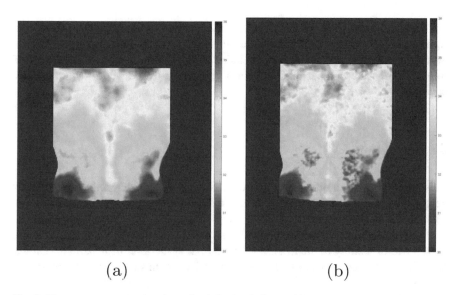

(a)   (b)

Fig. 3 Thermograms presenting the patient's back **a** before and **b** at the end of exercising

3.4 Thermal Image Analysis

The table below shows the summary of mode (Table 5) temperatures in individual ROIs at different moments of exercising—before, at the beginning, during and at the end.

In addition, to illustrate temperature changes, Fig. 3 shows the thermograms recorded during the exercises.

Table 6 Calculated EDA signal parameters

	Mean (μS)	Std	RPM	GSR	Amp (μS)
VFT before	19.95	**1.12**	9.96	10	20.72
DST before	**21.69**	0.32	**11.95**	12	**21.63**
Exercise	14.34	1.02	2	8	15.10
Psychological test	15.70	0.23	10.57	**17**	15.44
VFT after	14.92	0.30	5.98	6	15.23
DST after	14.27	0.17	5.98	6	15.54

3.5 Signal Processing

On the basis of the EDA signal analysis procedure described above, the parameters for the given time segments were determined as shown in Table 6, where *mean*—average signal value, *std*—standard deviation, *RPM*—number of GSR responses per minute, *GSR*—the number of GSRs for a given time period, *Amp*—average GSR energy.

4 Discussion

This article presents a procedure protocol that may serve to determine the patient's behavioural and physiological profile while therapeutic exercises. One person was examined with this protocol.

The results obtained by the subject in the STAI test (part X1), indicate a strong experience of anxiety at the time of examination, at the level of 8 stenium. On the other hand, the result obtained in the STAI-X2 confirm the occurrence of strong learned anxiety response. This means that the examined person is characterized by increased prediction of external or internal threats, manifested as anxiety, feeling of tension, constraint and danger.

The results of the JAWS test indicate strong intensification of emotions experienced in response to the training, both positive and negative. This suggests that the emotions experienced have a regulating and adaptive function, contributing to the optimization of the individual's performance in this particular situational context. This is confirmed by the high score in the HPHA subscale, which says that the researched person assesses the requirements set for him as positive and favorable (eustress). Among the emotions experienced, eagerness, hope and enthusiasm. The researched person expects that in spite of possible losses, he will obtain benefits thanks to the action taken.

The Verbal Fluency Tests was performed as a stressful situation and additionally checking the verbal fluency of the examined person. On the basis of the results obtained, a significant increase in the number of spoken words was observed after performing the exercises than before. The average time between successive spoken words also decreased. The above results may also be influenced by the popularity of individual letters. Statistical data showed that in the share of individual letters in all Polish words the letter R is 4.69%, while U.—2.5% [14]. The meta-analysis of Ahlskog et al. confirmed the neuroprotective effect of physical activity on cognitive performance, it is worthwhile to consider the current level of fluency in terms of its potential for change over time [15]. The same is true for executive functions, which are responsible for deliberate human behavior, especially in new, unusual situations [16]. However, based on the observation of the person during data acquisition, it could be seen that this test turned out to be a very stressful situation, which was reflected in the EDA signal.

The results of the Digit Symbol Tests performed before and after exercising differed. The examined person matched a total of 38 number–symbol pairs (38 correct) during the first attempt, and 10 more (47 correct) after the exercises. This changeability may result from better concentration of the patient, as well as greater awareness—getting rid of the so-called fear of the unknown. There are reports on the role of exercises in improving cognitive functions, including shortening stimulus response times, improving inference, recall and memory search [17].

Analyzing thermal imaging data, it was essential to note the small temperature variation in the individual ROI. The test person had always a higher temperature in the upper back areas. In Fig. 3 there is a noticeable drop in temperature in the 4th ROI (right-down)—the cold (blue) area increased. The use of a thermal imaging camera was applied to observe temperature changes in the back muscles (especially the spinal column) and to check the level of activation of individual muscle batches within the ROI during the exercises in the quantity approach. Traditional thermal imaging was used intentionally, instead of active, due to the non-invasive character of the study. Active thermovision may be an additional stress or pain factor, which could significantly affect the results and future modelling of the patient's behavioural and physiological profile during therapy.

The greatest variability in the obtained results can be noticed in the EDA signal analysis. The average signal value, number of RPM, GSR and average energy GSR, in individual time windows were the highest during The Digit Symbol Test. The highest number of galvanic responses (GSR) of the body, indicating the experiencing of certain emotions and increased psychogalvanic reaction of the skin, was recorded when filling psychological questionnaires after the exercises (JAWS).

The patient felt the highest stress at the beginning of the study, during the VFT and DST. The same elements performed after the exercises still stressed the patient, but to a lesser extent—the calculated parameters reached lower values. The VFT and DST tests were chosen deliberately because not only are they performed under time pressure, but also the desire to perform it as well as possible may be an additional stress factor. On the other hand, exercises performed in the Disc4spine system allowed the test person to calm down—the calculated parameters reached lower values in relation to the previously computed ones, obtained during the earlier steps.

All of the above components—tests and exercises—are components of the protocol, which with a larger set of data will allow to determine the patient's behavioural
and physiologic profile.

5 Summary

This article presents a procedure protocol that will allow to determine the behavioural
and physiological profile of the patient during therapeutic exercises. The whole protocol consists of several basic steps (psychological tests, DST, VFT, D4S exercises)
and the patient is monitored continuously using the Empatica E4 wristband. On the
basis of the collected data it was noticed that the most stressful situation for the
patient was performing the VFT and the DST, while exercises themselves proved
to be relaxing to some extent. The effect of the study was to formulate plans and
hypotheses for further research, this time in a quantitative approach.

Acknowledgements The study was realized within the project "DISC4SPINE dynamic individual
stimulation and control for spine and posture interactive rehabilitation" (grant no. POIR.04.01.02-
00-0082/17-00).

References

 1. Emery, C.F., Leatherman, N.E., Burker, E.J., MacIntyre, N.R.: Psychological outcomes of a
    pulmonary rehabilitation program. Chest **100**(3), 613–617 (1991)
 2. Ward, T., Maruna, S.: Rehabilitation. Routledge, Abingdon (2007)
 3. Watson, J.B.: Psychology as the behaviorist views it. Psychol. Rev. **20**(2), 158 (1913)
 4. Ganong, W.F.: Review of Medical Physiology. Mcgraw-hill, New York (1995)
 5. Filipiak, M., Paluchowski, W.J., Zalewski, B., Tarnowska, M.: Diagnoza psychologiczna: kom-
    petencje i standardy. Wybrane zagadnienia. Pracownia Testów, Warszawa (2015)
 6. Spielberger, C.D.: State-trait anxiety inventory for adults (1983)
 7. Wrześniewski, K., Sosnowski, T., Jaworowska, A., Fecenec, D., Inwentarz stanu i cechy lęku,
    S.T.A.I.: Polska adaptacja STAI. Podręcznik. Wydanie trzecie, rozszerzone [Polish adaptation
    of STAI. Manual, 3rd extended edition]. Pracownia Testów Psychologicznych PTP, Warszawa
    (2006)
 8. Boucsein, W.: Electrodermal Activity. Springer Science & Business Media, Berlin (2012)
 9. E4 Wristband User's Manual 20150608. Empatica Milano Italy, pp. 5–16 (2015)
10. Troyer, A.K., Moscovitch, M., Winocur, G., Leach, L., Freedman, M.: Clustering and switching
    on verbal fluency tests in Alzheimer's and Parkinson's disease. J. Int. Neuropsychol. Soc. **4**(2),
    137–143 (1998)
11. Sitek, E.J., Konkel, A., Międzobrodzka, E., Sołtan, W., Barczak, A., Sławek, J.: Kliniczne
    zastosowanie prób fluencji słownej w chorobie Huntingtona. Hygeia Public Health **49**(2),
    215–221 (2014)
12. Conn, H.O.: Trailmaking and number-connection tests in the assessment of mental state in
    portal systemic encephalopathy. Digestive Dis. Sci. **22**(6), 541–550 (1977)

13. Van Katwyk, P.T., Fox, S., Spector, P.E., Kelloway, E.K.: Using the Job-Related Affective Well-Being Scale (JAWS) to investigate affective responses to work stressors. J. Occup. Health Psychol. **5**(2), 219 (2000)
14. Przepiórkowski, A.: Narodowy korpus języka polskiego. Naukowe PWN (2012)
15. Ahlskog, J.E., Geda, Y.E., Graff-Radford, N.R., Petersen, R.C.: Physical exercise as a preventive or disease-modifying treatment of dementia and brain aging. In: Mayo Clinic Proceedings, vol. 86, No. 9, pp. 876–884. Elsevier (2011)
16. Banich, M.T.: Executive function. The search for an integrated account. J. Assoc. Psychol. Sci. **18**(2), 89–94 (2009)
17. Kamijo, K., McGowan, A.L., Pontifex, M.B.: Effects of physical activity on cognition in children and adolescents. In: Anshel, M.H., Petruzzello, S.J., Labbé, E.E. (eds.) APA Handbooks in Psychology Series. APA Handbook of Sport and Exercise Psychology, vol. 2. Exercise Psychology, pp. 331–343. American Psychological Association (2019)

Psychophysiological State Changes Assesment Based on Thermal Face Image—Preliminary Results

Marta Danch-Wierzchowska, Marcin Bugdol, and Andrzej W. Mitas

Abstract The analysis of the patient's psychophysiological condition is one of the key elements of properly conducted therapy. In the therapeutic tasks special attention is paid to monitoring the patient's condition. Our method proposed a robust for segmentation errors (based on median value) and an easily applied method for assessing the thermal profile of the face and its usage in psychophysiological state observation. The obtained results suggest that the central part of the face provides sufficient information to discriminate between an active and a non active individual, even during minor physical effort.

Keywords Behavioural biometrics · Human activity recognition · Thermal imaging · Physiotherapy

1 Introduction

The analysis of the patient's psychophysiological condition is the basis for properly conducted therapy and not only in the physiological context. In physiotherapeutic clinics the therapy is performed by trained medical staff who have knowledge about the way how the patient expresses its emotional state [2]. This applies especially to

M. Danch-Wierzchowska (✉) · M. Bugdol · A. W. Mitas
Faculty of Biomedical Engineering, Silesian University of Technology, Roosevelta 40, 41-800 Zabrze, Poland
e-mail: marta.danch-wierzchowska@polsl.pl

M. Bugdol
e-mail: marcin.bugdol@polsl.pl

A. W. Mitas
e-mail: andrzej.mitas@polsl.pl

E. Piętka et al. (eds.), *Information Technology in Biomedicine*, Advances in Intelligent Systems and Computing 1186, https://doi.org/10.1007/978-3-030-49666-1_14

activities related to fatigue during exercise and correction which requires significant patient involvement [9]. In the therapeutic tasks special attention is paid to monitoring the patient's condition in terms of reducing the risk of injury or inappropriate muscle compensation during exercises.

One of the proposed methods for evaluating the patient's condition in terms of the correctness of exercises and the adequacy of their intensity to the therapy complexity level is the analysis of the face thermal images [1]. The proposed measurement concept abstracts from measuring muscle activity, because it is assumed that physiotherapeutic activities will cause a non-specific thermal effect with a large influence of non-measurable input variables [13]. An interesting research thesis is the expected dependency between the patient's involvement during exercises and the distribution of his face temperature field. It is assumed that too small involvement of the exerciser will not change the face temperature and too high will lead to significant thermal changes, especially in nose, mouth and external parts of the ears. Related study presented in [11] justifies such approach. It was stated that thermal image analysis is becoming a common, non-invasive diagnostic method which is related to a drop of equipment price and the development of measuring technique. This gives the opportunity to apply and collect large datasets of various measurements which is required for machine learning algorithms. What is more, the morphological analysis of changes can be carried out in terms of assessment personalization [4], despite the fact that changes in the temperature field distribution are usually non-specific [6] even in areas as obvious as the nose. A prerequisite for increasing the reliability of measurements is to ensure the stability of the factors that affect the distribution of the temperature field such as: ambient temperature, ventilation, humidity or meals which determine the metabolism and heat exchange with the environment [11].

The literature mainly discuss classification methods that discriminate between basic emotions [5]. Another approach is to use thermal images for alcohol intoxication detection [3, 7]. Our work is focused on estimating a generic thermal profile of the face for assessing psychophysiological state changes during physiotherapeutic exercises. Monitoring of the homeostasis allows to infer about the physiology and the mental state. The response to emotional changes is very complex and the search for such behavioral biometrics is a separate scientific issue [4].

2   Materials and Methods

2.1   Thermal Images

The research group consists of 9 people (3 women and 6 men) who at the time of experiment were students of the Jerzy Kukuczka Academy of Physical Education in Katowice and Silesian University of Technology. Before starting the measurements, everyone was informed about the purpose of the test and gave their signed, written consent. Both technical staff and experienced physiotherapists supervised the entire process. The FLIR A300 camera with 320×240 pixel resolution, was chosen for thermal imaging. The emissivity factor ϵ was set to 0.95 and the accuracy of the camera is $\pm 2\,°C$. The distance between the patient and the camera was 2 m. 2 face photos was taken of each patient. The dataset contained 18 photos that were used for further analysis.

2.2 Data Acquisition

Data was obtained during personal physiotherapeutic session. An individual was asked to repeat ten times "Body Elongation" Exercises (BEE), which is a sequence of feet, knees and hips rotation, followed by a spinal cord elongation. The elongated posture was kept 10 s followed by 30 s of posture relaxation and new BEE was performed. The exercises were not challenging or exhausting. Before and after BEE sequence (10 repetition) the person was set down in front of a thermographic camera, then one was asked to look straight into the lens, and a facial image was taken. In the end the dataset consist of nine pairs of facial thermal images: one taken before and one after BEE sequence. Exemplary thermal images are presented in Fig. 1.

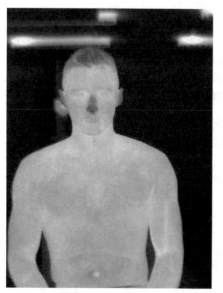
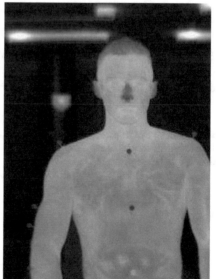

(a) before BEE   (b) after BEE

Fig. 1 Exemplary thermal image pair; the markers visible at the patient chest come from another examination, and have no influence on the results obtained during thermal imaging of the face

2.3 Data Preprocessing

For each obtained facial image the first preprocessing step was the transformation of gray-scale pixel values (0–255) into thermal values (in Celsius scale). Face Region of Interest (ROI) was segmented using basic thresholding (empirically set as 29.5 °C)—selecting human posture from background on thermal imaging is relatively simple task due to high temperature differences. There are photos on which the nose was colder than previously set threshold, nevertheless the specific localisation of the nasal hole in ROI binary mask allows to fill it without any sophisticated tools (Matlab *imfill* function). Any smaller object, that appears in the background were removed from ROI binary mask using morphological operations (Matlab *imdilate* following by *bwareaopen* functions).

2.4 Face Segment Descriptors

The face ROI was manually separated into 7 segments corresponding to face parts. The specified segments are presented in Fig. 2. For each face segment the mean and median values were estimated.

2.5 Statistical Data Analysis

For each image pair the differences of corresponding descriptors were calculated. In case of statistical significance differences denotation the normality of the descriptors difference distributions were verified using the Shapiro–Wilk test. The statistically

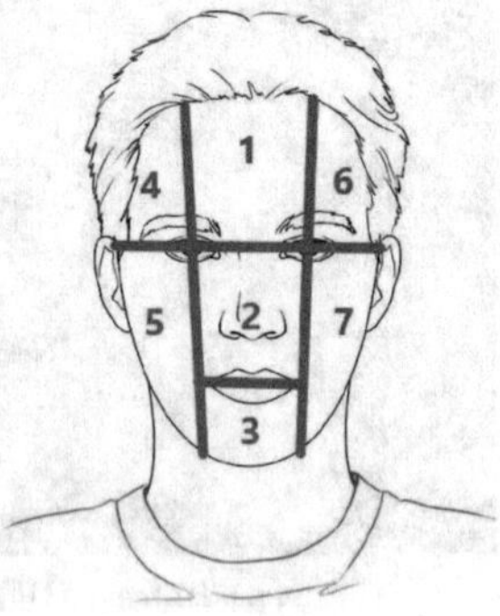

Fig. 2 Scheme of selected face segments for which the descriptors were estimated

significant differences were confirmed using the paired t-test or the Wilcoxon signed rank test, depending on the Shapiro–Wilk's test result (normally distributed, non-normally distributed respectively).

2.6 Data Classification

The descriptor values estimated from images were set as features for the Linear Discriminant Analysis (LDA). LDA was chosen due to its simplicity and facility of results interpretation. Classifier were validated using k-fold Cross-Validation. In order to find the most discriminating descriptor set between images before and after BEE, LDA with six different input sets was employed. Selected descriptor sets were specified as:

- mean values for all segments (Mn7)
- mean values for central segments (Mn3)
- mean values for lateral segments (Mn4)
- median values for all segments (Md7)
- median values for central segments (Md3)
- median values for lateral segments (Md4).

3 Results

3.1 Segments Descriptors

The differences between thermal images before and after BEE are easily visible. In Fig. 3 exemplary images of three individuals before and after BEE are presented. The face segments descriptors—set of mean and median, were estimated for each individual on the basis of temperature values inside respective segments. In Fig. 4 the distributions of face segments descriptors are shown, for face segments and for individuals respectively.

The differences between mean and median values for each individual in each face segment are presented in the form of multi-series histograms in Fig. 5. The differences are usually in the range of −0.2–0.2. The highest differences (higher than 0.5°) were observed for the central segment (2)—the nose segment. In most cases the median value is higher than the mean value.

3.2 Statistical Data Analysis

To prove statistically significant differences between the face temperature descriptors before and after BEE, the paired t-test and the Wilcoxon test were employed. The normality of the distribution of the descriptors differences was verified using the Shapiro–Wilk test. The normality test confirmed the non-normal distribution of descriptors in central forehead segment (1) in both mean and median distributions. Paired tests (t-test and Wilcoxon) showed significant statistical differences before and after BEE only for the chin segment (3) for both mean and median values. The normality test results are presented in Table 1. The results of paired t-test and Wilcoxon test are presented in Table 2. Each test was performed at significance level $\alpha = 0.05$.

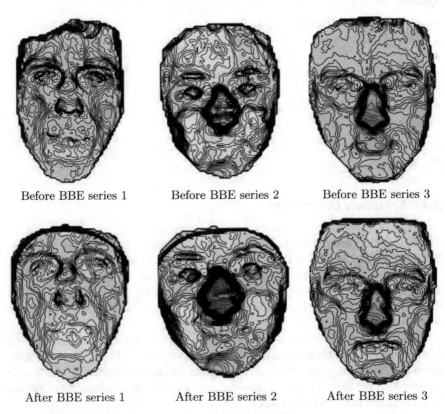

Before BBE series 1   Before BBE series 2   Before BBE series 3

After BBE series 1   After BBE series 2   After BBE series 3

Fig. 3 Thermal contour image before and after BEE for 3 individuals

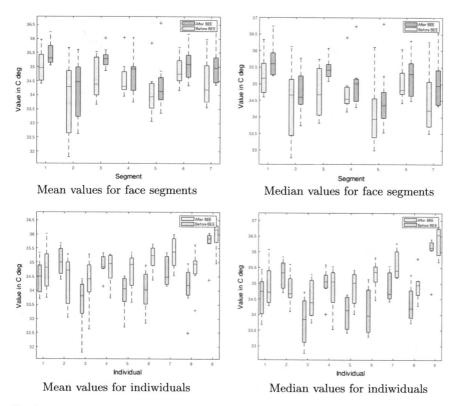

Mean values for face segments   Median values for face segments

Mean values for indiwiduals   Median values for indiwiduals

Fig. 4 Boxplots of mean and median values for face segments and for individuals before and after BEE

Table 1 Estimated p values for normality distribution of descriptors differences for face segments; bold values indicate cases for which the null hypothesis were reject in favor of the alternative; Mn—mean, Md—median

Segment	1	2	3	4	5	6	7
Mn p val	**0.02**	0.54	0.94	0.52	0.06	0.45	0.29
Md p val	**0.04**	0.75	0.80	0.51	0.05	0.46	0.77

3.3 Data Classification

The best results were obtained for classification with three segment from central face part as the input set. The classification results for each input set are presented in Table 3.

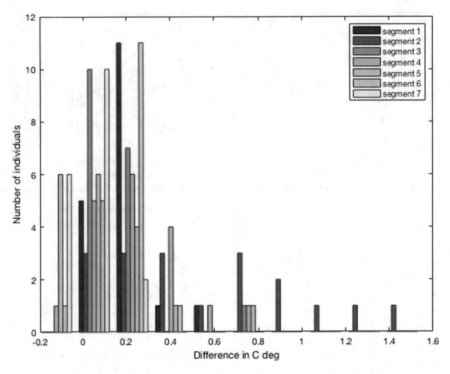

Fig. 5 Histogram of differences between median and mean values for segments, each color represents a different face segment (see Fig. 2)

Table 2 Estimated p values for matched pairs tests for face segments; bold values indicate cases for which the null hypothesis were reject in favor of the alternative; Mn—mean, Md—median

Segment	1	2	3	4	5	6	7
Mn p val	0.09	0.53	**0.01**	0.61	0.45	0.28	0.14
Md p val	0.09	0.39	**0.01**	0.47	0.31	0.40	0.18

Table 3 Classification efficiency for selected input set; ACC—Accuracy, TPR—True Positive Rate, TNR—True Negative Rate

Data set	ACC	TPR	TNR
Mn7	0.61	0.60	0.63
Mn3	**0.83**	**0.88**	**0.80**
Mn4	0.61	0.63	0.60
Md7	0.72	0.75	0.70
Md3	**0.89**	**1.00**	**0.82**
Md4	0.61	0.63	0.60

4 Conclusions and Discussion

In presented study we investigated whether the thermal changes on the person's face appears after non-intensive physiotherapeutic exercises. The estimated descriptors could constitute a generic thermal profile of the face [10].

The literature suggests that the mean value is a representative segment descriptor in thermal images analysis. In the presented study we proposed another descriptor—the median value. The difference between the mean and the median values are between −0.2 and 0.2 for most segments. The highest differences are observed for the nose segment, which is also the coldest area for all individuals. In most cases the median was higher than the mean, which could be caused by its insensitivity to incorrect segmentation, image artifacts or face covered by hairs, bands, etc. Mean value can be easier disturb by any outlier present in not perfectly segmented ROI. Therefore, the median appears to be more stable descriptor for thermal images than the mean.

More accurate classification were obtained for three central face segments (Mn3, Md3), and were significantly better than for the others. The obtained results suggest that lateral segments do not improve the classification results. Moreover, they introduce dispensable information. Observation and analysis of the central face part only can bring sufficient information.

The descriptors distributions suggest, that face temperatures are higher after BEE series, which is consistent with both, biological and physioterapeutical reports [8, 12]. Nonetheless, there were two individuals, whose faces were colder after exercises. This could be caused by increased skin perspiration, which introduce disturbances of temperature measurement in thermal images.

The classification methods presented in the literature are based on temperature measured in specific face points [3], specified face region (i.e. forehead, chin, cheeks, nose, maxillary) [5] or even convolutional neural networks [1]. Our method proposed robust for segmentation errors and easily applied method for assessing the thermal profile of the face and its usage in thermal changes detection.

5 Summary

The central face part provides sufficient information to discriminate between an active and a non active person, even during minor physical effort. The classification based on median values is more exact than the one based on mean values, yet the median is also more robust in terms of segmentation accuracy. We strongly recommend using median values as the new face segments descriptor during thermal images analysis. Assessing relative changes and coexisting trends, reflecting the time and intensity of the exerciser's reaction are interesting in the context of the conducted project and will be under our further investigation.

Ethics Approval and Consent to Participate
The study was presented to the Bioethical Commission of the Jerzy Kukuczka Academy of Physical Education in Katowice and approved in a statement (No. 3/2019). The research group consists of students of the Jerzy Kukuczka Academy of Physical Education in Katowice and Silesian University of Technology. Before starting the experiment, each student was informed about the purpose of the test and gave their signed, written consent.

   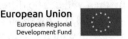

Acknowledgements The study was realized within the project "DISC4SPINE dynamic individual stimulation and control for spine and posture interactive rehabilitation" (grant no. POIR.04.01.02-00-0082/17-00).

References

1. Bordallo Lopez, M., Del-Blanco, C., Garcia, N.: Detecting exercise-induced fatigue using thermal imaging and deep learning. pp. 1–6 (2017). https://doi.org/10.1109/IPTA.2017.8310151
2. Goulart, C., Valadão, C., Delisle-Rodriguez, D., Caldeira, E., Bastos, T.: Emotion analysis in children through facial emissivity of infrared thermal imaging. PLOS ONE **14**(3), 1–17 (2019). https://doi.org/10.1371/journal.pone.0212928
3. Hermosilla, G., Verdugo, J.L., Farias, G., Vera, E., Pizarro, F., Machuca, M.: Face recognition and drunk classification using infrared face images. J. Sensors 5813514. https://doi.org/10.1155/2018/5813514 (2018)
4. Ioannou, S., Gallese, V., Merla, A.: Thermal infrared imaging in psychophysiology: potentialities and limits. Psychophysiology **51**(10), 951–963 (2014)
5. Ioannou, S., Morris, P., Mercer, H., Baker, M., Gallese, V., Reddy, V.: Proximity and gaze influences facial temperature: a thermal infrared imaging study. Front. Psychol. **5**, 845. https://www.frontiersin.org/article/10.3389/fpsyg.2014.00845 (2014). https://doi.org/10.3389/fpsyg.2014.00845
6. Kosonogov, V., De Zorzi, L., Honoré, J., Martínez-Velázquez, E.S., Nandrino, J.L., Martinez-Selva, J.M., Sequeira, H.: Facial thermal variations: a new marker of emotional arousal. PLOS ONE **12**, 1–15 (2017). https://doi.org/10.1371/journal.pone.0183592
7. Koukiou, G.: Intoxication identification using thermal imaging, p. 72128. https://www.frontiersin.org/article/10.3389/fpsyg.2014.00845 (2017). https://doi.org/10.5772/intechopen.72128
8. Quesada, J.I.P., Carpes, F., Bini, R., Palmer, R., Pérez-Soriano, P., de Anda, R.: Relationship between skin temperature and muscle activation during incremental cycle exercise. J. Therm. Biol. **48**, 28–35 (2015)
9. Sampaio, L., Bezerra, E., Paladino, K., dos Santos, J., Quesada, J., Rossato, M.: Effect of training level and blood flow restriction on thermal parameters: preliminary study. Infrared Phys. Technol. **79**, 25–31 (2016)
10. Sonkusare, S., Ahmedt-Aristizabal, D., Aburn, M., et al.: Detecting changes in facial temperature induced by a sudden auditory stimulus based on deep learning-assisted face tracking. Nat. Sci. Rep. **9**(4729) (2019)

11. Szentkuti, A., Kavanagh, H.S., Grazion, S.: Infrared thermography and image analysis for biomedical use. Period. Biol. **113**(4), 385–392 (2011)
12. Tanda, G.: Skin temperature measurements by infrared thermography during running exercise. Exp. Therm. Fluid Sci. **71**, 103–113 (2016)
13. Xu, X., Karis, A., Buller, M., Santee, W.: Relationship between core temperature, skin temperature, and heat flux during exercise in heat. Eur. J. Appl. Physiol. **113**(9), 2381–2389 (2013)

Application of Original System to Support Specialist Physiotherapy D4S in Correction of Postural Defects as Compared to Other Methods—A Review

Karol Bibrowicz, Tomasz Szurmik, Anna Lipowicz, and Andrzej W. Mitas

Abstract For years, body posture, its defects and methods of therapy have been the point of interest of specialists in many fields. The observed civilizational progress, sedentary lifestyle, and excessive use of electronic gadgets electronic gadgets are unfortunately associated with the growth of postural problems. This is associated with the increasing incidence of degenerative changes and pain in the musculoskeletal system and, in turn, decreasing quality of life. The paper presents the basic notions connected with the body posture, describes the existing concepts of postural defects therapy and based thereof, proposes a new model of diagnostic and therapeutic procedure. The DISC4SPINE system of dynamic individual stimulation and control for spine and posture interactive rehabilitation (D4S) is a modern system which uses professional knowledge and experience of experts in many fields. D4S is also an integrated biomechatronic system enabling: (a) diagnosis prior to rehabilitation, (b) real time therapy monitoring, and (c) personalization of therapeutic activities focusing on spinal conditions and postural disorders.

Keywords Posture · Postural defect correction · Examination · Methods of therapy · Diagnostics · Spine

K. Bibrowicz (✉)
Science and Research Center of Body Posture, Kazimiera Milanowska College of Education and Therapy, Poznań, Poland
e-mail: bibrowicz@wp.pl

T. Szurmik
University of Silesia in Katowice, Katowice, Poland
e-mail: info@orto-med.com.pl

A. Lipowicz
Department of Anthropology, Wrocław University of Environmental and Life Sciences, Wrocław, Poland
e-mail: lipowiczanna@gmail.com

A. W. Mitas
Department of Informatics and Medical Equipment, Faculty of Biomedical Engineering, Silesian University of Technology, Gliwice, Poland
e-mail: andrzej.mitas@polsl.pl

© The Editor(s) (if applicable) and The Author(s), under exclusive license to Springer Nature Switzerland AG 2021
E. Piętka et al. (eds.), *Information Technology in Biomedicine*, Advances in Intelligent Systems and Computing 1186, https://doi.org/10.1007/978-3-030-49666-1_15

1 Introduction

The problems of body posture, its defects and correction methods have been present both, in the public discourse and scientific writing for years [2, 4, 23]. This is due to the significance assigned to the correct body posture on the one hand and nuisance and problems caused by postural faults. Back pain, degenerative changes in joints and, in consequence, decreased quality of life is related to dysfunctions within the human postural system. There is also no single good answer to the question: should we correct or create the body posture? Or maybe, it is not a simple, dichotomous division? Perhaps, we need provide both, the conditions to facilitate modeling the correct posture and, at the same time, introduce correction procedures where necessary? For years, the world argues about the best definition of body posture, of what is considered correct posture and what is dysfunctional. Physiotherapists have different opinions, including the extreme claim that if something is common it cannot be treated as a defect. The specialist literature provides at least several dozen definitions of posture, correct posture or postural defects. Different criteria and conditions was used to describe posture quality [2, 4, 23, 26]. However, in addition to methods of examining and describing body posture, there was also a discussion of treatment methods that should be used correctly. Unfortunately, there is no consensus in this area either. There are at least as many correction methods as specialists in this field. However, one thing is unquestionable. There is no doubts that regardless of the complex nature of the problem, the role and significance of correct body posture, ensuring the right development of children and youth, decreasing the negative consequences of postural dysfunctions associated for example with epidemiological spread of spinal conditions in the population are large enough to be seriously addressed. The significance of the problem and determination to solve it motivated a group of specialists from different fields: biomechanics, IT engineers, medicine doctors, physiotherapists, anthropologists, psychologists and engineers-constructors attempt to develop a complex solution to the problem of diagnosis and therapy of postural dysfunctions. Thus, the D4S System of Dynamic Individual Stimulation and Control for Spine and Posture Interactive Rehabilitation was designed. The system is an attempt to set new diagnostic and therapeutic standards, and to meet the civilizational challenge of early prevention of postural defect in children and youth as well as pain within the musculoskeletal system in adults.

2 Objective

The goal of the work was draw attention to the importance and role of the straight posture, to present the main existing concepts for the treatment of postural dysfunction and to present possible applications of the new, original system D4S to support specialist physiotherapy in modeling body posture and correcting its defects.

3 Postural Defects—Epidemiology and Causes

From the clinical point of view, postural dysfunctions in the sagittal plane may be classified as non-structural or structural [6]. Structural pathologies include the following clinical items: idiopathic scoliosis, Scheuermann's disease (kyphosis), spinal birth defects, consequences of vertebral osteomyelitis, spondylolisthesis and other clinical diseases which cause postural dysfunctions. This term shows the occurrence of morphological malfunctions in bones and soft tissues (fascia, muscles, ligaments, tendons). In addition, structural alterations reveal more serious clinical problem, as they are less flexible and less correctable comparing to the non-structural dysfunctions. The most common types of non-structural postural changes in the sagittal plane in both, children and adults, are lordosis, kyphosis which may sometimes coexists with the lordosis (kyphosis-lordosis posture), flat back or "sway back" posture [6].

Postural disorders and their consequences as pain within the musculoskeletal system have become the epidemics of our times. However, we should emphasize that direct relationship between the posture irregularities and pain or wider, poorer health is not clear. There are publications which challenge such associations [5] and present completely different point of view [7]. Surely, further research are necessary to explain and determine clearly the role of postural deviations on health and pain within the musculoskeletal system. But we cannot ignore the epidemic scale of postural dysfunctions and pain conditions, which affect human population regardless of gender, age, ethnicity or place of living. According to the American Chiropractic Association, more than 80% of American population require medical assistance due to back pains. The costs of treatment of musculoskeletal pain conditions are many times higher than the costs of therapy of other chronic diseases such as diabetes, cancer or hearing diseases [3]. In the U.S. only, the costs of treatment amount up to 560 to 635 billion dollars USD [11].

According to American Posture Institute, one of the key determinants of the body posture are daily habits [2]. Other important factors which may influence how posture is shaped are: (1) repetitive patterns of professional movements, (2) sedentary lifestyle, (3) staying in sitting position for long time, (4) wrong position during lifting and carrying heavy loads, (5) asymmetric sitting position, (6) physical injuries, (7) wrong shoes, (8) asymmetric load on torso while standing, (9) lack of hygiene of rest and sleep. The most frequently described and diagnosed types of postural disorders related to the above listed factors are: (1) forward head posture, (2) rounded shoulders, (3) abducted scapulae, (4) thoracic kyphosis, (5) hyper lordotic lumbar spine, (6) lateral pelvic tilting, (7) knee/ankle deviations.

4 What Is More Important—Structure of Function?

Posture therapy has a long-standing tradition. During the years, different concepts emerged and therapeutic methods based on their assumptions. Because of their number, and various, often inter-related founding concepts, any attempts to classify and organize these methods may fail. However, we can develop more general classification based on the reductionist and holistic approach to body posture and body movements. The frequently used term "relaxed standing position" may suggest a static position. However, standing person is never static. So, even though vertical POSTURE is an important concept, Feldenkrais suggests that focusing on function and movement would provide a better description. In his opinion, ACTURE is a better word to describe the condition of a standing person [9]. Body posture and movement is a complex system of events involving many different body systems. Reductionist concepts involve dissecting the certain elements of posture and movement into smaller components which are then analyzed and treated in isolation. However, this approach did not allow for determination of mutual relations and dynamic interactions related to posture and movement. Therefore, it seems that these phenomena can be better understood using the holistic philosophy [10]. Already in the ancient times, Aristotle said that "the whole is greater than the sum of its parts" [1]. This implies that body posture and movement can be understood better when we view the musculoskeletal system as a whole, globally connected and complex system [8, 10].

However, until now, it is difficult to decide which of the above mentioned approach is better. Further, high quality research and more adequate evaluation tools are necessary to confirm the effects of these techniques [18]. According to the recommendations of the American College of Physicians [20], good therapeutic effects in the therapy o postural defects and back pain can be achieved by combining local therapies improving, for example, deep stabilization (e.g. Pilates) and exercises based on the concepts of global muscle and motor chains (e.g. Yoga, Tai-chi).

5 Principles of Selected Methods of Postural Therapy

5.1 Rolfing, or Structural Integration

As named by its founder Ida Rolf [21], focuses on working with the fascial structures. It uses original and regular, usually quite vigorous, manipulations of soft tissues. It was designed to extend the shortened tissues, which combined with the elements of positional and motor education, helps in the corrected fit and balance of the body. Ida Rolf assumed that structural changes as the key to functional improvement. She believed that structural reorganization of the body enables intelligent renegotiation of its relation with the gravity, so that new ways of standing, moving and being in general appear spontaneously [26]. The process of structural integration leads to the increase of individual potential, helps to deal with stress and recognize its symptoms, improves self-confidence and enables adaptation to changing circumstances [12].

5.2 Feldenkrais Method

Parallel to structural integration, Moshe Feldenkrais developed his own method of working with the body—functional integration. He believed that human structure gets formed through interactions taking place between our genetic heritage and the sum of all the movement our body makes during the whole life. Feldenkrais method focuses on the movement patterns which allow to discover how a person moves and then offers new movement options which may turn out more effective or comfortable. Finally, it helps to integrate the new options with wider movement repertoire. According to Feldenkrais, functional changes resulting from this method modify the body structure [19]. The methods includes individual work—Functional Integration and group sessions—Awareness Through Movement [26]. During both, individual and group therapy, the participants are guided with verbal instructions and specific movement sequences called the movement lesson. Movements are usually practiced when laying down or sitting, to the extent that suits individual patients, and the emphasis is put on experiencing the movements in self and self in the movement. Sessions may focus on movements from different developmental periods, for example rolling, crawling or standing up. They may be related with certain function like posture, walking or breathing. The sessions may also focus on experiencing own motor abilities connected with certain muscles, joints, whole movement patterns or experiments with imagination [5].

5.3 Pilates

The method was developed by Joseph Pilates at the beginning of the 20th century and was originally called Contrology. It is a universal postural training to ensure correct posture through stimulation and strengthening deep postural muscles. It is a system of exercises to help postural muscles function in a balanced way, support the spine and raise awareness of the spine in the neutral position. It is also used in prevention and therapy of back pain. Exercises help to increase the awareness of own body, which allows better functioning in both, static positions and locomotion. Therapy uses mainly the so called clinical Pilates which is based on the following principles: (1) right breathing, inhaling through nose and mouth during certain phase of an exercise, (2) concentration, total focus on the movement performed, (3) centering, every movement begins in the "center" of the body, that is from the deep muscles and reaches outside, (4) control based on conscious movement combined with breathing, (5) fluency of movements, (6) coordination and precision of movement. The method is used, among others, by physiotherapists, osteopaths, personal trainers and fitness instructors, in patients at every level of mobility [12, 14, 16].

5.4 Methods of Work Based on the Muscle Chain Concepts

Recently, these methods have become more and more popular. One of the first people to emphasize their role during therapy of weakened muscles was Herman Kabat (PNF Proprioceptive Neuromuscular Facilitation). According to him, the brain does not recognize single muscles but movement patterns. One of the first people to talk about muscular chains and use them in postural treatment was Francoise Mezieres. She developed a method which uses exercises stretching whole groups of muscles at the same time. She called such groups of muscles muscular chains. She had many followers who with time modified the structures of muscle chains, added more muscles and developed their own methods. Godelive Dennys-Struyf GDS, Souchard RPG, Busquet [22–24, 26] and others focused mainly on work with muscular chains responsible for the static aspect of human posture. Piret and Bezieres [22, 24] were one of the first ones to explain the mechanics of the spiral chains. They focused on movements patterns rather than static posture. The concept which tries to explain the whole spiral structure of movement is Spiraldynamik developed by Yolanda Deswarte and Christian Larsen [15, 16]. They were interested primarily in the relationships between the anatomy, three-dimensional systems and gravity. They considered spiral as the basic structural component in the universe. This refers both, to form and function. Only three-dimensional connections of spiral structures in the whole body ensure harmony of movements [15, 16]. Spiral chains and spiral movement concept are also the key element of Spiral Stabilization Method—SMSYSTEM. The methods was developed by Czech medicine doctor, Richard Smišek [25]. According to his concept, restoration of balance in the muscular-ligamentous apparatus, improvement of the posture patterns and the quality of walking may be achieved through activation of the spiral muscular chains. Smišek says that most of the back pains is related to distorted functioning of these chains. He identified to basic mechanisms of stabilization of the spine and joints: (1) vertical, relax stabilization and (2) spiral stabilization during movement. He suggests exercises which combine a complex functional training and movement control using the central nervous system. The main assumption of this method is activation of the spiral muscular chains thanks to which spinal traction is achieved.

6 D4S System of Individual Stimulation and Control for Spine and Posture Interactive Rehabilitation

The article presents functionalities of the D4S System of Dynamic Individual Stimulation and Control for Spine and Posture Interactive Rehabilitation. D4S is an integrated biomechatronic system enabling: (a) diagnosis prior to rehabilitation, (b) real time therapy monitoring, and (c) personalization of therapeutic activities focusing on spinal conditions and postural disorders.

From the technical and medical point of view, the diagnostic and rehabilitation system D4S has a diagnostic module (to detect potential postural defect, its parameters and potential risk factors) and a therapeutic module (enabling performing a series of correction exercises in the standing position, based on the latest modern developments, in particular stabilizing exercises based on the training of short, one-joint muscles responsible for motor control). D4S is based on the original algorithms of work of the diagnostic and rehabilitation set, developed upon the original concept of methodology which is adapted to developmental age and patient's physique, and considers the effectiveness of exercises, analysis of the psycho-physical condition of the patient and the principles of virtual gamification. D4S is complemented with an online platform to operate the computer aided measuring system which registers anthropometric, behavioral, diagnostic and therapeutic data.

Diagnostic module consists of the measuring systems to perform noninvasive assessment of the degree of postural and spinal deviation. Rehabilitation modules have measuring systems to observe the therapy, and executive systems. Therapeutic actions can be monitored (observation of physiological parameters and psychical condition) in the real time. The telework module enables continuous activity and provides access to the dispersed warehouse of the diagnostic data. The Diagnostic Module (DM) allows fast and precise detection of defect included in the catalogue of the diagnosed diseases, determination of its degree, then it helps to define the therapy, monitor it and collect data for research. Potential online access to the data enables validation using big data sets and confrontation with similar cases. TOF (Time-of-Flight) cameras, thermal camera with detectors to measure moments of forces and localization of the selected anthropometric points, and special podoscope with the function of measuring foot load enable complete assessment of the biomarkers necessary for the diagnosis, therapy development and monitoring of the results. The function of physiological and behavioral analysis through monitoring the HRV (Heart Rate Variability), pulse wave, galvanic skin response, respiratory capacity and the scale of pain and psychological questionnaires is a unique support in the complex assessment of patient's condition before, during and after the treatment. It has the following advantages over the traditional techniques (manual measurement environment): (1) option of using biocybernetic feedback and gamification in the extended diagnostics; (2) ability to control and evaluate the degree of spinal and lumbo-pelvic-hip curves; (3) control of the body symmetry in the frontal and transverse plane; (4) assessment of temperature distribution on the surface of the back as the element of correction training quality control; (5) evaluation of psychophysical condition with particular focus on physical condition during the exercises, which determines patient's activity and engagement; (6) immediate access to the wide spectrum of diagnostic parameters to detect threats, design and evaluate the therapy; (7) use of behavioral biometrics in therapy and to navigate the gamification module. Introduction of completely new measuring techniques significantly improves the quality of diagnosis.

Using the D4S diagnostic module enables:

1. Diagnosis of posture in children and youths during screening tests performed in kindergartens, schools, summer camps, sanatoriums;
2. Diagnosis of posture in children and youths during diagnostic examinations in doctors' and physiotherapists' offices. Such diagnostics will allow to assess:

   - projection of the center of the body mass on the supporting plane, foot arch,
   - position of the heel bones in the frontal plane to detect valgus and varus deformity,
   - positioning of knees in frontal, sagittal and horizontal plane,
   - the degree of pelvic tilt in sagittal plane and the degree of torsion,
   - the value of curvatures of the spine in sagittal and frontal plane,
   - the degree of rotation of spine and ribs,
   - positioning of the head in all planes,
   - the degree of activation of anterior abdominal muscles,
   - shape and mobility of the thorax,
   - the degree of body symmetry.

3. Determination of norms for measurements performed with D4S;
4. Development of the patient's profile and calculation, based on its parameters (like age, gender, body built, maturity, potential inherited traits), of probability of developing postural defect within the next 2 years and scheduling the date of the next visit;
5. Creation of database with information about the postures of children and youths, which would enable creation of standards and centiles describing the ranges of correct values obtained in D4S measurements;
6. Identification of critical moments to the development of postural defects and identification of prodromes (sudden changes in the body mass, vertebral asymmetry, change of spine curvature in sagittal plane etc.);
7. Regular monitoring development of children and youths in order to identify the moment critical for developing postural defect.

Therapeutic module for therapy and exercises in the standing position is equipped in components to assess functioning of lower limbs, pelvis, pectoral girdle, head and spine. The lower part of the device is used to evaluate for the foot arch in widely accepted and proven tests, the performance of which will be verified for the D4S using known measurements. It is also used to evaluate functioning of the lower limbs muscles by measuring the forces resulting from the contact between feet and the floor. The unique, innovative construction enables activation of the spiral mechanism of the lower limbs, which is one of the key elements of positioning lower body part, including pelvis.

The measuring components on the platforms to measure the pressure of feet on the ground, and the software allow the performance of looped exercises and constant assessment of the quality of movement and objective evaluation of patient's commitment and progresses. Thank to this approach, the patient may observe on the terminal (patient's screen) the results of their actions in the independent feedback and engages in improving thereof, while the therapist may observe the quality of patient's activities in the real time. Another therapeutic achievement is the innovative pelvis measuring clip. The original system of fixing the clip on the pelvis allows constant monitoring its angular position in sagittal, frontal and horizontal plane. The clip controls and supports optimal positioning of the pelvis in sagittal plane and during the therapy, it gradually restricts this movement increasing the lumbar-pelvic-hip stability. The measuring sensors and the gamification system are the components activating motor abilities of the pelvis, especially in terms of improving its stability, strength and functioning of pelvic floor muscles and muscles controlling the position of the pelvis.

Shoulder clip enables summary evaluation, activation and therapy of the upper parts of torso and head. The elements of this clip are equipped in sensors to measure the angular positioning of the pectoral girdle and evaluate the functioning of muscles in the torso area. Collaboration of the clip components with the lower clip and the ground will allow to optimize the position of the body. In this way, we can activate muscles responsible for reversing kyphosis and strengthen the paraspinal structures which regulate the relations between the pectoral sector of the spine and scapulae. The ability to generate small movements enables activation of deep stabilizers which can be treated in a way similar to NEURAC method. Posture rehabilitation module is the therapeutic cage to perform the set of correction exercises in the standing position, based on the latest solutions, in particular biofeedback with computer acquisition and data processing (biocybernetic feedback). Regular performance of the series of stabilizing exercises based on the training of short, one-joint muscles responsible for motor control and training of posture control systems. The evidence base for functioning of the station is building and then consolidating the posture, starting from the lower body parts, through positioning of feet and knees, optimization of the pelvis position, anti-gravity activation of the spine and positioning the thorax and the head. The original concept of static and dynamic exercises using the biocybernetic feedback in the therapy of postural dysfunctions may influence the course of rehabilitation and optimize the therapy in many ways. The device construction enables evaluation and training of moments of forces acting on the area of pectoral gridle, head and lumbo-pelvic-hip complex, along with monitoring the intra-abdominal pressure. The advantages are: targeted application and diverse diagnostic during the therapy, access to successively updated data warehouse, reasoning based on the original mathematic models, validation in the original data acquisition system and verification of diagnoses in the computer aided decision making system. The ability to monitor the effectiveness of the training with multi-plane assessment of the positioning of the pectoral gridle, thorax and lumbo-pelvic-hip complex. Greater effectiveness (expected as shorter rehabilitation time with the same durability of results) will be achieved thanks to optimization of the working conditions. These conditions are ensured by: assessment of the moments of forces of muscles responsible for the mobility of the lumbo-pelvic-hip complex and pectoral girdle, forces rotating the lower limbs inside and outside, muscles stabilizing the position of the head and influencing the range of neck mobility, assessment of functioning of muscles actively expanding the spine and evaluation and control of intra-abdominal pressure and its role in spinal stabilization and activity of anterior and lateral abdominal muscles.

Application of the therapeutic module allows to:

1. Correct postural defects;
2. Support rehabilitation process;
3. Optimize therapeutic procedure;
4. Introduce special set of exercises for children in corsets and after surgeries;
5. Use special exercise program for children prepared to surgeries, through preparation and optimization of thoracic functions, strengthening muscles which stabilize the posture, especially at anti-gravity level;
6. Verify the adequacy of exercises early and on the regular basis;
7. Monitor the quality and effectiveness of the correction methods used;
8. Correct scoliosis:

   – resistance-based reduction of scoliotic curvatures;
   – stretching muscles cramped on the concave side of spine curvature.

7 Summary

D4S System of Dynamic Individual Stimulation and Control for Spine and Posture Interactive Rehabilitation is an ultra innovative, world-class product. Until now, we found no other, so complex devices (market analysis, patent clearance) which would perform diagnostic and therapeutic functions for postural defects and, at the same time, include an advanced IT platform to support the decision making process of therapists by personalizing and standardizing procedures applied to patients (Table 1). The project assumptions included using the latest solutions in both, the diagnostic and therapeutic module. In addition to the whole spectrum of anthropometric and medical measurements, the system offers the possibility to use behavioral biometrics to design the therapy and evaluate psychophysical condition of patients. Exercises based on biocybernetic feedback or controlled gamification module have wide application. The therapy also uses the latest, well documented therapeutic concepts such as: activating the spiral functional mechanism of the lower limbs, strengthening muscles responsible for deep stabilization, activating muscles responsible for the extension mechanism, activating primary spine stabilizers, stabilizing exercises based on the training of short, one-joint muscles responsible for motor control and training of posture control systems, activation of anti-gravity muscles responsible for the quality of posture at all functional levels, functional therapy based on the concepts of musculofascial chains. So far on the market, only diagnostic (e.g. Diers, Diasu, Mora) [14] or only therapeutic (e.g. FED or Skolas) [13, 17] systems have been available. The advantage of D4S is the relatively low purchase cost and the unique diagnostic and therapeutic functionalities. The authors are convinced that the system will contribute to the development of new diagnostic and therapeutic standards, and will meet the civilizational challenge of early prevention of postural defect in children and youth as well as pain within the musculoskeletal system in adults.

Table 1 Selected functionalities of therapeutic and diagnostic methods

Method	Built-in diagnostics	Monitoring of parameters during therapeutic session	Active database	Muscular chain stimulation, movement habits	Segment exercises	Static exercises	Locomotor exercises	Three plane effect	Deep stabilization exercises	Exteroreceptor training
D4S	+	+	+	+	+	+	+	+	+	+
Mezieres	-	-	-	+	+	+	+	+	-	-
Feldenkrais	-	-	-	+	-	+	+	+	+	-
Pilates	-	-	-	+	+	+	+	+	+	+
Rolfing	-	-	-	-	+	+	-	+	-	-
Spiraldynamik	-	-	-	+	+	+	+	+	+	+
Spiral stabilization	-	-	-	+	+	-	+	+	+	-
Diers	+	+	+	-	-	-	-	-	-	-
Diasu	+	+	+	-	-	-	-	-	-	-

8   Conclusions

The widely understood problem of human health, functionality of our body and brain is inseparable from the quality of body posture and the way we express ourselves through movement. Postural changes and increasingly frequent postural disorders are connected with the observed civilizational progress. The results of sedentary lifestyles, excessive use of electronic gadgets contribute to the occurrence of postural problems and more frequent degenerative changes and pain within the musculoskeletal system and all its consequences. Correction of posture and our mobility patterns becomes the growing challenge of our times. The model of diagnostic and therapeutic procedure based on the **D4S System of Dynamic Individual Stimulation and Control for Spine and Posture Interactive Rehabilitation** is an attempt to set new diagnostic and therapeutic standards, and to meet the civilizational challenge of early prevention of postural defect in children and youth as well as pain within the musculoskeletal system in adults. It is the modern system which utilizes professional knowledge and experience of experts in many fields. D4S is an integrated biomechatronic system enabling: (a) diagnosis prior to rehabilitation, (b) real time therapy monitoring, and (c) personalization of therapeutic activities focusing on spinal conditions and postural disorders. The D4S system is currently in the course of clinical trials.

Acknowledgements The study was realized within the project "DISC4SPINE dynamic individual stimulation and control for spine and posture interactive rehabilitation" (grant no. POIR.04.01.02-00-0082/17-00).

References

1. Arystoteles, P.: Fizyka. O niebie. O powstaniu i niszczeniu. Meteorologika. O świecie. Metafizyka. In: Dzieła wszystkie, vol. 2. PWN (In Polish) (2003)
2. Burns, K., Wade, M.: The Posture Principles: Posture by Design not by Circumstance. Rethink Press Great Britain (2018)
3. Crow, W.T., Willis, D.R.: Estimating cost of care for patients with acute low back pain: a retrospective review of patient records. J. Amer. Osteopath. Assoc. **109**(4), 229–233 (2009)
4. Carini, F., Mazzola, M., Fici, C., Palmeri, S., Messina, M., Damiani, P., Tomasello, G.: Posture and posturology, anatomical and physiological profiles: overview and current state of art. Acta bio-medica: Atenei Parmensis **88**(1), 11 (2017)
5. Christensen, S.T., Hartvigsen, J.: Spinal curves and health: a systematic critical review of the epidemiological literature dealing with associations between sagittal spinal curves and health. J. Manip. Physiol. Ther. **31**(9), 690–714 (2008)
6. Czaprowski, D., Stoliński, Ł., Tyrakowski, M., Kozinoga, M., Kotwicki, T.: Non-structural misalignments of body posture in the sagittal plane. Scoliosis Spinal Disord. **13**(1), 6 (2018)
7. Deed, H., DC1, Betz, J,. Ferrantelli, J.: Sagittal spinal curves and health. J. Vertebr. Subluxation Res. **31**, 1–8 (2009)
8. Dischiavi, S.L., Wright, A.A., Hegedus, E.J., Bleakley, C.M.: Biotensegrity and myofascial chains: a global approach to an integrated kinetic chain. Med. Hypotheses **110**, 90–96 (2018)

9. Feldenkrais, M.: Body and Mature Behaviour: A Study of Anxiety, Sex, Gravitation and Learning. Routledge, Abingdon (2013)
10. Silva Filho, J.N.D., Gurgel, J.L., Porto, F.: Effects of stretching exercises for posture correction: systematic review. Man. Ther. Posturol. Rehabil. J. **12**, 265–272 (2015)
11. Simon, L.S.: Relieving pain in America: a blueprint for transforming prevention, care, education, and research. J. Pain Palliat. Care Pharmacother. **26**(2), 197–198 (2012)
12. Jacobson, E.: Structural integration: origins and development. J. Altern. Complement. Med. **17**(9), 775–780 (2011)
13. Kamelska-Sadowska, A.M., Protasiewicz-Fałdowska, H., Zakrzewska, L., Zaborowska-Sapeta, K., Nowakowski, J.J., Kowalski, I.M.: The effect of an innovative biofeedback SKOL-AS^R on the body posture and trunk rotation in children with idiopathic scoliosis-preliminary study. Medicina **55**(6), 254 (2019)
14. Książek-Czekaj, A., Wiecheć, M., Śliwiński, G., Śliwiński, Z.: Monitoring the results of scoliosis improvement using the Diers system. Fizjoter Pol **16**(3), 124–134 (2016)
15. Larsen, C.: Footloose and Pain Free: Spiraldynamik ^{R}: a long term strategy to Keep your feet healthy. Georg Thieme Verlag (2013)
16. Larsen, C., Miescher, B.: Spiraldynamik^R Becoming and remaining pain-free and flexible. Georg Thieme Verlag (2009)
17. Nisser, J., Smolenski, U., Sliwinski, G. E., Schumann, P., Heinke, A., Malberg, H., Werner M., Elsner S., Drossel W. G., Sliwinski Z., Derlien, S.: The FED-Method (Fixation, Elongation, Derotation)-a Machine-supported Treatment Approach to Patients with Idiopathic Scoliosis-Systematic Review. Zeitschrift für Orthopädie und Unfallchirurgie (2019)
18. Paolucci, T., Attanasi, C., Cecchini, W., Marazzi, A., Capobianco, S.V., Santilli, V.: Chronic low back pain and postural rehabilitation exercise: a literature review. J. Pain Res. **12**, 95 (2019)
19. Peterson, J.: Teaching Pilates for postural faults, illness and injury: a practical guide, 1e (2009)
20. Qaseem, A., Wilt, T.J., McLean, R.M., Forciea, M.A.: Noninvasive treatments for acute, sub-acute, and chronic low back pain: a clinical practice guideline from the American College of Physicians. Ann. Int. Med. **166**, 514–530 (2017)
21. Rolf, I.P.: Rolfing: The integration of human structures. D. Landman Pub. (1977)
22. Rosario, J.L.: Understanding muscular chains-a review for clinical application of chain stretching exercises aimed to correct posture. EC Orthop. **5**(6), 209–234 (2017)
23. Rosario, J.L.: What is Posture? A review of the literature in search of a definition. EC Orthop.**6**, 111–133 (2017)
24. Richter, P., Hebgen, E., Safrończyk, K., Gieremek, K.: Punkty spustowe i łańcuchy mięśniowo-powięziowe w osteopatii i terapii manualnej. Galaktyka (In Polish) (2014)
25. Smíšek, R., Smíšková, K., Smíšková, Z.: Muscle chains. Manual techniques, Movement Therapy (2016)
26. Smith, J.: Strukturalna praca z ciałem. WSEiT (In Polish) (2014)

Methods of Therapy of Scoliosis and Technical Functionalities of DISC4SPINE (D4S) Diagnostic and Therapeutic System

Tomasz Szurmik, Karol Bibrowicz, Anna Lipowicz, and Andrzej W. Mitas

Abstract Evidence is being found for the diversity of factors which can cause scoliosis. These factors range from a lifestyle to genes and intracellular phenomena taking place in human body. To treat idiopathic scoliosis, different equipment and kinesiotherapy exercises are used. If preventive methods prove ineffective, or sometimes parallel to them, orthopedic solutions are applied, such as innovative braces or less and less invasive surgeries and materials which grow with the patient and allow to avoid next surgical interventions in the future. In this paper D4S method is presented. It enables active therapy of scoliosis and postural disorders in three planes. It includes a diagnostic module for complex diagnosis of the body posture and scoliosis, using a wide range of parameters. It also allows to monitor the patient during the therapeutic session and the "Database" module enables archiving and optimization of therapy procedure, which may improve its effectiveness.

Keywords Idiopathic scoliosis · Vertebral rotation · Therapeutic methods · Disc4Spine · D4S

T. Szurmik (✉)
University of Silesia in Katowice, Katowice, Poland
e-mail: info@orto-med.com.pl

K. Bibrowicz
Science and Research Center of Body Posture, Kazimiera Milanowska College of Education and Therapy, Poznań, Poland
e-mail: bibrowicz@wp.pl

A. Lipowicz
Department of Anthropology, Wrocław University of Environmental and Life Sciences, Wrocław, Poland
e-mail: LipowiczAnna@gmail.com

A. W. Mitas
Department of Informatics and Medical Equipment, Faculty of Biomedical Engineering, Silesian University of Technology, Gliwice, Poland
e-mail: andrzej.mitas@polsl.pl

© The Editor(s) (if applicable) and The Author(s), under exclusive license to Springer Nature Switzerland AG 2021
E. Piętka et al. (eds.), *Information Technology in Biomedicine*, Advances in Intelligent Systems and Computing 1186, https://doi.org/10.1007/978-3-030-49666-1_16

1 Introduction

With the development of expertise and as a result of scientific discoveries, we can observe how definitions of scoliosis evolve [1]. Scoliosis is considered a sideways curve of the spine with accompanying spinal and thoracic twist and disturbed sagittal profile [2, 3]. It is also known that scoliosis is not limited to the frontal plane and is described as "three-dimensional deformity of the spinal column and thorax". It causes spinal curvatures in the frontal plane, axial twist and disturbance of curves in the sagittal plane [4, 5]. Among many known and described classifications of scoliosis, the simplest one is into: idiopathic and non-idiopathic. It is believed that *"scoliosis is a general term covering a heterogenous group of diseases involving alterations in the shape and positioning of the spine"*. Due to the lack of precise definition of *scoliosis*, it is recommended to use it together with a relevant describing adjective. Thus, we can identify the following types of scoliosis:

- **functional scoliosis**—the cause is secondary and beyond the spine, this may be due, for example, result from a shorter lower limb or asymmetric tone of the paraspinal muscles. It usually subsides or decreases when the cause is removed (e.g. when lying) [6];
- **structural scoliosis**—characterized by fixed liaisons in the built, structure and position of the vertebrae and intervertebral discs and fixed liaisons within the muscular-ligamentous apparatus [7];
- **idiopathic scoliosis** (spontaneous)—type of structural scoliosis with no clear causal factor [8–10]. Some of the characteristics are: spinal deformity in three planes, distortion of physiological lumbar lordosis and thoracic kyphosis, vertebral rotation and rib prominence. Other diagnostic features of idiopathic scoliosis include: development during adolescence, tendency to worsening during growth spurts, more frequent occurrence in girls. Untreated, it may lead to severe deformations of the body as well as limited chest functioning and exercise capacity. They can significantly decrease the quality of life. Regardless of type, scoliosis is diagnosed when deformation of the spine is at least 100 in Cobb scale [6, 7, 11, 12].

Research into the causes of idiopathic scolioses cover different aspects [13–23]. Relationships are investigated between scoliosis and genetic [24–26] or hormonal [27] factors, connective tissue disorders [28] and structural and functional disorders of certain parts of the locomotor system [3, 29–31].

The aim of the paper is to present methods used in treatment of scoliosis using the therapeutic functionalities of the innovative methods called Dynamic Individual Stimulation and Control For Spine and Posture Interactive Rehabilitation—D4S.

2 Definitions of Key Therapeutic Needs

Inability to identify clear causal factor for scoliosis results in mainly symptomatic treatment being applied, which focuses mainly on the biomechanical and neurophysiological aspects of defects. In 2004, an international Society of Scoliosis Orthopedic Rehabilitation and Treatment (SOSORT) [7], gathering all groups of therapists engaged in scoliosis treatment was founded. It focuses on the development of preventive methods of scoliosis therapy, unification of training curricula based on medical evidence and development of therapeutic guidelines. At present, therapeutic programs in the majority of the so called "schools" or methods of conservative treatment of scoliosis are compliant with the SOSORT principles and fulfill a joint mission to provide the best orthopedic, physiotherapeutic, orthotic and psychosocial care for people with lateral scoliosis and their families. According to SOSORT guidelines, exercises used in therapy of scoliosis are described as physiotherapy specific scoliosis exercises (PSSE). Their effectiveness is constantly evaluated. The results show that PSSE may be an effective therapy method for patients with mild and moderate defects [32–36].

SOSORT has defined the main goals of the complex conservative treatment of idiopathic scoliosis:

1. To stop curve progression at puberty (or possibly even reduce it);
2. To prevent or treat respiratory dysfunction;
3. To prevent or treat spinal pain syndromes;
4. To improve aesthetics via postural correction.

SOSORT experts agree that PSSE should include:

1. Auto-correction in 3D;
2. Training in activities of daily living (ADL);
3. Stabilizing the corrected posture;
4. Patient education.

Therapists in many countries develop their own conservative treatment methods and procedures. But they all accept the guidelines set by SOSORT. Poland has contributed significantly to the process of developing and implementation of methods of conservative treatment of scoliosis. These methods are: Dobomed [37], Individual Functional Therapy of Scoliosis FITS [38] and recently developed therapy using the D4S system.

3 Therapeutic Methods and Approach to Patients in the Context of Selected Causes of Spinal Disorders

Therapy of lateral spinal dysfunctions is still relevant and unsolved medical issue. On the one hand, we can observe the development of more and more advanced surgery techniques, on the other hand, there is a strong emphasis on the conservative treatment of scolioses. The "wait and observe" concept recommended by part of the orthopedic community raises doubts when it comes to therapy of children. Waiting and observing how a minor curve of 10–25° develops until a surgery is possible, meets with the protests of parents of sick children as well as practitioners, physiotherapists and orthotics specialists, involved in the treatment process [35].

4 Non-surgical Scoliosis Treatment and Rehabilitation Methods—Characteristics of Selected Methods of Scoliosis Therapy

In severe spinal curvatures, surgery may be applied [39]. The goal is to stop the progressing scoliosis. Other, non-surgical treatment method is bracing. Improvement of brace structures and surgical procedures is a separate and quite wide field which develops along with the increasing state of knowledge. Braces are ever lighter, surgeries involving placing implants in the spine evolve towards implant which grow with the patient as to avoid future surgical interventions.

In non-surgical therapy and rehabilitation of scolioses, one or more of the following therapeutic methods can be used:

1. Lyon Method (France)—is one of the oldest therapeutic methods [40]. Its most recent history dates back to the middle of the 20th century. Constantly modernized and developed, it combines kinesitherapy and bracing. New types of braces are designed, such as ARTbrace (Asymmetrical Rigid Torsion Brace). Kinesitherapy involves three-dimensional mobilization of the spine, mobilization of the iliopsoas muscle (lumbar scoliosis) and daily activity training including correction of sitting position. The Lyon method also aims at improving patient's emotional condition, strengthening motivation, education, improving the movement range, neuromuscular control, better coordination and strengthening spine stabilizers.
2. Schroth Method (Germany)—developed in 1920 by Katherina Schroth, the most popular method in Germany [41]. It is one of the most known and documented of conservative scoliosis treatment methods. Studies revealed many positive results of therapy using this specific approach to scoliosis. Due to its dynamic development and over 2,500 certified therapists, is has its advocates all over the world. Schroth system is based on the classification of the body into the so called "blocks". They show deformations of torso as alteration of this geometrical form: from rectangular into trapezoid. This classification is the grounds for designing the therapy. The principles of using Schroth method in therapy base on the SOSORT guidelines. The goal of individual and group exercises is:

   – proactive spinal corrections to avoid surgery,
   – postural training to avoid or decelerate progression,
   – information to support a decision-making process,
   – teaching a home-exercise program,

- support self-correction,
- prevention and coping strategies for pain.

An important element is special, specific breathing method—Rotation Angular Breathing (RAB).

3. SEAS Method (Scientific Exercises Approach to Scoliosis) (Italy)— individualized scientific approach to conservative scoliosis treatment developed based on the latest research and constantly evolving as new results are published in the literature [42]. It originates from the Lyon concept. It was invented by Michele Romano and Alessandra Negrini from Instituto Scientifico Italiani Colonna Vertebrale (ISICO). The method focuses on regaining postural control and improving spinal stability through exercises and active, three-dimensional correction. The main therapeutic goal of SEAS is to improve spinal stability. Other objectives are: improvement of postural balance, preserving the physiological positioning of the spine in sagittal plane, preventing curve progression, improved functioning of the respiratory system and improved quality of patients' life. The most visible difference between SEAS and other methods is the fact that no exercise is considered better than others. The goal of SEAS method is not only curvature correction but also complex postural rehabilitation. Muscle endurance strengthening exercises, training to maintain correct position, development of balance reactions and neuromotor integration is combined with exercises on unstable grounds, orthoptic exercises involving binocular vision or correction during global movement, for example when patients learn to walk properly.

4. BSPTS Method (Barcelona Scoliosis Physical Therapy School) (Spain)—concept derived from the principles developed by Katherina Schroth [43]. The treatment is based on integral scoliosis care which involves specific education, observation and intervention, bracing according to Rigo-Cheneau principles and surgical procedure. BSPTS may be described as the plan of therapy through cognitive, sensory-motor and kinesthetic training to teach patients how to correct posture and curvatures.

5. Dobomed Method (Poland)—developed in 1979 by Prof. Krystyna Dobosiewicz [37, 44]. It originated from the principles of Klapp and Schroth methods. It is a biodynamic three-dimensional self-correction method based on the pathomechanics of idiopathic scoliosis. The main Dobomed concept is active correction involving original mobilization of a curvature, with particular focus on "kyphotization" of the thoracic spine and/or "lordotization" of the lumbar spine. The goal is to stabilize and correct spinal deformations and to prevent progression and/or reduce the curvature, improve general functioning, especially of the respiratory system, thanks to carefully selected techniques of asymmetrical breathing.

6. Side Shift (United Kingdom), created by Tony Betts, conservative treatment method is based on the approach by Dr. Min Mehta who said that scoliosis can be stabilized through lateral trunk shifts. Side Shift approach also uses the assumptions of the Schroth method and SOSORT guidelines. The goal of the method is active correction of spinal curve through side shifts movements of the trunk

towards the concavity. Breathing exercises used in Schroth method are included as well as myofascial release techniques [45].

7. Functional Individual Therapy of Scoliosis (FITS) (Poland)—based upon integration of elements selected from various therapeutic approaches that have been adapted and modified to form a different scoliosis treatment concept [38]. The most important FITS exercise mechanisms are:

   (a) Sensory-motor balance training to improve nervous system control over muscle function;
   (b) Mobilization and release of myofascial structures that limit three-plane corrective movements;
   (c) Three-plane corrective breathing to improve derotation and breathing mechanism;
   (d) Neuromuscular re-education;
   (e) Auto-correction in activities of daily living.

8. Global postural re-education GRP (France)—developed by Philippe E. Souchard, this therapeutic approach sees human body in general [46]. The method aims at reduction of postural deformations, regaining symmetry of back muscles and correct posture through active muscle stretching, control exercises and sensory integration. It includes both, -recreating the static function which determines body posture and dynamic function. The key to this method is global work with harmoniously acting muscles which form neuromuscular coordination chains. Stretching a muscle or a group of muscles creates compensations and forces global tension.

5   D4S in Therapy—Methods, Duration and Technical Grounds in the Context of Therapeutic Expectations

D4S (Poland)—guidelines for conservative treatment for idiopathic scoliosis developed by SOSORT experts as well as thorough analysis of the existing therapeutic achievements and evaluation of the threats related to postural correction and conservative treatment for scoliosis motivated specialists from the Faculty of Biomedical Engineering of the Silesian University of Technology, Faculty of Physiotherapy of the Jerzy Kukuczka Academy of Physical Education in Katowice and Meden-InMed company to design a complex diagnostic and therapeutic system for widely understood therapy of postural disorders and scolioses (D4S). The system was developed based fully on SOSORT guidelines and its functionalities include:

1. Full diagnostics and constant therapy monitoring;
2. Correction of static postural disorders in sagittal plane;
3. Three-dimension scoliosis correction;
4. Functional correction during daily activities (walking, sitting);
5. Stabilization of the corrected posture;

6. Correction of dysfunctions connected with distorted binocular vision and dysfunctions of the temporomandibular joints;
7. Education of patients.

D4S system is developed by an interdisciplinary team of specialists. D4S device combines diagnostic and therapeutic functions and enables monitoring of movements in the real time. Its modular structure allows gradual implementation of different functions depending on the needs and capacity of a given therapy unit. The first module is clearly diagnostic, based on the latest scientific findings. It enables quick diagnosis of potential defects and identification of its parameters which are then used for further monitoring and collecting the scientific data. The second module is a therapeutic cage for correction exercises performed in the standing position. The exercises address mainly dysfunctions in sagittal plane and have been designed based on the latest solutions, especially stabilizing exercises involving training of short, one-joint muscles responsible for motor control. The third module is a station for advanced exercise based on the "Pression" concept, performed while kneeling on all fours. These exercises are original Polish contribution to conservative treatment for scoliosis [47]. The modules, single or as a set, facilitate effective therapy applied under the supervision of physiotherapists or orthopedists. As for the technical side, D4S may be used within telemedicine networks, as they not only allow to explore huge amounts of data but also provide remote access to specialist help.

Measurement results stored in its database will be used to:

1. Monitor progress of the therapy;
2. Determine postural characteristics of persons at greater risk of postural defects;
3. Adapt individual set of rehabilitation exercises according to the psychosomatic profile of the patient;
4. Identify epidemiologically dominating developmental postural disorders;
5. Search for causal relationships to apply proper prevention procedures.

Successively expanded database will allow to determine the range of variability of the certain body and posture parameters, mobility and how they change during the therapy. Data exploration performed as data mining will reveal previously hidden correlations, which will facilitate selection of right exercises for the next patients. D4S is based on the original algorithms of work of the diagnostic-rehabilitation set, developed upon the original concept of methodology which is adapted to developmental age and patient's physique, and considers the effectiveness of exercises, analysis of the psycho-physical condition of the patient and the principles of virtual gamification. The system includes an online platform to operate the computer aided measuring system which registers anthropometric, behavioral, diagnostic and therapeutic data. Legally secured data warehouse will be successively updated with the results of longitudinal and cross-sectional research, thus functioning as an IT database for individual treatment and therapy monitoring. Patient assumes the kneeling position which eliminates the action of gravity on the spinal axis. Active heads are positioned accordingly on the tops of curvature arches to derotate and correct through moments released from the forces. For S-curve scoliosis, it is possible to treat two curvatures in three planes at the same time, what improves therapy effectiveness. Additional advantage is breathing during exercise, which stimulated the position of chest.

Comparing the selected functionalities of therapeutic methods, we can conclude that patient management evolves with the development of knowledge about the causes of idiopathic scoliosis. Other important factor are test results which show the tangible benefits of the properly chosen conservative treatment. All the methods described above use exercises to activate muscle chains, exercises performed in three planes, exercises of the certain body segments and proprioceptive stimulation. Several of them, including D4S, enable therapy applied in movement, which yields the desired results during the daily activities. However, only D4S has a built-in diagnostic module used to determine the type of disorder and measure its parameters. It also provides the unique opportunity to monitor and evaluate different parameters during the therapeutic sessions. In addition, the function of collecting and storing the data obtained allows to design individual therapy according to the needs of the patient. The above description indicates that interdisciplinary approach to both, diagnostics and therapy is the natural direction of the development of research and therapeutic practice. In the age of civilizational development, an additional advantage of this trend is the collaboration of specialists from different fields, which facilitates multi-aspect therapeutic activities and, consequently, more effective prevention of locomotor system and posture disorders and scolioses.

6 Summary

To summarize, methods used to treat idiopathic scoliosis involve stopping or decreasing the symptoms, neuromuscular stimulation through activation of the muscular chains and proprioceptive, respiratory and mechanical stimulation of the vertebral bodies. This results from the known symptoms of scoliosis. D4S methods offers all functions of other therapeutic methods used in conservative treatment for idiopathic scolioses (Table 1). It includes the mechanical aspect of spinal dysfunctions in three planes, using specially designed heads. It also enables simultaneous correction of 2 curves in three planes. The standing module facilitates selective or complex exercises of postural muscles through proprioceptive stimulation. Various sensors register muscle strength, tone and temperature and spatial positioning of the spine and the whole motor system. This provides the opportunity to design therapy programs for different dysfunctions, based on the data collected in the database. The D4S system is currently in the course of clinical trials.

Table 1 Selected functionalities of therapeutic and diagnostic methods

Method	Built-in diagnostics	Monitoring of parameters during therapeutic session	Active database	Muscular chain stimulation, movement habits	Segment exercises	Static exercises	Locomotor exercises	Three plane effect	Proprioception
D4S	+	+	+	+	+	+	+	+	+
Lyon	−	−	−	+	+	+	−	+	+
Schroth	−	−	−	+	+	+	−	+	+
SEAS	−	−	−	+	+	+	+	+	+
BSTS	−	−	−	+	+	+	−	+	+
Dobomed	−	−	−	+	+	+	−	+	+
Side shift	−	−	−	+	+	+	−	+	+
FITS	−	−	−	+	+	+	+	+	+
GRP	−	−	−	+	+	+	+	+	+

7 Conclusions

1. Early diagnosis and therapy is crucial for idiopathic scoliosis therapy.
2. Multi-aspect treatment including neuromotorics, movement habits, muscle chains and proprioception enables complex reaction to this undesirable body condition.
3. Due to the use of various sensors, D4S is an innovative diagnostic tool.
4. Measuring different parameters during the therapy allows constant and long-term validation and proper selection of therapeutic parameters.

Acknowledgements The study was realized within the project "DISC4SPINE dynamic individual stimulation and control for spine and posture interactive rehabilitation" (grant no. POIR.04.01.02-00-0082/17-00).

 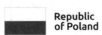 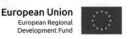

References

1. Kohler, R., Rey, J.C., Zayni, R.: Historical survey of scoliosis treatment. In: Mary, P., Vialle, R., Guigui, P. (eds.) La scoliose idiopathque de l'enfant, pp. 1–15. Elsevier Masson, Paris (2009)
2. Stokes, I.A.F.: Die Biomechanik des Rumpfes. In: Weiss, H.R. (ed.) Wirbelsäulendeformitäten – Konservatives Management, pp. 59–77. Pflaum, München (2003)
3. Stokes, I.A., Burwell, R.G., Dangerfield, P.H.: Biomechanical spinal growth modulation and progressive adolescent scoliosis - a test of the 'vicious cycle' pathogenetic hypothesis: summary of an electronic focus group debate of the IBSE. Scoliosis **1**, 16 (2006). https://doi.org/10.1186/1748-7161-1-16. [PMID: 17049077]
4. Grivas, T.B., Vasiliadis, E.S., Rodopoulos, G., Bardakos, N.: The role of the intervertebral disc in correction of scoliotic curves. A theoretical model of idiopathic scoliosis pathogenesis. Stud. Health Technol. Inform. **140**, 33–36 (2008)
5. Somerville, E.W.: Rotational lordosis: the development of the single curvature. J. Bone Jt. Surg. **34B**, 421–427 (1952)
6. Kotwicki, T., Durmała, J., Czaprowski, D., Głowacki, M., Kołban, M., Snela, S., Śliwiński, Z., Kowalski, I.M.: Zasady leczenia nieoperacyjnego skolioz idiopatycznych - wskazówki oparte o zalecenia SOSORT 2006 (society on scoliosis orthopaedic and rehabilitation treatment). Ortop. Traumatol. Rehabil. **11**(5), 379–412 (2009)
7. Negrini, S., Grivas, T.B., Kotwicki, T., Maruyama, T., Rigo, M., Weiss, H.R.: Why do we treat adolescent idiopathic scoliosis? What we want to obtain and to avoid for our patients. SOSORT 2005 consensus paper. Scoliosis **1**, 4 (2006)
8. Negrini, S., Aulisa, A.G., Aulisa, L., Circo, A.B., de Mauroy, J.C., Durmala, J., Grivas, T.B., Knott, P., Kotwicki, T., Maruyama, T., Minozzi, S., O'Brien, J.P., Papadopoulos, D., Rigo, M., Rivard, Ch.H., Romano, M., Wynne, J.H., Villagrasa, M., Weiss, H.R., Zaina, F.: 2011 SOSORT guidelines: orthopaedic and rehabilitation treatment of idiopathic scoliosis during growth. Scoliosis **7**, 3 (2012). https://doi.org/10.1186/1748-7161-7-3. Accessed 20 Jan 2012
9. Parent, S., Newton, P.O., Wenger, D.R.: Adolescent idiopathic scoliosis: etiology, anatomy, natural history and bracing. Instr. Course Lect. **54**, 529–536 (2005)
10. Roaf, R.: The basic anatomy of scoliosis. J. Bone. Jt. Surg. Br. **48**(4), 786–792 (1966). [PMID: 5953815]

11. Lenke, L.G., Edwards, C.C., Bridwell, K.H.: The Lenke classification of adolescent idiopathic scoliosis: how it organizes curve patterns as a template to perform selective fusions of the spine. Spine 28(20), S199–S207 (2003)
12. Weiss, H.R., Negrini, S., Hawes, M.C., Rigo, M., Kotwicki, T., Grivas, T.B., Maruyama, T., Members of the SOSORT.: Physical exercises in the treatment of idiopathic scoliosis at risk of brace treatment - SOSORT consensus paper. Scoliosis 1, 6 (2006). https://doi.org/10.1186/1748-7161-1-6. Accessed 11 May 2006
13. Beaulieu, M., Toulotte, C., Gatto, L., Rivard, C.H., Teasdale, N., Simoneau, M., et al.: Postural imbalance in non-treated adolescent idiopathic scoliosis at different periods of progression. Eur. Spine J. 18, 38–44 (2009)
14. Cheung, J., Halbertsma, J.P., Veldhuizen, A.G., Sluiter, W.J., Maurits, N.M., Cool, J.C., et al.: A preliminary study on electromyographic analysis of the paraspinal musculature in idiopathic scoliosis. Eur. Spine J. 14, 130–137 (2005)
15. Fadzan, M., Saltikov, J.B.: Etiological theories of adolescent idiopathic scoliosis: past and present. Open Orthop. J. 11(Suppl-9, M3), 1466–1489 (2017)
16. Fleming, A., Keynes, R.J., Tannahill, D.: The role of the notochord in vertebral column formation. J. Anat. 199, 177–180 (2001)
17. Patten, S.A., Moldovan, F.: Could genetic determinants of inner ear anomalies be a factor for the development of idiopathic scoliosis? Med. Hypotheses 76, 438–440 (2011)
18. Shi, L., Wang, D., Chu, W.C., Burwell, R.G., Freeman, B.J., Heng, P.A., et al.: Volume-based morphometry of brain MR images in adolescent idiopathic scoliosis and healthy control subjects. AJNR Am. J. Neuroradiol. 30, 1302–1307 (2009)
19. Shi, L., Wang, D., Chu, W.C., Burwell, G.R., Wong, T.T., Heng, P.A., et al.: Automatic MRI segmentation and morphoanatomy analysis of the vestibular system in adolescent idiopathic scoliosis. Neuroimage 54(Suppl 1), S180–S188 (2011)
20. Simoneau, M., Lamothe, V., Hutin, E., Mercier, P., Teasdale, N., Blouin, J.: Evidence for cognitive vestibular integration impairment in idiopathic scoliosis patients. BMC Neurosci. 10, 102 (2009)
21. Siu King Cheung, C., Tak Keung Lee, W., Kit Tse, Y., Ping Tang, S., Man Lee, K., Guo, X., et al.: Abnormal peripubertal anthropometric measurements and growth pattern in adolescent idiopathic scoliosis: a study of 598 patients. Spine (Philadelphia, PA, 1976) 28, 2152–2157 (2003)
22. White, A.A., Panjabi, M.M.: Practical biomechanics of scoliosis and kyphosis. Clinical Biomechanics of the Spine, 2nd edn. pp. 128–168. J.B. Lippincott Co., Philadelphia (1990). ISBN 0-397-50720-8
23. Yang, Z.D., Li, M.: There may be a same mechanism of the left-right handedness and left-right convex curve pattern of adolescent idiopathic scoliosis. Med. Hypotheses 76, 274–276 (2011)
24. Alden, K.J., Marosy, B., Nzegwu, N., Justice, C.M., Wilson, A.F., Miller, N.H.: Idiopathic scoliosis: identification of candidate regions on chromosome 19p13. Spine (Philadelphia, PA, 1976) 31, 1815–1819 (2006)
25. Edery, P., Margaritte-Jeannin, P., Biot, B., Labalme, A., Bernard, J.C., Chastang, J., et al.: New disease gene location and high genetic heterogeneity in idiopathic scoliosis. Eur. J. Hum. Genet. 19, 865–869 (2011)
26. Weiss, H.R.: Idiopathic scoliosis: how much of a genetic disorder? Report of five pairs of monozygotic twins. Dev. Neurorehabil. 10, 67–73 (2007)
27. Barrios, C., Cortes, S., Perez-Encinas, C., Escriva, M.D., Benet, I., Burgos, J., et al.: Anthropometry and body composition profile of girls with non surgically-treated adolescent idiopathic scoliosis. Spine 36(18), 1470–1477 (2011)
28. Hadley-Miller, N., Mims, B., Milewicz, D.M.: The potential role of the elastic fiber system in adolescent idiopathic scoliosis. J. Bone Jt. Surg. Am. 76, 1193–1206 (1994)
29. Czaprowski, D., Kotwicki, T., Pawłowska, P., Stoliński, L.: Joint hypermobility in children with idiopathic scoliosis: SOSORT award 2011 winner. Scoliosis 6, 22 (2011). https://doi.org/10.1186/1748-7161-6-22. [PMID: 21981906]

30. Hristova, G.I., Jarzem, P., Ouellet, J.A., Roughley, P.J., Epure, L.M., Antoniou, J., et al.: Calcification in human intervertebral disc degeneration and scoliosis. J. Orthop. Res. **29**, 1888–1895 (2011)
31. Kouwenhoven, J.W., Vincken, K.L., Bartels, L.W., Meij, B.P., Oner, F.C., Castelein, R.M.: Analysis of preexistent vertebral rotation in the normal quadruped spine. Spine (Philadelphia, PA, 1976) **31**, E754–E758 (2006)
32. Kuru, T., Yeldan, İ., Dereli, E.E., Özdinçler, A.R., Dikici, F., Çolak, İ.: The efficacy of three-dimensional Schroth exercises in adolescent idiopathic scoliosis: a randomised controlled clinical trial. Clin. Rehabil. **30**(2), 181–190 (2016)
33. Monticone, M., Ambrosini, E., Cazzaniga, D., Rocca, B., Ferrante, S.: Active self-correction and task-orientated exercises reduce spinal deformity and improve quality of life in subjects with mild adolescent idiopathic scoliosis. Results of a randomized controlled trial. Eur. Spine J. **23**(6), 1204–1214 (2014)
34. Negrini, S., et al.: 2016 SOSORT guidelines: orthopaedic and rehabilitation treatment of idiopathic scoliosis during growth. Scoliosis Spinal Disord. **13**, 3 (2018). https://doi.org/10.1186/s13013-017-0145-8
35. Schreiber, S., Parent, E.C., Hedden, D.M., Hill, D., Moreau, M.J., Lou, E., Watkins, E.M., Southon, S.C.: The effect of Schroth exercises added to the standard of care on the quality of life and muscle endurance in adolescents with idiopathic scoliosis - an assessor and statistician blinded randomized controlled trial: "SOSORT 2015 award winner". Scoliosis **10**, 24 (2015)
36. Williams, M.A., Heine, J.P., Williamson, E.M., Toye, F., Dritsaki, M., Petrou, S., Crossman, R., Lall, R., Barker, K.L., Fairbank, J., Harding, I., Gardner, A., Slowther, A.M., Coulson, N., Lamb, S.E.: Active treatment for idiopathic adolescent scoliosis (ACTIvATeS): a feasibility study. Health Technol. Assess. **19**(55) (2015)
37. Durmała, J.: Metoda Dobosiewicz (DoboMed). Rehabilitacja w Praktyce **1**, 25–27 (2009)
38. Białek, M.: Mild angle early onset idiopathic scoliosis children avoid progression under FITS method (functional individual therapy of scoliosis). Medicine (Baltimore) **94**(20), e863 (2015). https://doi.org/10.1097/MD.0000000000000863
39. Cardoso, M., Keating, R.F.: Neurosurgical management of spinal dysraphism and neurogenic scoliosis. Spine (Philadelphia, PA, 1976) **34**, 1775–1782 (2009)
40. De Mauroy, J.C., Journe, A., Gagaliano, F., Lecante, C., Barral, F., Pourret, S.: The new Lyon ART brace versus the historical Lyon brace: a prospective case series of 148 consecutive scoliosis with short time results after 1 year compared with a historical retrospective case series of 100 consecutive scoliosis; SOSORT award 2015 winner. Scoliosis **10**, 26 (2015). https://doi.org/10.1186/s13013-015-0047-6
41. Weiss, H.R.: The method of Katharina Schroth - history, principles and current development. Scoliosis **6**, 17 (2011)
42. Romano, M., Negrini, A., Parzini, S., Tavernaro, M., Zaina, F., Donzelli, S., Negrini, S.: SEAS (scientific exercises approach to scoliosis): a modern and effective evidence based approach to physiotherapic specific scoliosis exercises. Scoliosis **10**, 3 (2015). https://doi.org/10.1186/s13013-014-0027-2
43. Rigo, M., Quera-Salvá, G., Villagrasa, M., Ferrer, M., Casas, A., Corbella, C., Urrutia, A., Martínez, S., Puigdevall, N.: Scoliosis intensive out-patient rehabilitation based on Schroth method. Stud. Health Technol. Inform. **135**, 208–227 (2008)
44. Durmała, J., Kotwicki, T., Piotrowski, J.: Stabilization of progressive thoracic adolescent idiopathic scoliosis using brace treatment and DoboMed physiotherapy. Scoliosis **4**(Suppl 2), O29 (2009)
45. Muruyama, T., Takeshita, K., Kitagawa, T.: Side-shift exercise and hitch exercise. Stud. Health Technol. Inform. **135**, 246–249 (2008)
46. Souchard, P.E., Meli, O., Sgamma, D., Pillastrini, P.: Rieducazione posturale globale EMC (Elsevier Masson SAS, Paris). Med. Riabil. **16**(3), 1–10 (2009). https://doi.org/10.1016/S1283-078X(09)70207-X
47. Szurmik, T.: Koncepcja zachowawczego leczenia pacjentów ze skoliozą z użyciem specjalistycznych urządzeń. Zeszyty naukowe. BWST Żywiec. **T3**(1), 203–217

Methods for Assessing the Subject's Multidimensional Psychophysiological State in Terms of Proper Rehabilitation

Anna Mańka, Patrycja Romaniszyn, Monika N. Bugdol,
and Andrzej W. Mitas

Abstract The background of the work presented in this article is a method of monitoring the subject's psychophysical state during exercises. The essential context is the creation of a mechanism to prevent hyperactivity. Therefore, in the designed diagnostic and rehabilitation system continuous subject observation over time with the use of precise, not-burdening, and non-invasive measuring devices (Empatica E4) is proposed. For this purpose, a set of parameters was selected for Electrodermal Activity, Blood Volume Pulse, Heart Rate and Inter-Beats Interval signals to determine the subject's multimodal psychophysiological state.

Keywords Subject monitoring · Psychophysiological state · EDA · BVP · HR · Physiotherapy

1 Introduction

During physiotherapy sessions with significant subject participation both in the sense of intellectual activity and physical exercises, especially in motor-cognitive therapy, there is a serious problem of maintaining a proper state of mental balance. Exercises in

A. Mańka (✉) · P. Romaniszyn · M. N. Bugdol · A. W. Mitas
Faculty of Biomedical Engineering, Silesian University of Technology, Roosevelta 40, 41-800
Zabrze, Poland
e-mail: anna.manka@polsl.pl

P. Romaniszyn
e-mail: patrycja.romaniszyn@polsl.pl

M. N. Bugdol
e-mail: monika.bugdol@polsl.pl

A. W. Mitas
e-mail: andrzej.mitas@polsl.pl

© The Editor(s) (if applicable) and The Author(s), under exclusive license
to Springer Nature Switzerland AG 2021
E. Piętka et al. (eds.), *Information Technology in Biomedicine*, Advances in Intelligent
Systems and Computing 1186, https://doi.org/10.1007/978-3-030-49666-1_17

the presence of a trainer or therapist are a cause of stress, even when the circumstances of the therapy are obvious or well known, because there is a natural problem of matching the level of investment of own effort to the expected benefits assessed by a subjective caregiver. It is a phenomenon similar to the white apron effect described by doctors. The multitude of variants of the subject's reaction mechanism results from the number of degrees of freedom (e.g. health status, personality type, age, mood, character, level of education, external conditions). The common element is the effectiveness of the therapy, understood by the authors as an effect adequate to the effort put in at a minimum cost, involving the expected result.

In case of a multidimensional random variable which individual dimensions are continuous or discrete, and many are fuzzy, analysis is simply not feasible. In rehabilitation practice, decision-making is usually in the hands of a therapist who defines qualitatively and quantitatively the exercise without being able to assess the subject's level of effort. On the other hand, the risk of therapy failure depends heavily on the commitment of both subject and therapist. Usually, the optimal solution is to achieve an efficiency level about $\frac{2}{3}$ of maximum performance. This ensures, that there is a safe margin to increase effort and at the same time the level of activation is satisfactory.

The background of the work presented in this article is a method of monitoring the subject's psychophysical state during exercises. The essential context is the creation of a mechanism to prevent hyperactivity. Lazy performance of therapeutic tasks will at most bring no results in the expected time, while overzealous performance of them will bring a new unpredictable risk of damage. Therefore, in the designed diagnostic and rehabilitation system continuous subject observation over time with the use of precise, not-burdening, and non-invasive measuring devices is proposed. The basic problem is the selection of physical quantities that most clearly describe the subject's condition and commonly occur in people in a similar health situation.

The aim of the presented study was to determine the parameters that can be used to monitor the subject during specific rehabilitation exercises. The course of research provides a series of measurements commonly considered representative of stress levels. The task to be solved is the selection of a minimal set of variables covering the adopted set of psychophysiological features. The creation and ongoing analysis of such behavioral profile is a condition of safe physiotherapy, and for the person leading the subject is undoubtedly support in the decision-making process.

2 Materials and Methods

The entire presented protocol is a part of the DISC4SPINE project, which aims to develop a system of Dynamic Individual Stimulation and Control For Spine and Posture Interactive Rehabilitation.

The research group consisted of 9 students (3 women, 6 men)—7 from the J. Kukuczka Academy of Physical Education and 2 students from the Silesian University of Technology. Their average age was 23.3 years (min 22, max 23). Before the examination, the participant was informed about the purpose of the study and gave written consent to it.

2.1 Data Aquisition

During the experiment, the Empatica E4 was used to acquire biomedical signals. This device allows recording raw data saved in the .csv format on an external server. The first obtained signal was the skin Electrodermal Activity (EDA), with a sampling rate of 4 Hz. The second recorded signal was Blood Volume Pulse (BVP) acquired using a photoplethysmograph at 64 Hz. On the basis of the BVP, the mean Heart Rate (HR) and Inter-Beats Interval (IBI) values were computed.

At the beginning of the study, the examined person was told to put the device on his or her left wrist in a proper location [1]. The device was on the wrist throughout the whole examination. The subject was asked to relax and calm down due to the need to stabilize the values of individual signals. After about 15 min, the examined person started performing appropriate exercises under physiotherapist supervision. In the initial position, the subject stood free, with feet parallel to each other. Then the individual elements of the subject's body were determined in the corrected position:

- in order to activate muscles acting on the so-called short and long foot,
- to activate muscles acting on the ankle, knee and hip joints,
- to activate muscles acting on the posterior pelvic tilt,
- to activate muscles of the anterior abdominal wall, including the transverse abdominal muscle,
- to retract arms and shoulders,
- to correct head and cervical alignment,
- for elongation execution.

2.2 Signal Processing

2.2.1 EDA

The electrodermal activity is a signal that allows the analysis of the subject's condition on the basis of changes in skin electrical conductivity. It reflects the level of stress, pain, involvement, fatigue and other sensations [2].

Based on the collected data and literature sources, the signal was analyzed by determining basic statistical parameters [3, 4]. The processing of electrodermal activity, for each subject separately, consisted of several basic stages.

The first step of the EDA signal processing was Z-Score normalization, which is based on the mean and standard deviation (SD):

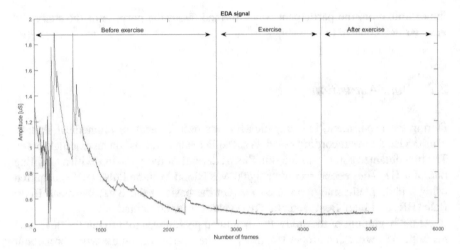

Fig. 1 EDA signal example with timestamps for one individual

$$V' = \frac{V - mean}{SD},$$

where V is the original signal and V' is the signal after normalization. Next signal denoising using a wavelet transform with a maximum level of decomposition of $log_2 N$ was done, where N is the number of signal samples. Then, the detection of Galvanic Skin Response (GSR) was performed, which are sudden, leaping changes in skin electrical conductivity. For this purpose, Matlab toolbox distributed under the free GNU GPL license for EDA processing and analysis—EDA-master—was used. The last stages were the framing of the EDA signal (30s frame) with overlay (5s) and dividing the signal into selected fragments corresponding to the individual stages of the test, according to the following timestamps—before (instruction), during and after exercise (Fig. 1).

A regression line was also determined for individual signal segments. On the basis of the above information, the following parameters were determined in the mentioned time periods:

1. average value (EDA.mean),
2. standard deviation (EDA.SD),
3. 20th percentile (EDA.20th),
4. 80th percentile (EDA.80th),
5. number of response (EDA.GSR),
6. number of response per minute (EDA.rpm),
7. average energy of GSR (EDA.enGSR),
8. number of significant GSR—higher than $1.5\,\mu S$ (EDA.GSR1.5),
9. average energy of significant GSR (EDA.enGSR1.5),
10. number of crossing with the regression line (EDA.crl).

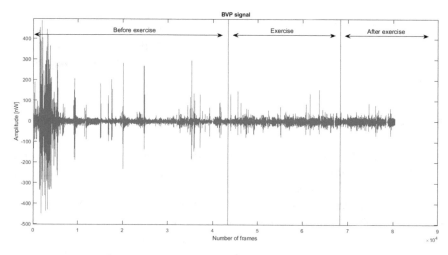

Fig. 2 BVP signal example with timestamps for one individual

2.2.2   BVP

Cardiac signals were used to assess the emotional state of the subject. The Empatica E4 device provides a Blood Volume Pulse signal based on data from a plethysmographic sensor. Individual values of BVP inform about the light signals that were reflected from vessel and went back to the sensor. This signal was presented without units because it was derived from the combination of two different measures of the amount of light from green and red exposure [1].

The signal was analyzed for each subject separately according to steps proposed in literature [3]. Preprocessing of the BVP signal included trimming to essential data and dividing into segments corresponding to a specific stage of the study (before, during, and after exercising). Each signal fragment (Fig. 2) was saved in a separate matrix and was further analyzed.

The noisy BVP signal was obtained during a period of increased subject mobility, so the outliers had to be cleaned. The winsorization was performed for the 2% range. The aim of this approach was to limit extreme values below the 2nd and above the 98th percentile of the data. As a result of this operation, the data were filtered by trimming the signal extremes. Then, windows with a duration of 30 s and an overlay of 5 s was designated. On the basis of literature [3, 5, 6], the following statistical parameters were computed for the mentioned time periods:

1. average value (BVP.mean),
2. standard deviation (BVP.SD),
3. 20th percentile (BVP.20th),
4. 80th percentile (BVP.80th),
5. quartile deviation (BVP.QD),
6. peak-to-peak amplitude variation (BVP.amp),

7. first and second signal derivative (BVP.der1 and BVP.der2).

No frequency parameters have been determined for the BVP signal because signal acquisition time was shorter than the recommended minimum signal length which is 5 min [6].

2.2.3   HR

From BVP, the HR signal was determined by the algorithm proposed by Empatica E4, which also prefiltered the data. Each HR sample contains average heart rate values computed in spans of 10 s [1].

    The first step was to divide the signal into fragments, according to timestamps (Fig. 3). Next, the preprocessing was performed to determine the first and last second for each frame. Based on this information, the signal was cutted into frames—the first value was the sum of HR values starting from the first second to the given frame and the last value was the sum of HR values up to the last second belonging to the given frame. A regression line was also determined for each frame. In the last step, the following statistical parameters were calculated for each frame of the HR signal in the time domain [3, 6]:

1. average value (HR.mean),
2. standard deviation (HR.SD),
3. 20th percentile (HR.20th),
4. 80th percentile (HR.80th),
5. quartile deviation (HR.QD),
6. linear regression coefficients (HR.a and HR.b),
7. number of crossing with linear regression line (HR.cross).

2.2.4   IBI

The BVP signal was the input signal to Empatica E4 algorithm that provides the IBI signal. On the basis of diastolic peaks, the algorithm removed false peaks and detected heart beats. As a result, the final signal containing information about the time and length of the peaks was obtained [1]. Finally, the signal was determined for periods of low activity of the subject. By the way the signal was obtained, it is recommended to analyze this signal in experiments where movements were static. Due to the low mobility of the subject during the study, we decided to include this signal into the analysis. Nevertheless, the mechanism rejecting empty signal frames has been implemented.

    Since IBI signal is not continuous, it is impossible to determine frames perfectly corresponding to those for BVP. To be able to simultaneously analyze parameters for IBI and BVP signal, the IBI signal was divided into frames almost corresponding to the frames calculated for the BVP signal. A matrix with the times of subsequent

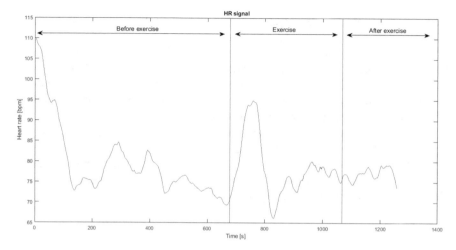

Fig. 3 HR signal example with timestamps for one individual

BVP signal samples was determined. For each BVP frame, a series of IBI samples, which time of occurrence was in this frame, were calculated. IBI and BVP frames did not start at the same time and were not of equal length due to the way the IBI signal was obtained.

The duration and content criteria of including IBI frames into analysis were implemented according to the signal characteristic. A frame that contained samples with a time of occurrence between adjacent samples greater than 3 s was not subjected to further analysis. In this case, the frame was divided in order to select the longest fragment. Finally, all frames containing less than 10 samples were rejected. The following parameters were determined for each frame of the IBI signal in the time domain [3, 6]:

1. mean value of duration of heartbeat (IBI.mean),
2. standard deviation of duration of heart beat (IBI.SD),
3. percentage of differences between consecutive IBI samples differing by 20, 50 and 70 ms (IBI.p20, IBI.p50 and IBI.p70),
4. percentage of frames that met the duration and content inclusion criteria (IBI.%all).

Due to the characteristics of the received signal frames, it was impossible to perform frequency analysis.

2.3 Statistical Data Analysis

The set of analyzed parameters to all signals included parameters mentioned above. The parameters calculated for three time intervals were compared: before, during, and after exercising. For each time interval descriptive statistics were calculated: mean, standard deviation, quartiles, quartile range, minimum, and maximum. First, the assumptions required to proceed ANOVA for repeated measurements were verified (normality—Shapiro-Wilk test, equal-size groups—chi-squared test, homogeneous sphericity—Mauchly's test). If the assumptions were fulfilled, ANOVA for repeated measurements with Huynh and Feldt correction was carried out, otherwise the Friedman test was employed. When the obtained p-value was less than 0.05, the pairwise Wilcoxon test with Holm–Bonferroni correction was computed.

The IBI parameters were not statistically analyzed due to the low efficiency of determining the coefficients for exercise interval—only for two subjects the designated frames met the duration and content inclusion criteria. This limitation results from the increased mobility of the examined person and the implemented method in Empatica E4 of determining IBI signal samples.

3   Results

3.1   EDA

Table 1 shows the most important EDA parameters. In Table 2 the results of the analysis of statistical significance of differences between individual parameters before, during, and after the exercises were presented.

Table 1 Descriptive statistics of selected EDA parameters

ID		1	2	3	4	5	6	7	8	9
EDA.mean (μS)	Before	0.321	0.624	0.796	16.70	5.103	0.343	0.188	2.026	15.031
	During	0.339	1.962	0.481	36.753	4.728	0.551	0.219	1.926	23.768
	After	0.343	3.909	0.507	34.461	4.201	0.681	0.234	2.256	19.531
SD	Before	0.004	0.016	0.062	0.976	0.181	0.006	0.003	0.051	0.375
	During	0.003	0.106	0.004	0.339	0.071	0.022	0.007	0.097	0.199
	After	0.006	0.125	0.015	0.442	0.206	0.023	0.003	0.040	0.321
EDA.GSR	Before	55	24	21	4	26	20	12	7	1
	During	55	11	78	19	3	36	48	35	21
	After	9	19	8	16	15	15	47	22	14
rpm	Before	0.031	0.027	0.031	0.004	0.039	0.024	0.016	0.002	0.001
	During	0.157	0.032	0.135	0.052	0.074	0.094	0.115	0.114	0.054
	After	0.069	0.107	0.055	0.137	0.135	0.118	0.332	0.149	0.062
EDA.crl	Before	77	10	10	9	24	129	359	13	6
	During	253	37	148	2	48	54	257	42	12
	After	42	28	40	15	21	25	147	20	43

Table 2 Statistical significance of differences for selected EDA parameters

Variable	Test	p-value
EDA.mean	Friedman	0.169
EDA.SD	Friedman	0.2359
EDA.GSR	Friedman	0.1653
EDA.rpm	**Friedman**	**0.0018**
EDA.crl	**ANOVA**	**0.054**

3.2   Cardiac Signals

The results of BVP and HR parameters selected on the basis of statistical analysis were presented in Tables 3 and 4 for BVP and HR, respectively. In Table 5 information about analysis of statistical significance of differences between individual parameters for each study stage were presented for both signals.

4   Discussion

This article presents an analysis of selected parameters calculated for physiological signals: EDA, BVP, HR, and IBI. Due to small diversity between groups only selected parameters are presented.

During the analysis of the EDA signal, changes in signal parameters at different time points were noticed. In almost all cases (excluding subjects no 3, 5 and 8) an increase in the average signal value (EDA.mean) during the exercises was observed in comparison to the value before exercise. The variation of the standard deviation of the average signal value was individual. The influence of the exercises on noticeable changes of this value (larger or smaller fluctuations of the value) cannot be clearly stated. A significant increase of the GSR during exercising, indicating experiencing certain emotions and increased psychogalvanic response of the skin, was noticed each time (with the exception of the 2nd and 5th subjects)—both before and after exercising these values were lower. The parameter describing the frequency of skin galvanic response per minute (EDA.rpm) reached higher values during the exercises than before for each examined person, which also indicates increased activity of sympathetic nervous system to eccrine sweat glands, which is a measure of stress [2]. Similarly, in case of EDA.crl parameter, on the basis of the analysis it can be stated, that in 6 out of 9 cases (for the exception of subjects 4, 6 and 7) an increase in the number of intersections with the EDA signal regression line during exercise was observed.

By performing a statistical analysis of the above parameters, only in case of the EDA.rpm coefficient the multiple groups comparison test turned out to be statistically significant (at significance level 0.05). The median value of GSR before exercising

Table 3 Descriptive statistics of selected BVP parameters (b—before, d—during, a—after)

ID		1	2	3	4	5	6	7	8	9
BVP.SD	b	8.860	47.962	68.260	39.797	32.609	30.868	21.805	40.090	29.628
	d	10.121	14.193	11.067	16.825	11.478	5.692	10.153	63.942	27.667
	a	35.112	23.843	22.610	43.135	40.598	20.711	22.839	33.391	47.996
BVP 20th	b	−5.379	−18.235	−48.594	−21.906	−15.458	−14.745	−12.650	−28.031	−21.973
	d	−8.030	−8.210	−9.140	−9.117	−9.495	−3.718	−5.844	−26.530	−16.659
	a	−38.533	−14.423	−14.086	−24.388	−24.289	−14.235	−11.549	−18.629	42.159
BVP 80th	b	5.823	21.691	45.524	25.944	13.209	13.418	12.847	26.689	21.628
	d	8.254	8.900	9.075	9.967	9.891	4.422	6.726	30.238	16.862
	a	31.598	4.842	14.127	23.522	25.306	12.382	11.685	18.785	37.484
BVP QD	b	4.360	13.354	36.372	17.317	10.858	10.000	8.913	21.083	16.325
	d	5.734	6.615	7.249	7.109	7.785	3.051	4.739	21.475	12.716
	a	29.211	10.679	11.295	8.149	18.651	10.534	9.134	14.170	31.203
BVP amp	b	54.951	318.370	355.929	219.132	213.077	198.884	124.404	227.581	144.469
	d	43.710	93.130	52.718	100.789	55.719	29.505	60.210	394.955	154.234
	a	228.748	143.961	136.436	270.331	228.620	126.122	137.103	218.753	261.220

Table 4 Descriptive statistics of selected HR parameters

ID	HR.SD			HR.a		
	Before	During	After	Before	During	After
1	1.444	1.451	2.572	0.105	0.105	0.239
2	1.687	1.628	1.461	0.143	0.090	0.172
3	1.359	1.446	2.095	0.137	0.040	0.223
4	1.092	1.011	1.365	0.049	0.052	0.194
5	0.852	1.176	1.096	−0.002	−0.060	−0.004
6	0.974	1.156	1.059	0.007	0.001	0.044
7	1.790	1.388	2.290	−0.070	−0.057	−0.089
8	2.756	2.345	4.062	0.210	0.220	0.298
9	1.491	2.092	1.938	0.129	0.070	−0.033

Table 5 Statistical significance of differences for selected cardiac parameters

Variable	Test	p-value
BVP.SD	Friedmans	0.0701
BVP.20th	**Friedman**	**0.0251**
BVP.80th	Friedman	0.0626
BVP.QD	Friedman	0.0527
BVP.amp	Friedman	0.0743
HR.SD	**ANOVA**	**0.0326**
HR.a	ANOVA	0.0721

was statistically different from the ones during and after exercising (p-value equal to 0.023 and 0.012, respectively). In case of EDA.crl, the p-value for ANOVA was 0.054, therefore no post-hoc analyses were carried out, however the obtained p-value is not much higher than the significance level.

Changes in cardiac parameters were observed during individual stages of the study. For 7 out of 9 cases BVP standard deviation decreased during the exercise stage and later increased. This may mean that the exercises can be burdensome for those subjects, because the functioning of the heart was more regular, which is an undesirable phenomenon. The proper work of the heart is irregular and is characterized by high variability in parameters, which reflects the body's ability to adapt to changing conditions [7]. A similar observation occurs for the BVP.amp parameter. The difference between the largest and smallest values for the frame decreased during the exercise stage for 7 cases. This is due to the fact that the BVP waveform was more regular during exercises, which again may mean a significant load on the heart. There was an increase in the BVP.20th for the exercise phase for 8 cases. Reverse observations can be seen for the BVP.80th since this parameter in this study phase has decreased in 7 cases. The BVP.QD value decreased for the exercise phase compared to the first phase for 7 out of 9 subjects. In case of the remaining BVP parameters, no significant changes were noted during all experiment stages.

In case of heart rate parameters, there is a different relationship for HR.SD than the one observed for BVP.SD. HR.SD was greater during the exercises for 5 subjects and greater after the exercises for 8 out of 9 subjects indicating high variability of HR during and after exercising. An increase in heart rate during exercising is a normal response of the body [8]. The HR.a parameter was greater in the last study stage compared to the previous one for 6 subjects. No clear impact of the exercises on other HR parameters was observed.

The multiple groups comparison test shows that parameters differentiating the three study intervals were BVP.20th for the BVP signal and HR.SD for the HR signal. In case of BVP.20th, the post-hoc test showed a significant difference between the first and second time interval. For HR.SD there was a significant difference between means calculated for the first and third examination step. P-value between 0.05 and 0.1 was obtained for BVP.SD, BVP.80th, BVP.QD, BVP.amp and HR.a. In case of BVP.QD, the p-value for Friedman's test was 0.0527, therefore no further analysis was carried out. Nevertheless, the obtained p-value is slightly higher than the set significance level and it can be assumed, that with a larger group BVP.QD would prove to be statistically significant.

The experiment has several limitations. The study was conducted over several days, which made it impossible to maintain the same experimental conditions. The determined time intervals were of different lengths for each subject, which resulted in a different number of frames, which could affect the received parameters. It would be advisable to set the recommended length of the signal recording, which would allow to determine important parameters. The lack of access to the pure signal waveforms was caused by the use of a selected device. Empatica E4 performs initial data processing and determines HR and IBI signals right after data acquisition [1]. Performing these steps according to own algorithms could result in obtaining different results. The lack of information about the type of changes performed by Empatica E4 may also limit the possibility of comparing our results with other works. Bigger population with a higher variety of health and age is needed to confirm the obtained results. In order to improve the analysis, it would be necessary to determine and examine the dependencies for frequency-domain parameters.

Despite these limitations, it was possible to determine the parameters differentiating specific study groups. The observed changes in parameters may indicate that some elements of the exercise were more strongly negatively or positively perceived by the subject because they disturbed the momentary state of parameters balance. Stress is subjective, felt differently by each person [3]. We can observe changes in parameters and, based on them, suppose what is happening with the subject. It is difficult to assess it directly. The psychophysiological state of the subject is a multidimensional phenomenon that requires the inclusion of additional elements in the analysis, such as the assessment of emotional state or behavior. Use of EDA and cardiac features for stress detection task can be limited since extracted parameters are related to each individual and different arousal of signal depends on the different stimulus. Those signals can be used to assess subject's state but stress and emotions templates as well as additional parameters need to be gathered to perform precise analysis of the subject's condition. Nevertheless, those parameters can be used to monitor the subject's condition during rehabilitation exercises, which can be used in the created rehabilitation system in the DISC4SPINE project.

 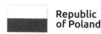 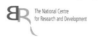 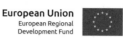

Acknowledgements This study was conducted as a part of the 'DISC4SPINE dynamic individual stimulation and control for spine and posture interactive rehabilitation' project (grant no. POIR.04.01.02-00-0082/17-00).

References

1. E4 wristband user's manual 20150608. Empatica, Milano, Italy, pp. 5–16 (2015)
2. Liu, M., Fan, D., Zhang, X., Gong, X.: Human emotion recognition based on galvanic skin response signal feature selection and SVM. In: 2016 International Conference on Smart City and Systems Engineering, pp. 157–160. IEEE (2016)
3. Gjoreski, M., Luštrek, M., Gams, M., Gjoreski, H.: Monitoring stress with a wrist device using context. J. Biomed. Inform. **73**, 159–170 (2017)
4. Ragot, M., Martin, N., Em, S., Pallamin, N., Diverrez, J.M.: Emotion recognition using physiological signals: laboratory vs. wearable sensors. In: International Conference on Applied Human Factors and Ergonomics, pp. 15–22. Springer, Cham (2017)
5. Handouzi, W., Maaoui, C., Pruski, A., Moussaoui, A.: Short-term anxiety recognition from blood volume pulse signal. In: 2014 IEEE 11th International Multi-conference on Systems, Signals and Devices (SSD14), pp. 1–6. IEEE (2014)
6. Camm, A.J., Malik, M., Bigger, J.T., Breithardt, G., Cerutti, S., Cohen, R.J., Lombardi, F.: Heart rate variability: standards of measurement, physiological interpretation and clinical use. Task force of the European society of cardiology and the North American society of pacing and electrophysiology (1996)
7. Shaffer, F., Ginsberg, J.P.: An overview of heart rate variability metrics and norms. Front. Public Health **5**, 258 (2017)
8. Genovesi, S., Zaccaria, D., Rossi, E., Valsecchi, M.G., Stella, A., Stramba-Badiale, M.: Effects of exercise training on heart rate and QT interval in healthy young individuals: are there gender differences? Europace **9**(1), 55–60 (2007)

Multimodal Signal Acquisition for Pain Assessment in Physiotherapy

Aleksandra Badura, Maria Bieńkowska, Aleksandra Masłowska, Robert Czarlewski, Andrzej Myśliwiec, and Ewa Pietka

Abstract Pain monitoring during physiotherapy is an important factor determining the course of therapy. However, current pain scales are subjective and do not feature a unified level of pain that indicates the required interruption of the therapy. Hence, in this study a multimodal platform with wearable devices for monitoring and objective assessment of pain is presented. In the case study, six patients with neck pain underwent fascial therapy with simultaneous recording of signals. For classification we used electrodermal activity, electromyography, and respiration signals. The decision relies on the occurrence of signal distortion surrounding the onset of the pain in a specified time period.

Keywords Pain in physiotherapy · Pain assessment · Pain monitoring · Physiotherapy · Manual therapy

A. Badura (✉) · M. Bieńkowska · E. Pietka
Faculty of Biomedical Engineering, Silesian University of Technology, Roosevelta 40, 41-800 Zabrze, Poland
e-mail: aleksandra.badura@polsl.pl

M. Bieńkowska
e-mail: maria.bienkowska@polsl.pl

E. Pietka
e-mail: ewa.pietka@polsl.pl

A. Masłowska · A. Myśliwiec
Institute of Physiotheraphy and Health Science, Academy of Physical Education in Katowice, Mikołowska 72a, 40-065 Katowice, Poland
e-mail: a.maslowska@onet.com.pl

A. Myśliwiec
e-mail: a.mysliwiec@awf.katowice.pl

R. Czarlewski
APA Sp. z o.o., Tarnogórska 251, 44-105 Gliwice, Poland
e-mail: robert.czarlewski@apagroup.pl

E. Piętka et al. (eds.), *Information Technology in Biomedicine*, Advances in Intelligent Systems and Computing 1186, https://doi.org/10.1007/978-3-030-49666-1_18

227

1 Introduction

Pain level assessment is a substantial element of medical procedures that determines not only the outcome but also the commencement of physiotherapeutic treatment. Active and passive therapeutic actions are strongly connected with pain which can be seen as the guardian of the tissue. Still, the pain and associated discomfort may limit the treatment significantly. The absence of pain indicates a too conservative approach, whilst using too much force may result in additional injuries. Adaptation of physical therapy applied to a suffering patient seems to be a challenging task due to the multidimensional and subjective aspect.

Subjective 0–10 point ratings are commonly used to estimate the intensity of pain. Its level depends on the gender, environmental factors, social conditions [20] and may be based on experience of the patient having a disturbed pain processing in the human nervous system. That all makes self-report rating highly subjective and indicates the need to develop automatic pain monitoring systems.

The problem of pain assessment is being considered by both commercial companies and scientists. One of the known commercial systems is the PainChek [26]. It is dedicated to people with communication difficulties allowing recording patient's facial expressions while caregivers can complete data based on the observations. The PMD-200 monitoring device by Medasense [27] employed in operating rooms and critical care settings for patients under general anesthesia uses a non-invasive finger sensor collecting pulse wave, galvanic skin response, temperature, and acceleration. The last noted commercial system is the PainMonitor Index [25] designed for clinical use as well. It is based on the skin conductance level measurement, where pain level is determined according to the number of signal peaks during a predefined time unit.

Zhang et al. [22] presented an approach based on a 3D video recording to assess the pain during cold stimulation. Another commonly used modalities reflecting the pain occurrence are electrocardiography (ECG), electromyography (EMG) and electrodermal activity (EDA) [16–18], electroencephalography (EEG) [17] and respiration (RSP) [16] signals. Mostly, the heat is used as a pain stimulant. Another ways for evoking pain sensations are electrical stimulation with functional near-infrared spectroscopy (fNIRS) data acquisition [10, 11] and chromatic RGB, depth and thermal video data (RGBDT) [6]. Approaches to pain assessment during blood collection stimuli [3], in patients with chronic diseases with saturation [21] and in patients after surgery [9] were examined either.

The stimulant of known intensity, beginning time and duration is common for mentioned surveys. On the other hand, physiotherapy is a complicated process where a therapist has to adjust force of hardly measurable intensity. There are many works [8, 15, 19] basing on UNBC-McMaster database [13] gathering data from patients with shoulder pain. The study protocol assumed active and passive range-of-motion tests. Lee et al. [8] triggered typical back pain by exacerbating maneuvers (such as toe touches, back arches, and facet-joint loading twists) in patients with chronic low back pain. Fear-avoidance behavior research related to physical exercises was carried out [1, 14] with the use of EMG sensors. Nevertheless, our research reveals the lack of surveys into the automatic pain monitoring in physiotherapy session. To the best of our knowledge, no such dedicated tools were developed so far.

The overall goal of the project is to develop a multimodal platform for pain assessment during physiotherapy. In the current study an acquisition setup has been developed and a pilot test has been performed. Patients suffering from the neck pain have been subjected to a physiotherapeutic procedure. The acquisition system archives data from four devices including Empatica E4 wristband, RespiBAN Professional, K-FORCE Grip, and USB camera. Acquired data is synchronized in time. Since the response to the pain inducement is patient-dependent, data processing algorithm relies on the analysis of the entire multimodal set of signals.

The chapter is arranged as follows: Sect. 2 presents the acquisition system. Description of pilot study is included in Sect. 3, while Sect. 4 presents signal processing, classification, and results. Finally, Sect. 5 concludes the paper.

2 Acquisition System

The system consists of three wireless devices for collecting biomedical and physiological signals and an external camera recording therapy scene and patient's voice integrated with PainMonit software platform (Fig. 1). All of the devices have their own software to conduct the visualization and analysis, whereas the PainMonit platform synchronizes all acquired signals and allows for multi-visualisation. In the synchronization process, individual samples obtained from ResiBAN and K-FORCE are marked with a common time stamp just upon receipt. The Empatica wristband first sends the samples to its own server, and after applying time stamps sends them to the platform. As a result, a synchronised set of signals marked with time stamps is delivered and displayed on a physiotherapist's screen. In the future, a user-friendly interface will indicate severe pain occurrence.

2.1 Empatica E4 Wristband

E4 wristband [23] is a wearable device for real-time physiological data acquisition. It includes pulse plethysmography and EDA sensor. Additionally, it contains infrared thermopile and triaxial accelerometer not used in this study. During examination the wristband is placed on the non-dominant hand according to manufacturer's guidelines. The band is tightened firmly, yet not to constrict the blood flow.

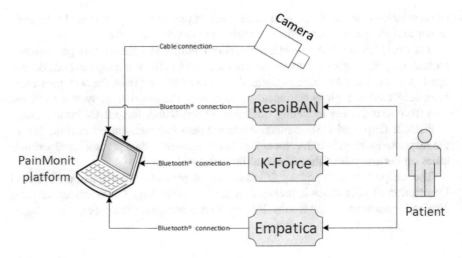

Fig. 1 Scheme of the acquisition system

2.2 RespiBAN Professional

Respiban professional [28] produced by Biosignalsplux is a wearable device with an integrated inductive respiratory sensor and triaxal accelerometer. Its main part is a hub mountable on the chest with a strip. The hub allows connecting up to eight analog inputs, i.e. electromyography, electrodermal activity, electrocardiography, electroencephalography, temperature, or force sensors. The sampling frequency can be customized. For data acquisition, the center of the strip is placed over the chest and is fastened firmly. EDA electrodes are placed on the index and ring finger tips of the non-dominant hand, while EMG electrodes are placed on the forehead to register signals from corrugator supercilii muscles [5]. Both types of sensors are connected to the hub.

2.3 K-FORCE Grip

K-force grip [24] is a manual dynamometer for the measurement of the grip strength. It weighs 200 g and measures force with a sampling frequency of 75 Hz. The patient keeps the K-FORCE grip in his dominant hand and squeezes it while the pain occurs. Since the patient is not informed about it, the measurement is spontaneous.

3 Materials

The signal acquisition starts before the patient is subjected to the physiotherapy. The fascial technique is used during the therapy. International guidelines do not impose specific methods for the treatment of pain. Referring to the literature, it is an effective method that decreases the pain, as well as significantly improves the quality of life [2]. Based on the medical record, the therapist applies an appropriate therapy, painful to the patient. The therapy takes about 10 to 15 min and depends on the number of pressed points. The procedure causes the tissue inflammation, which disappears within several days, and results in pain relief. Two types of pain level monitoring are applied. In the conventional mode, the patient speaks out a number in the range of 0–10 to indicate the pain level. Additionally, the multimodal platform registers the signals (as discussed in Sect. 2).

4 Recognition Approach

The current preliminary study is to detect abnormalities in EDA, RSP, and EMG signals resulting from a severe pain incident [7, 12, 15] and relate them to the patient response. Two main difficulties make the task nontrivial. Firstly, the pain may occur unexpectedly, thus the patient reaction is spontaneous and often delayed. Secondly, the signal deformation is patient-dependent and only selected signals reflect the pain incident.

4.1 Selected Signals and Preprocessing

The electrodermal activity (EDA), the respiration wave (RSP) and the electromyography (EMG) are subjected to the analysis.

For **EDA** analysis, the model proposed by Greco et al. [4] is used. It assumes the EDA signal as the sum of three terms—tonic, phasic, and noise components. The tonic component is responsible for slow drifts of the baseline skin conductance level, while the phasic one (p_{EDA}) reflects the short-time response to the stimulus. In this survey, rapid reactions to the therapy are essential. Thus, the phasic factor is processed. The shape of a single phasic response is modeled with the Bateman function:

$$h(\tau) = \left(e^{-\tau/\tau_0} - e^{-\tau/\tau_1}\right) u(\tau), \tag{1}$$

where τ_0 is the slow time constant, τ_1 is the fast time constant and $u(\tau)$ is the unitary step function. The Laplace transform followed by the discrete-time approximation gives the autoregressive–moving-average model, which represent phasic component p_{EDA} used in further processing. First, the Gaussian-weighted moving average filter

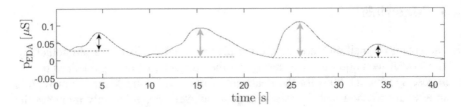

Fig. 2 Selection of peaks in p'_{EDA} signal. Green arrows indicate differences between corresponding local minimum and maximum greater than t_{EDA} threshold

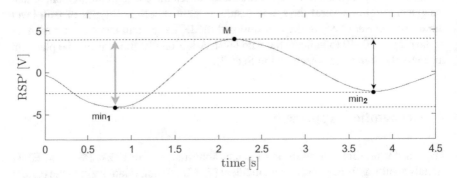

Fig. 3 Relative amplitude in RSP'. The difference between peak (M) and selected local minimum min_1 ($M - min_1 > M - min_2$) is marked by a green arrow. Peak is detected if this value exceeds t_{RSP}

with a frame width of 1 s is applied to this component yielding p'_{EDA}. Next, relevant peaks higher than adjacent local minima by the extent of $t_{EDA} = k_{EDA} \cdot \max(p'_{EDA})$ (relative amplitude, Fig. 2) are selected, where $k_{EDA} = 0.15$ is a coefficient determined experimentally.

Low-pass filter is applied to the **RSP** signal resulting in RSP'. Since the breathing signal contains the inhale and the exhale waveforms, two consecutive minima are found. The larger amplitude gives the result (Fig. 3). Data peaks with relative amplitude over $t_{RSP} = k_{RSP} \cdot \max(RSP')$ are selected ($k_{RSP} = 0.58$ was chosen experimentally).

EMG signal is filtered with Gaussian-weighted moving average filter (2 s frame width) giving EMG'. Then, the 1st derivative is determined. All samples of $\frac{dEMG'}{d\tau}$ with values over t_{EMG} are marked. The threshold is determined as:

$$t_{EMG} = Q_{0.98}\left(\left|\frac{dEMG'}{d\tau}\right|\right),\tag{2}$$

where $Q_{0.98}$ indicates the 98th percentile.

Two pain markers are recorded during the therapy. First, the patient pronounces the pain level. Independently, patient's pain feelings based on the therapy video recording is marked offline by an operator. Moreover, video allows painful moments not expressed by the patient verbally (other sounds could be heard, patient moves suddenly, frowns) to be noticed. These patient's feelings are subjectively rated in the range of 0–10 and marked by an operator.

4.2 Classification

Because of a sudden onset of pain, the data is divided into 4–6 s frames with a 20% overlap. The decision rule is applied to each single frame. If at least two of three signals (EDA, RSP, EMG) indicate some abnormalities on one or more already selected samples, it is marked as a *pain* frame (Fig. 4).

The correctness of the classification is assessed on the basis of subjectively expressed pain level. Furthermore, a pain cut-off threshold is used to exclude irrelevant (too low) indicators. For each patient, the cut-off value may differ. Moreover, it is set to be lower than the maximum pain level value expressed by the subject. Only indicators over the threshold are taken into consideration. Finally, binary (*pain* versus *no pain*) classification approach is applied.

Since the patient informs about the pain verbally with some delay, a backward shift (0 to 5 s) of pain markers is applied.

4.3 Results

The preliminary evaluation is based on the analysis of data registered during a physiotherapy of six patients. Table 1 shows the results. For Patients #1, #2, #4, and #6 two sets are presented. The one with higher pain threshold gives better classification results, however very few frames are considered as *pain* frames (restrictive selection). In Patient #3 and Patient #4 any change is noticed between the highest and subsequent threshold value. Due to a short time of the pain events in comparison with the entire therapy time, sensitivity is an important evaluation factor. Figure 5 presents confusion matrices for *pain-no pain* classification results.

4.4 Discussion

Preliminary pain recognition study confirms the presence of abnormalities in EDA, RSP and EMG signals during a painful physiotherapy. It can be noticed that the multimodal platform recognizes the onset of acute pain. However, the moments between patient's verbal labels, so far considered to be *no pain*, may affect the classification results. As observed, patients get used to painful feeling and frequently do not express it. Thus, this approach may be improved by finding a way to obtain complete pain feeling level labels in the future.

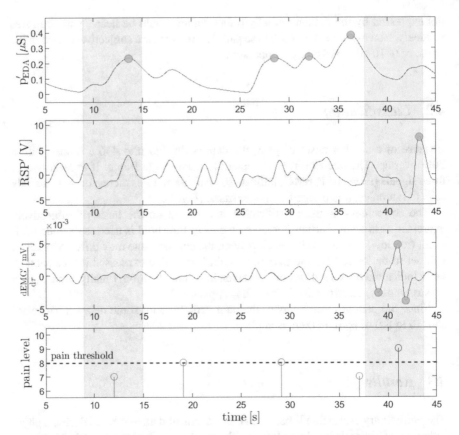

Fig. 4 Decision rule performance. Green dots indicate selected peaks in p'_{EDA}, RSP' and $\frac{dEMG'}{d\tau}$ signals. Pain level chart reflects the patient's assessment. Values under the threshold are skipped in the classification process. Sample blue highlighted frame (width 6 s) corresponds to *no pain* label. Sample red highlighted frame, where two of three signals (RSP' and $\frac{dEMG'}{d\tau}$) indicated selected samples occurrence, is marked as *pain*

Time between pain onset and imparting it by the patient was disregarded by applying the time shift factor and sufficient frame width. The best results were obtained for Patient #2 (83%, 73%, and 73% for sensitivity, specificity, and accuracy respectively) with 1–2.5 s shift and 6 s frame width. An about 4 s shift was applied for Patients #3, #4, #6 as well. This leads to the conclusion that body's response to pain could occur faster than verbal expression.

As for now, only severe pain (above the individual threshold) was considered. It may be noticed, that for several subjects an increasing pain threshold value results in higher classification outcomes. Moreover, a few subjects (Patient #4 and Patient #6) have already undergone the therapy in the recent past, so for them pain is easier to bear or it even it is not addressed (the maximum pain level expressed by both patients is 6). The threshold is adjusted to the maximum patient's pain level. For low

Table 1 The best results of the *pain* versus *no pain* classification for six patients. Differences in time shift and pain threshold values (subjectively noted) indicate patient-dependent reactions to pain

Patient	Frame width (s)	Time shift (s)	Pain threshold	Sensitivity	Specificity	Accuracy
#1	4.5	0.0	8	0.67	0.87	0.87
	4.5	0.0	9	1.00	0.87	0.87
#2	6.0	1.0–2.5	8	0.83	0.73	0.73
	6.0	1.0–2.5	9	1.00	0.71	0.72
#3	6.0	4.0–4.5	7	0.57	0.68	0.67
#4	5.5	4.0	4	0.33	0.84	0.80
#5	5.0	0.0	6	0.75	0.96	0.94
	5.0	0.0	7	1.00	0.94	0.94
#6	4.5	4.0	4	0.30	0.93	0.90
	4.5	4.0	5	0.67	0.92	0.92

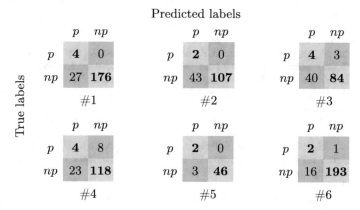

Fig. 5 Confusion matrices. Values correspond to the number of *pain* (*p*) and *no pain* (*np*) frames

values (i.e. Patients #4 and #6) the recognition system is less sensitive, because the signals do not indicate the existence of pain. Individual reactions for pain have been observed. For Patient #3 the pain level made him speechless. Thus, classification results may be affected by missing *pain* labels. Facial expression may be significant in some patients, whereas unnoticeable in others (i.e. Patient #1). This indicates a patient-dependent approach to the problem. In general, the imbalance between *pain* and *no-pain* events may skew the classification results since many false positives can be noticed in confusion matrices. However, obtaining high sensitivity is relevant at this stage of the study.

In our further work, we plan to distinguish more pain levels with particular emphasis on acute pain. Such information is essential to the physiotherapist. A universal recognition system requires examining more patients with the inclusion of a wider signal pool.

5   Conclusion

In this study a new multimodal platform for pain monitoring in physiotherapy was presented. Stability and good quality of recording devices is crucial for proper pain assessment. Coincident signals abnormalities occurring simultaneously with the pain feeling have been confirmed. In order to make the platform more robust, a significantly larger number of patients will be involved in the study.

Acknowledgements This work was supported by The National Centre for Research and Development (grant number WPN-3/1/2019).

References

1. Aung, M.S.H., Bianchi-Berthouze, N., Watson, P., Williams, A.C.d.C.: Automatic recognition of fear-avoidance behavior in chronic pain physical rehabilitation. In: Proceedings of the 8th International Conference on Pervasive Computing Technologies for Healthcare, PervasiveHealth '14, pp. 158–161. ICST (Institute for Computer Sciences, Social-Informatics and Telecommunications Engineering), Brussels, BEL (2014)
2. Branchini, M., Lopopolo, F., Andreoli, E., Loreti, I., Marchand, A., Stecco, A.: Fascial manipulation® for chronic aspecific low back pain: a single blinded randomized controlled trial. F1000Research **4** (2015). https://doi.org/10.12688/f1000research.6890.1
3. Erel, V.K., Özkan, H.S.: Thermal camera as a pain monitor. J. Pain Res. **10**, 2827 (2017)
4. Greco, A., Valenza, G., Lanata, A., Scilingo, E.P., Citi, L.: cvxEDA: a convex optimization approach to electrodermal activity processing. IEEE Trans. Biomed. Eng. **63**(4), 797–804 (2016)
5. Gruss, S., Geiger, M., Werner, P., Wilhelm, O., Traue, H.C., Al-Hamadi, A., Walter, S.: Multimodal signals for analyzing pain responses to thermal and electrical stimuli. JoVE (Journal of Visualized Experiments) (146), e59,057 (2019)
6. Haque, M.A., Bautista, R.B., Noroozi, F., Kulkarni, K., Laursen, C.B., Irani, R., Bellantonio, M., Escalera, S., Anbarjafari, G., Nasrollahi, K., et al.: Deep multimodal pain recognition: a database and comparison of spatio-temporal visual modalities. In: 2018 13th IEEE International Conference on Automatic Face & Gesture Recognition (FG 2018), pp. 250–257. IEEE (2018)
7. Jafari, H., Courtois, I., Van den Bergh, O., Vlaeyen, J.W., Van Diest, I.: Pain and respiration: a systematic review. Pain **158**(6), 995–1006 (2017)
8. Lee, J., Mawla, I., Kim, J., Loggia, M.L., Ortiz, A., Jung, C., Chan, S.T., Gerber, J., Schmithorst, V.J., Edwards, R.R., et al.: Machine learning–based prediction of clinical pain using multimodal neuroimaging and autonomic metrics. Pain **160**(3), 550–560 (2019)
9. Lim, H., Kim, B., Noh, G.J., Yoo, S.K.: A deep neural network-based pain classifier using a photoplethysmography signal. Sensors **19**(2), 384 (2019)
10. Lopez-Martinez, D., Peng, K., Lee, A., Borsook, D., Picard, R.: Pain detection with fnirs-measured brain signals: a personalized machine learning approach using the wavelet transform and bayesian hierarchical modeling with dirichlet process priors. In: 2019 8th International Conference on Affective Computing and Intelligent Interaction Workshops and Demos (ACIIW), pp. 304–309. IEEE (2019)
11. Lopez-Martinez, D., Peng, K., Steele, S.C., Lee, A.J., Borsook, D., Picard, R.: Multi-task multiple kernel machines for personalized pain recognition from functional near-infrared spectroscopy brain signals. In: 2018 24th International Conference on Pattern Recognition (ICPR), pp. 2320–2325. IEEE (2018)

12. Lopez-Martinez, D., Picard, R.: Multi-task neural networks for personalized pain recognition from physiological signals. In: 2017 Seventh International Conference on Affective Computing and Intelligent Interaction Workshops and Demos (ACIIW), pp. 181–184. IEEE (2017)
13. Lucey, P., Cohn, J.F., Prkachin, K.M., Solomon, P.E., Chew, S., Matthews, I.: Painful monitoring: automatic pain monitoring using the unbc-mcmaster shoulder pain expression archive database. Image Vis. Comput. **30**(3), 197–205 (2012)
14. Olugbade, T.A., Aung, M.H., Bianchi-Berthouze, N., Marquardt, N., Williams, A.C.: Bi-modal detection of painful reaching for chronic pain rehabilitation systems. In: Proceedings of the 16th International Conference on Multimodal Interaction, ICMI '14, p. 455–458. Association for Computing Machinery, New York, NY, USA (2014)
15. Tavakolian, M., Hadid, A.: A spatiotemporal convolutional neural network for automatic pain intensity estimation from facial dynamics. Int. J. Comput. Vis. **127**, 1413–1425 (2019)
16. Velana, M., Gruss, S., Layher, G., Thiam, P., Zhang, Y., Schork, D., Kessler, V., Meudt, S., Neumann, H., Kim, J., et al.: The senseemotion database: a multimodal database for the development and systematic validation of an automatic pain-and emotion-recognition system. In: IAPR Workshop on Multimodal Pattern Recognition of Social Signals in Human-Computer Interaction, pp. 127–139. Springer (2016)
17. Walter, S., Gruss, S., Ehleiter, H., Tan, J., Traue, H.C., Werner, P., Al-Hamadi, A., Crawcour, S., Andrade, A.O., da Silva, G.M.: The biovid heat pain database data for the advancement and systematic validation of an automated pain recognition system. In: 2013 IEEE international conference on cybernetics (CYBCO), pp. 128–131. IEEE (2013)
18. Werner, P., Al-Hamadi, A., Gruss, S., Walter, S.: Twofold-multimodal pain recognition with the X-ITE pain database. In: 2019 8th International Conference on Affective Computing and Intelligent Interaction Workshops and Demos (ACIIW), pp. 290–296. IEEE (2019)
19. Werner, P., Al-Hamadi, A., Limbrecht-Ecklundt, K., Walter, S., Gruss, S., Traue, H.: Automatic pain assessment with facial activity descriptors. IEEE Trans. Affect. Comput. 286–299 (2016). https://doi.org/10.1109/TAFFC.2016.2537327
20. Wiesenfeld-Hallin, Z.: Sex differences in pain perception. Gend. Med. **2**(3), 137–145 (2005)
21. Yang, F., Banerjee, T., Narine, K., Shah, N.: Improving pain management in patients with sickle cell disease from physiological measures using machine learning techniques. Smart Health **7**, 48–59 (2018)
22. Zhang, X., Yin, L., Cohn, J.F., Canavan, S., Reale, M., Horowitz, A., Liu, P., Girard, J.M.: Bp4d-spontaneous: a high-resolution spontaneous 3D dynamic facial expression database. Image Vis. Comput. **32**(10), 692–706 (2014)
23. E4 wristband. https://www.empatica.com/en-int/research/e4/
24. K-force grip. https://k-invent.com/produit/k-force-grip/
25. Medstorme, the painmonitor index. https://med-storm.com/products/the-pain-monitor/
26. Painchek, intelligent pain assessment. https://www.painchek.com/how-it-works/
27. Pmd-200, monitoring physiological pain response to optimize analgesia. https://medasense.com/pmd-200
28. Respiban professional. https://plux.info/biosignalsplux-wearables/313-respiban-professional-820202407.html

Classification of Heat-Induced Pain Using Physiological Signals

Philip J. Gouverneur, Frédéric Li, Tibor M. Szikszay, Waclaw M. Adamczyk, Kerstin Luedtke, and Marcin Grzegorzek

Abstract Objectively assessing the pain level of a patient is crucial in various medical situations. Until now the gold standard is represented by questionnaires which have different drawbacks. To continuously assess pain, questionnaires must be answered repeatedly which is time consuming for medical stuff and prone to errors. Thus, pain automatic classification systems could improve health care, especially when patients are unable to communicate their pain level. Previous works based on heat-based pain induction predominantly tried to predict the applied temperature stimuli itself. In contrast, our work is presenting an approach to predict self-reported pain as well. Therefore, a small dataset of 10 subjects was acquired using a thermode to induce pain. Subjects were asked to rate their pain perception on a computerised visual analogue scale (CoVAS). Different classifiers were trained using both temperature and CoVAS labels. Our experiments showed the superiority of the CoVAS labels for pain recognition.

Keywords Pain recognition · Machine learning · Deep-learning · Physiological signals · Pain perception

P. J. Gouverneur (✉) · F. Li · M. Grzegorzek
Institute of Medical Informatics, University of Luebeck, Luebeck, Germany
e-mail: gouverneur@imi.uni-luebeck.de

F. Li
e-mail: li@imi.uni-luebeck.de

M. Grzegorzek
e-mail: grzegorzek@imi.uni-luebeck.de

T. M. Szikszay · W. M. Adamczyk · K. Luedtke
Department of Health Sciences, Academic Physiotherapy, Pain and Exercise Research Luebeck (P.E.R.L), University of Luebeck, Luebeck, Germany
e-mail: tibormaximilian.szikszay@uksh.de

W. M. Adamczyk
e-mail: waclaw.adamczyk@uksh.de

K. Luedtke
e-mail: kerstin.luedtke@uni-luebeck.de

© The Editor(s) (if applicable) and The Author(s), under exclusive license to Springer Nature Switzerland AG 2021
E. Piętka et al. (eds.), *Information Technology in Biomedicine*, Advances in Intelligent Systems and Computing 1186, https://doi.org/10.1007/978-3-030-49666-1_19

239

1   Introduction

Pain is a subjective feeling and an essential compound of our lives. It is defined as an "unpleasant sensory and emotional experience associated with actual or potential tissue damage, or described in terms of such damage" according to the *International Association for the Study of Pain (IASP)* [9]. It serves as natural protective mechanism against harm of the body and can be indicative of health problems. It is a particularly important factor for medicine and health care, as pain can be both a symptom and a disease [3]. Moreover, correct pain management is a fundamental part of the work in hospitals. Wrong treatment, including over-usage of opioids, can lead to severe health issues as addiction to certain drugs and reduced breathing which may result in stopped respiration and thus death. Whereas an under-dose of medication causes ongoing pain and may even prolong hospital stay. For good pain management, accurate pain assessment is indispensable. But there is no simple solution to objectively measure pain. The current gold-standard for pain assessment is self-report [10] where patients report the intensity of their perceived pain. One of the simplest and most common possibilities is the Eleven-point Numeric Rating Scale (NRS-11). The subject is asked to express its pain as a number between 0 and 10, where zero represents "no pain" and ten constitutes "highest pain imaginable".

While these self-expressed pain values give an insight about the patient's current status, they come with major drawbacks. **(1)** First, pain is always a subjective experience [1]. Communicated pain intensities are therefore strongly dependent on the individual person and in particular his or her perception and tolerance of pain. Thus, outcomes of self-report have a large variance across individuals which can make comparison difficult. In addition, it was shown that patients tend to overestimate recalled pain compared to current pain [2, 12], which further weakens the reliability of such tools. **(2)** Pain assessment through self-reports cannot continuously measure pain. Establishing a self-report is a time-consuming action for patients and medical staff. As a result, it can only be performed occasionally. **(3)** The patient must be conscious and able to state their experience. This requirement is not fulfilled in various medical scenarios where the subject cannot communicate or is not able to give a detailed and accurate description (e.g. coma or dementia patients, kids, etc).

The aforementioned points highlight the clear need for an objective continuous assessment of pain which would not depend on the subject or medical staff's action. In the past, works have tried to obtain such system using machine learning techniques. The latter usually train classifiers for binary classification of specific tasks, like no pain versus a certain pain level. Several approaches exist to acquire the labelled dataset needed to train such classifiers, but the most popular is heat-based pain induction. Although the stimulus temperature is normally used as label during the training, these values do not represent the true pain level of the participants. The subjective perception of the participant is not encoded. Our paper therefore proposes to evaluate the difference between temperature and self-reported pain levels using machine learning approaches. A small dataset of heat-induced pain including both the temperature and the subjects individual perceived pain level, measured with a computerised visual analogue scale (CoVAS), was recorded. Our preliminary study includes the training of a random forest using hand-crafted features and a deep neural network. The models were evaluated on both labelling approaches.

This work is structured as follows. First, a review of the state-of-the-art using physiological data to classify pain is given in Sect. 2. Afterwards, the proposed classification approach is explained in Sect. 3. Section 4 summarises the results, which are discussed in Sect. 5. Finally, a conclusion and outlook are given in Sect. 6.

2   Related Work

Recent works in the field of automated pain classification mainly differ in the experimental setup (for example, sensor modalities, implemented pain stimuli or number of subjects used) and the pattern recognition approach (for example, the pre-processing methods, features or machine learning algorithms used).

While the building of such system is a complex procedure, one of the most crucial steps is the acquisition of a dataset. Many works have attempted to build sets of physiological sensor data labelled with pain information such as **X-ITE** pain [4], **Sense Emotion** [15] and **BP4D**+ [19] databases. But the most important and widely used by far remains the **BioVid** Heat Pain [17]. During its acquisition, a thermode[1] was used to apply heat stimuli to the forearm of 90 subjects. Electrodermal activity (EDA), electrocardiogram (ECG) and electromyogram (EMG) of three pain related muscles were recorded. Moreover, video data of the participants were observed as well. Heat stimuli were calibrated per person during an initial calibration phase. Therefore, the pain threshold (sensation from warmth to pain) and tolerance (unacceptable pain) temperatures for each individual were estimated. Heat stimuli were induced at those two temperatures to get examples of low and high pain respectively. In addition, two intermediate pain levels were introduced, resulting in 4 pain classes. Apart from this, 1 non-painful class with a baseline temperature of $32\,°C$ exists. During the induction process, each pain level was applied 20 times using 4 s stimuli each. Inter-stimuli intervals at the baseline temperature lasted 8–12 s.

Past works carrying out studies on the BioVid dataset are numerous. Walter et al. [16] were the first ones to evaluate the performance of a classifier exclusively based on the physiological modalities of the BioVid Heat Pain database. A pre-processing step, including a Butterworth filter for EMG and ECG signal, an Empirical Mode Decomposition technique and a detection of "bursts of activity via the EMG using the Hilbert Spectrum" [16] was conducted. Features measuring amplitude, frequency, stationarity, entropy, linearity, and variability of the signals were extracted. A forward and backward selection as feature selection part was tested. A support vector machine (SVM) was trained and evaluated in a 10-fold cross validation scheme. It could be shown that the forward selection outperformed the backward selection in any task with a best accuracy of 94.73% for the task Baseline versus highest pain (B vs.

---

[1]http://medoc-web.com/products/pathway/.

T4) using a 10-fold cross-validation. Furthermore, a leave-one-subject-out (LOSO) evaluation resulted in a best accuracy of 77.05% for B versus T4. Kächele et al. [5] were the first to transform the task into a regression problem, so to predict a continuous pain level instead of a class. Moreover, they evaluated a subject clustering approach, where people were grouped based on similar physiological responses. A random forest classifier was then specialised according to the found cluster of people. It could be shown that this personalisation step improved the performance of the system.

More recent studies attempted to use deep neural networks for their ability to learn features autonomously. Lopez et al. [6] were the first to evaluate neural networks on the BioVid dataset. A multi-task neural network was implemented to define a task for each subject. While classical machine learning approaches try to solve one task at a time, multi-task learning (MTL) aims at training models to solve several tasks simultaneously. A DNN with layers shared between tasks, and task-specific layers was chosen. One commonly shared and one person specific hidden layer resulted in an output for each subject. Thus, the network has commonly shared layers and splits up into task specific layers, each with an individual classification output. Using a 10-fold cross validation a maximum accuracy of 82.75% for the task B versus P4 could be achieved. It could be shown that their MTL approach outperforms traditional single-task-learning (SVM or DNN) ones. Thiam et al. [13] could further demonstrate the power of deep learning models. Using a pre-processing phase similar to Walter et al. [16] they trained convolutional neural networks on input data of all modalities and models trained for each modality separately (early and late fusion). Using a late fusion method with learnable parameters assigning a weight to each modality, it could be shown that the late fusion performs best, and the EDA signal is mainly contributing to the classification result. Using a LOSO evaluation for the B versus T4 task an accuracy of 84.40% and 84.57% could be achieved for the late fusion and a uni-modal EDA model respectively.

3   Materials and Methods

3.1   Data Acquisition

The data of 10 healthy subjects was acquired. Pain was induced by applying thermal stimuli using a Pathway CHEPS (Contact Heat—Evoked Potential Stimulator) via a 27 mm diameter contact surface attached with a Velcro strap (Medoc, Ramat Yishai, Israel) to the non-dominant forearm (10 cm below the elbow). Participants were in comfortable siting position. Data acquisition was divided into two phases: calibration and pain induction phase.

3.1.1 Calibration

Before calibration started, participants were familiarised with the computerised visual analogue scale (CoVAS; Medoc, Ramat Yishai, Israel). The CoVAS is a slider that allows to collect pain ratings in real time. After instruction participants underwent a staircase procedure which aim was to determine the temperature that evoked pain at the level of 50 (*pain50*) measured on the scale ranging from 0 ("no pain") to 100 ("unbearable pain"). Participants received a series of stimuli of increasing temperature starting from 32 °C to the first limit of 40 °C. Every subsequent trial had a temperature limit higher by of 1 °C, but the highest possible temperature was 49 °C. Each stimulus lasted 10 s (30 °C/s raise and fall rates). Participants were asked to continuously evaluate their pain intensity during each 10 s period using CoVAS. After identification of the *pain50* level the best suited stimulation interval (a–e) was selected accordingly:

(a) Pain50: 42–43 °C resulted in a paradigm including the temperatures 40–45 °C
(b) Pain50: 43–44 °C resulted in a paradigm including the temperatures 41–46 °C
(c) Pain50: 44–45 °C resulted in a paradigm including the temperatures 42–47 °C
(d) Pain50: 45–46 °C resulted in a paradigm including the temperatures 43–48 °C
(e) Pain50: 46–47 °C resulted in a paradigm including the temperatures 44–49 °C

Lastly, a calibration check procedure was performed to adjust the temperature if necessary. The following two stimuli were applied for 10 s each: the lowest and the highest temperature of the stimulation interval (e.g. stimulation interval A corresponds to 40 °C and 45 °C). Calibration check was successful if the lowest stimulus (e.g. 40 °C) was rated as non-painful and the highest stimulus as tolerable but corresponded to at least 80 out of 100. If this assumption was not fulfilled, the temperature interval was then adjusted.

3.1.2 Pain Induction

After identifying the appropriate stimulus interval, six different whole-number temperatures in the range of the corresponding interval were applied eight times in a random order (total 48 stimuli per subject) for 10 s (30 °C/s raise and fall rates) each. Inter-stimuli intervals at a baseline temperature of 32 °C had a random duration between 20 to 30 s. The total duration of the data acquisition was about 30 min.

3.1.3 Sensors

Sensor data of the wearables *Empatica E4*[2] and *RespiBan*[3] were collected during the pain induction phase to record 10 sensor modalities. The Empatica E4 is a wristband,

---

[2]https://www.empatica.com/research/e4/.
[3]https://plux.info/biosignalsplux-wearables/313-respiban-professional-820202407.html.

worn on the non-dominant hand, measuring blood volume pulse (BVP) from which heart rate (HR) and inter-beats-interval (IBI) are computed, electrodermal activity (EDA) and skin temperature. The RespiBan is a small wearable worn with a chest strap measuring respiration (Resp) and configurable sensors. We decided to use a similar setup to the BioVid dataset with following sensors: EDA signal was measured at the fingertips of the non-dominant arm. The heart activity was recorded using an electrocardiogram (ECG) with positive electrode at the upper left, negative electrode at the upper right pectoral and a reference electrode placed at the right waist. Two surface electromyography (sEMG) sensors were used to track the activity of the *trapezius* and *zygomaticus* muscles that are associated with the perception of pain. A reference electrode was placed above the 7th cervical vertebrae.

3.2 Data Pre-processing and Segmentation

Sensor data of the different modalities were synchronised with the temperature stimulus of the Pathway system and the CoVAS rating as well. In addition, the data were re-sampled to a fixed frequency of 100 Hz. Modalities with a lower initial frequency were up sampled by linear interpolation. To reduce the time during learning and help the model converge faster, the data has been standardised for the deep neural network approach initially. For each sensor channel of each subject the *standard score*, also referred to as *z-score*, was computed. No further pre-processing or cleaning of the data was implemented.

After the acquisition process there were one recording of sensor modalities and temperature and CoVAS values for each participant. Therefore, two individual segmentation processes were implemented. Windows of data were segmented using the temperature stimulus itself and the CoVAS ratings respectively. For both approaches, the onset and offset of a pain window were detected using a simple threshold-based rule. Afterwards, a fixed window of 10 s was centred around the middle of the on- and offset. The data of all sensor modalities was segmented using this time interval. Intermediate data between pain stimuli was used to find as many non-overlapping "no-pain" windows as possible. Although previous works have shown that distinguishing no pain versus high pain is the simplest task [6, 7, 11, 14, 18, 20], we decided to go for a non-standard "pain" versus "no pain" problem. This decision was made because of the small size of our dataset. Categorising pain examples by intensity would indeed have led to classes with too few examples and therefore unrepresentative results. Segmenting sections of 10 s of the 10 sensor channels with a frequency rate of 100 Hz results in time windows of shape 1000×10.

Figure 1 shows an example of data segmentation. A section of both CoVAS (orange) and heater (blue) data are shown for one subject. The segmentation for both approaches is highlighted in green and red respectively. Note the differences in similar heater stimuli and the perceived pain (CoVAS). This subjective perceived component is lost using an approach based on the pain stimulus exclusively.

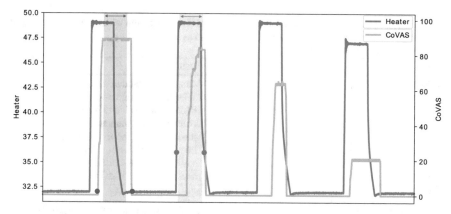

Fig. 1 Example of temperature (heater) and CoVAS ratings. A possible window using the temperate approach is visualised in green, a possible window for the CoVAS approach in red. On and offset are highlighted as dots in their respective colour as well

1365 windows for the heater and 1410 windows for CoVAS approach were extracted. Since the baseline inter-stimulus intervals last between 2 to 3 times longer than the pain stimuli, more "no pain" windows are obtained than pain leading to an unbalanced dataset. Pain examples account for approximately one third and one fourth of the heater and CoVAS datasets respectively.

3.3 Machine Learning Approaches

3.3.1 Hand Crafted Features

Instead of training classifiers on the raw data, models (like a random forest) are normally built based on hand crafted features. This step of extracting features using our dataset included the calculation of mostly statistical features (for example mean, standard deviation, min, max) computed on the time and frequency domains, raw and normalised signals as well of the first order derivative. These specific features for each sensor channel were taken from different sources in the literature [8, 14, 18]. In total 141 features for each window have been computed. Table 1 summarises the computed features for each sensor modality individual.

3.3.2 Deep Neural Network

Deep learning models have the capability to automatically learn features from given data. Therefore, models are trained in an end-to-end manner, which means that the raw data is directly mapped to a class output using a neural network model. Differ-

Table 1 The used features for every sensor channel and the source from which they were retrieved from. Note: For the features processed by the Empatica E4(HR, IBI) no complex, but simple statistical features were computed

Sensors	Source	Features
EDA/ EMG/ ECG	[18]	Max, range, standard deviation (std), inter-quartile range, root mean square (RMS), mean value of local maxima, mean absolute value, mean of the absolute values (mav) of the first differences (mavfd), mavfd on standardised signal, mav of the second differences (mavsd), mavsd on standardised signal
HR/IBI	–	Mean, std, max, min
Other (BVP, Resp)	[14]	On the raw and normalised signal: 1st order derivative and 2nd order derivative: mean, mean of absolute values, std On the raw signal: max peak, peak range (max-min), mean value of maxima, mean value of minima, skewness, kurtosis On the power spectrum of the signal: mean, std, area (sum), median, spectral entropy

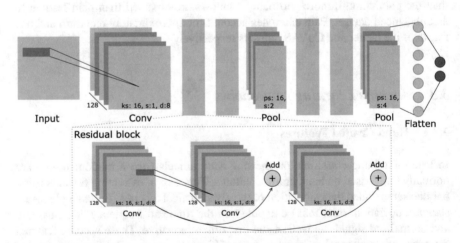

Fig. 2 Deep classification architecture of the CNN using residual blocks (highlighted in blue)

ent architectures as multi-layer perceptron (MLPs), convolutional neural networks (CNNs) and residual CNNs were tested. Preliminary results showed that the residual CNN worked best, thus this model is referred to the DNN approach from now on. Figure 2 shows the implemented architecture with its individual layers and used hyper-parameters, as number of kernels, kernel size (**ks**), pool size (**ps**), stride length (**s**) and dilation rate (**d**). The classification outcome of the network is obtained by a softmax activation in the last fully connected layer after an flatten operation.

Table 2 Classification performances averaged over the LOSO folds for the presented approaches (HCF and DNN using temperature and CoVAS labels) using accuracy and F_1 score. The best performing method for each metric is depicted in bold

	Acc (%)		AF_1 (%)	
	HCF	DNN	HCF	DNN
CoVAS	**75.57**	66.49	56.01	**59.10**
T°C	**66.91**	58.54	52.73	**56.27**

	CoVAS				Temperature		
HCF	Confusion matrix(%)		Estimated labels		Confusion matrix(%)		Estimated labels
			No Pain	Pain			No Pain	Pain
	True labels	No Pain	90.85	9.15	True labels	No Pain	89.72	10.28
		Pain	77.14	**22.86**		Pain	78.70	**21.30**
DNN	Confusion matrix(%)		Estimated labels		Confusion matrix(%)		Estimated labels
			No Pain	Pain			No Pain	Pain
	True labels	No Pain	70.19	29.81	True labels	No Pain	59.89	40.11
		Pain	43.71	**56.29**		Pain	43.26	**56.74**

Fig. 3 Performance of the presented approaches visualised by 4 confusion matrices

4 Results

It was decided to evaluate the models in a subject independent way using a *leave-one-subject-out* (LOSO) cross validation. Since the dataset is limited in size and a class imbalance is existing, *accuracy* and F_1 score were chosen as evaluation metrics. The main advantage of using a LOSO scheme is that the model's performance is evaluated in a subject-independent way. The data of one person is in either the training or the testing set. Thus, the evaluation of the classifier provides a more realistic estimation of how good the classifier is working for data of never seen subjects.

The performance evaluation of the presented approaches is summarised in Table 2 and the confusion matrices for HCF and DNN using both CoVAS and temperature labels are shown in Fig. 3. The HCF approach tends to predict "no pain" more often, the approach has a higher accuracy and *false negative* rate compared to the DNN approach. On the contrary the DNN has better recognition of pain to the detriment of no pain, resulting in a higher F_1 score but also *false positive* rate. For all computed tests, the approach using temperature labels was outperformed by CoVAS labels.

5 Discussion

While both classification approaches do not yield outstanding results compared to previous works, using CoVAS labels obtain better results compared to the temperature label. This seems to confirm our assumptions that the subjective perceived component is lost using approaches based on the pain stimulus exclusively. Furthermore, a direct comparison between the presented results and previous works cannot be drawn. In distinction to methods performed on the BioVid dataset no fine granular task like "no pain" versus "high pain" was implemented, but the task "no pain" versus "pain". Therefore, a lower performance compared to these tasks is to be expected because various pain states are summarised as one. Previous works stated performance rates around chance and 80% accuracy for the tasks "no pain" versus "low pain" and "no pain" versus "high pain". These results would lead to the assumption that the combined task settles in between. Achieving a best accuracy rate of 75.57% and best F_1 score of 59.10%, this assumption can be confirmed.

In order to understand why the achieved performances are only mediocre, we computed T-distributed Stochastic Neighbour Embedding (t-SNE) plots of the HCF and DNN features for further analyse. 4 different labels were attributed for the data of each subject using the temperature labels. Data acquired during stimuli of the two lowest temperatures of the stimulation interval were labelled as "low pain". The two intermediate and two highest temperatures were used to label data as "medium" and "high" pain respectively. Data acquired during induction at the baseline temperature were labelled as "no pain". Afterwards, the 144 presented hand-crafted and DNN features (outputs of the last-but-one fully connected layer of the network) for each data sample were computed. These characteristics were extracted for every participant of the dataset individually and fed to the t-SNE algorithm, which computes a low-dimensional representation of high dimensional data. For both feature types, two groups of subjects could be distinguished based on visual examination of their t-SNE embeddings. For some subjects, the t-SNE plots show separable classes, while for the others, features from all classes are mixed. The features of 2 and 1 out of 10 subjects yielded t-SNE embeddings with clear distinction between no pain and pain classes for HCF and DNN respectively. Figure 4 provides examples of t-SNE embeddings of features computed for subjects from each cluster, for both HCF and DNN. On the left plots, no clusters are visible. On the right plots, "no pain" can be separated from "pain" quite good. These results underline the assumption that there are different groups of (physiological) reactions of participants when confronted with pain and that they can be clustered as such. Previous papers have already shown that clustering subjects outperforms traditional single-task-learning methods for pain recognition. Thus, approaches relying on clustering will be evaluated in the future.

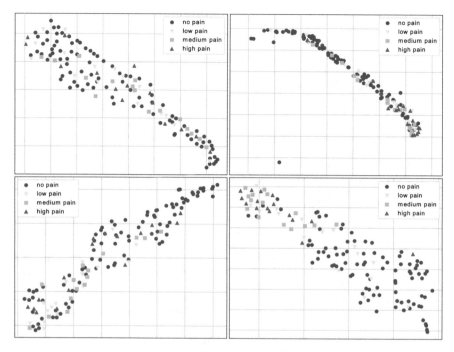

Fig. 4 Examples of t-SNE plots for the HCF (upper plots) and DNN (lower plots) features of four subjects

6 Conclusion

This work explored the use of both temperature and self-report label to classify heat-induced pain. A small dataset including physiological sensor modalities of 10 subject was acquired and analysed. A random forest based on hand-crafted features and a deep neural network were trained and evaluated on this set. While previous works using machine learning algorithms were mainly based on the pain stimulus itself (for example a temperature label), our results lead to the conclusion that the self-perceived intensity rating (for example using a CoVAS slider) as label is a far better choice. This finding could possibly lead to improvements in the field of automated pain recognition.

Nevertheless, those promising results must be further evaluated considering the very small size of the dataset we used. Therefore, a new dataset with increased number of subjects and further sensor modalities (like RGB cameras) is planned. Having a larger dataset, more refined pain classes could be defined. In addition, in previous works elaborated subject clustering methods will be implemented to increase the classification performance of our system.

Acknowledgements This work was funded by the German Federal Ministry of Education and Research (BMBF) in the frame of the project *PainMonit* (grant number: 01DS19008A).

References

1. Armati, P., Chow, R.: Pain: The Person, the Science, the Clinical Interface. IP Communications Pty, Limited, Melbourne (2015)
2. Brink, M.V.D., Bandell-Hoekstra, E., Abu-Saad, H.H.: The occurrence of recall bias in pediatric headache: a comparison of questionnaire and diary data. Headache **41**(1), 11–20 (2001)
3. Davies, H., Crombie, I., Macrae, W.: Where does it hurt? Describing the body locations of chronic pain. Eur. J. Pain **2**(1), 69–80 (1998)
4. Gruss, S., Geiger, M., Werner, P., Wilhelm, O., Traue, H.C., Al-Hamadi, A., Walter, S.: Multi-modal signals for analyzing pain responses to thermal and electrical stimuli. JoVE (J. Vis. Exp.) **2019**(146), e59057 (2019)
5. Kächele, M., Thiam, P., Amirian, M., Schwenker, F., Palm, G.: Methods for person-centered continuous pain intensity assessment from bio-physiological channels. IEEE J. Sel. Top. Signal Process. **10**(5), 854–864 (2016)
6. Lopez-Martinez, D., Picard, R.: Multi-task neural networks for personalized pain recognition from physiological signals. In: 2017 7th International Conference on Affective Computing and Intelligent Interaction Workshops and Demos (ACIIW), pp. 181–184. IEEE (2017)
7. Lopez-Martinez, D., Picard, R.: Continuous pain intensity estimation from autonomic signals with recurrent neural networks. In: 2018 40th Annual International Conference of the IEEE Engineering in Medicine and Biology Society (EMBC), pp. 5624–5627. IEEE (2018)
8. Lopez-Martinez, D., Rudovic, O., Picard, R.: Physiological and behavioral profiling for nociceptive pain estimation using personalized multitask learning (2017). arXiv preprint arXiv:1711.04036
9. Merskey, H.: Pain terms: a list with definitions and notes on usage. Recommended by the IASP subcommittee on taxonomy. Pain **6**, 249–252 (1979)
10. Pasero, C., McCaffery, M.: Pain Assessment and Pharmacologic Management - E-Book. Elsevier Health Sciences, Amsterdam (2010)
11. Salah, A., Khalil, M.I., Abbas, H.: Multimodal pain level recognition using majority voting technique. In: 2018 13th International Conference on Computer Engineering and Systems (ICCES), pp. 307–312. IEEE (2018)
12. Stone, A.A., Broderick, J.E., Shiffman, S.S., Schwartz, J.E.: Understanding recall of weekly pain from a momentary assessment perspective: absolute agreement, between- and within-person consistency, and judged change in weekly pain. Pain **107**(1), 61–69 (2004)
13. Thiam, P., Bellmann, P., Kestler, H.A., Schwenker, F.: Exploring deep physiological models for nociceptive pain recognition. Sensors **19**(20), 4503 (2019)
14. Thiam, P., Kessler, V., Amirian, M., Bellmann, P., Layher, G., Zhang, Y., Velana, M., Gruss, S., Walter, S., Traue, H.C., et al.: Multi-modal pain intensity recognition based on the senseemotion database. IEEE Trans. Affect. Comput. (2019)
15. Velana, M., Gruss, S., Layher, G., Thiam, P., Zhang, Y., Schork, D., Kessler, V., Meudt, S., Neumann, H., Kim, J., et al.: The senseemotion database: a multimodal database for the development and systematic validation of an automatic pain-and emotion-recognition system. In: IAPR Workshop on Multimodal Pattern Recognition of Social Signals in Human-Computer Interaction, pp. 127–139. Springer (2016)
16. Walter, S., Gruss, S., Limbrecht-Ecklundt, K., Traue, H.C., Werner, P., Al-Hamadi, A., Diniz, N., da Silva, G.M., Andrade, A.O.: Automatic pain quantification using autonomic parameters. Psychol. Neurosci. **7**(3), 363–380 (2014)
17. Werner, P., Al-Hamadi, A., Niese, R., Walter, S., Gruss, S., Traue, H.C.: Towards pain monitoring: facial expression, head pose, a new database, an automatic system and remaining challenges. In: Proceedings of the British Machine Vision Conference, pp. 1–13 (2013)
18. Werner, P., Al-Hamadi, A., Niese, R., Walter, S., Gruss, S., Traue, H.C.: Automatic pain recognition from video and biomedical signals. In: 2014 22nd International Conference on Pattern Recognition, pp. 4582–4587. IEEE (2014)

19. Zhang, Z., Girard, J.M., Wu, Y., Zhang, X., Liu, P., Ciftci, U., Canavan, S., Reale, M., Horowitz, A., Yang, H., et al.: Multimodal spontaneous emotion corpus for human behavior analysis. In: Proceedings of the IEEE Conference on Computer Vision and Pattern Recognition, pp. 3438–3446 (2016)
20. Zhi, R., Yu, J.: Multi-modal fusion based automatic pain assessment. In: 2019 IEEE 8th Joint International Information Technology and Artificial Intelligence Conference (ITAIC), pp. 1378–1382. IEEE (2019)

Modeling and Simulation

Flow in a Myocardial Bridge Region of a Coronary Artery—Experimental Rig and Numerical Model

Bartlomiej Melka, Marcin Nowak, Marek Rojczyk, Maria Gracka, Wojciech Adamczyk, Ziemowit Ostrowski, and Ryszard Bialecki

Abstract The myocardial bridge is a coronary abnormality in which one of the coronary arteries tunnels through the myocardium rather than resting on top of it. During the heart systole this artery is contracted disturbing the normal blood flow. The paper focuses on the modeling of the flow in a developed experimental rig mimicking the myocardial bridge. The results of the CFD simulations of a periodically compressed elastic conduit were presented as pressure and velocity fields.

Keywords CFD · Blood flow · Coronary artery · Myocardial bridge

1 Introduction

The coronary abnormality in which one of the epicardial coronary arteries is partially covered by the heart muscle is called the myocardial bridge (MB). During the heart

B. Melka · M. Nowak · M. Rojczyk · M. Gracka · W. Adamczyk · Z. Ostrowski (✉) · R. Bialecki
Biomedical Engineering Lab., Department of Thermal Engineering, Silesian University of Technology, Konarskiego 22, 44-100 Gliwice, Poland
e-mail: ziemowit.ostrowski@polsl.pl

B. Melka
e-mail: bartlomiej,melka@polsl.pl

M. Nowak
e-mail: marcin.nowak@polsl.pl

M. Rojczyk
e-mail: marek.rojczyk@polsl.pl

M. Gracka
e-mail: maria.gracka@polsl.pl

W. Adamczyk
e-mail: wojciech.adamczyk@polsl.pl

R. Bialecki
e-mail: ryszard.bialecki@polsl.pl

E. Piętka et al. (eds.), *Information Technology in Biomedicine*, Advances in Intelligent Systems and Computing 1186, https://doi.org/10.1007/978-3-030-49666-1_20

contraction, heart muscles are contracting the segment of the coronary artery under the MB and the lumen of this blood vessel is decreasing. The reduced internal volume of this artery causes a reversed flow of the blood from the aforementioned region into the proximal segments of the blood coronary system. As the majority of the literature sources claim, the MB was firstly described by Reyman in 1737 during the autopsy [7]. However, some sources point that MB was firstly described by Cranicianu in 1922 [3] and that MB was firstly investigated using the angiography technique by Portman and Iwing in 1960 [2]. The most common region of this pathology is located in the middle of the left anterior descending artery (LAD) [4, 8]. The blood flow disturbances could foster the atherosclerosis plaque deposition [1]. Therefore, patients with MB could be more often threatened by coronary heart disease [5]. Moreover, authors in [9] claim that MB could affect to myocardia ischemia even without significant atherosclerotic stenosis.

One of the ways for the non-invasive investigation techniques in the case of flow through the MB is the Computational Fluid Dynamics (CFD). This approach, based on the computer modeling, yields results for the wide spectrum of the geometries. However, the implementation of the dynamic movement of the blood vessel during the systole and artery contraction is a challenging task. Advanced methods of mesh manipulation, such as mesh deformation or dynamic re-meshing, are necessary to reflect the real behavior of the blood vessel distortion in numerical modeling.

Results coming from numerical modeling of the new and advanced approaches should be validated on the base of experimental research to make them credible. Therefore, introducing the new numerical approaches or investigating new cases requires often the creation of a dedicated test rig. The example of the experimental research based on the measurement of the flow behavior in a channel with a dynamic throat could be [6].

The paper deals with the numerical investigation reproducing the rapid pressure changes accompanied by the significant pipe distortion. The CFD investigation reflected the model of MB developed during experimental activities.

2   Description of the Experiment

The object of the research during the experimental investigation was a propylene tube mimicking the MB section. The dynamic, periodic contraction effect on the tube was implemented by increasing the pressure outside the tube. This happened in a closed cylindrical chamber enclosing the tube. Increasing the pressure in the chamber contracts the tube similarly as the heart muscle contracts the MB artery during the systole. The described construction is presented in Fig. 1.

The presented research object was a part of the larger test rig that mimicked the human blood circulatory system which is presented in Fig. 2. The mass flow of the medium in the system was generated by a pulsatile pump (Harvard Apparatus).

The damping elements were installed at the outlet of the pump and in three more locations, presented in Fig. 2. They were used to avoid medium pulsation and to

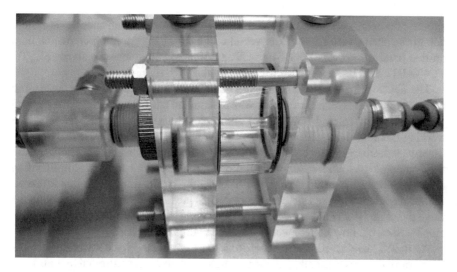

Fig. 1 Artificial myocardial bridge design

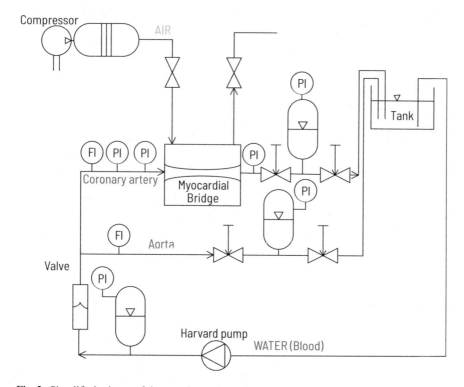

Fig. 2 Simplified scheme of the experimental test rig

simulate the energy accumulation potential occurring in the human circulation system due to the elastic distortion of the vessels. In each of the damping elements, both on-line pressure sensors (DB SENSOR, DMP343) and solenoid valves (FESTO VOVG-B12-M32C-AH-F-1H2) were installed.

The developed rig contains dampers containing air above the water level. The pressure of the air inside the damper was maintained constant. In Fig. 2, the applied pressure transducers and flow meters are depicted as PI and FI respectively. The working medium during the experiments was water. Downstream the MB section, water was discharged into a tank, that is an open to the environment. Though there is no analogue of such a reservoir real blood circulation, this kind of simplification is often made in experiments in order to close the circulation. From this reservoir water was pumped by the Harvard pump. As it is presented in Fig. 2 after passing the valve the main flow is split into two sections: aorta and the coronary artery. In each blood vessel, the flow meters were installed (Endress+Hauser).

As it was mentioned, the silicone tube was contracted by air which is transferred from the pressure tank. An open-and-close period was controlled by Lab View (National Instruments) application, where times of openings were defined using NI procedure. Data acquisition was performed on the computer using NI cRIO-9074 and NI 9265 analog output.

As it was mentioned, the investigated MB section represented by the synthetic pipe was under the influence of the external pressure within the chamber. This pressure was changing during the cycle and caused the pipe distortion mimicking the contraction effect in the MB. The shape of the investigated pipe during the cycle was recorded by camcorder with a frequency of 500 frames per second. The acquisition of the pipe shape was conducted in two perpendicular views covering the maximum distortions. In those two views, the default pipe shape without over-pressure within the MB chamber is presented at the top level in Fig. 3a, b. The maximum distortions are presented on the bottom level in Fig. 3c, d. Additionally, the external dimensions of the pipe in specific views were presented in this figure. The internal shape was estimated by subtracting the pipe wall thickness reaching 0.8 mm at each side. As it is visible in the presented figure, in the first view the measuring length is decreasing while in the second view the controlling dimension is increasing. However, the effective area of the lumen was reduced during the contraction progress.

3   Numerical Model

The numerical domain corresponds to the already described contracted section of the tube. Additionally, the 19 cm section was added before the MB and 13 cm section was added behind the MB. At each end of the described additional sections, pressure sensors were located.

The mesh, used in the numerical model, was built with additional inlet and outlet sections using hexahedral elements. Tetrahedral elements were used in the artery section where the vessel deformation (MB) occurs. These type of elements was used

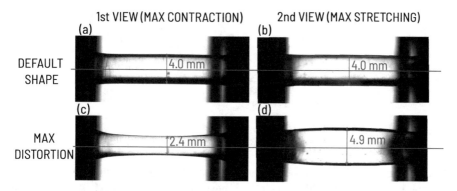

Fig. 3 Shape acquisition of the investigated MB section

the simulate the flow with dynamic mesh settings, covering the mesh deformation and re-meshing options between each of the time steps. Therefore, together with the re-meshing procedure, the number of elements varied, especially in the MB artery section. The implemented numerical mesh consisted of approx. 80 k elements.

A set of mass and momentum conservation equations Eqs. (1), (2) was solved within the computational domain using ANSYS FLUENT, a commercial CFD solver. The mesh changes were introduced by in-house User Defined Functions,

$$\frac{\partial p}{\partial t} + \nabla \cdot (\rho \boldsymbol{v}) = 0 \tag{1}$$

where p is the pressure, t is the time, ρ is the density and $\boldsymbol{v}$ is the velocity vector.

$$\frac{\partial}{\partial t}(\rho \boldsymbol{v}) + \nabla \cdot (\rho \boldsymbol{v} \boldsymbol{v}) = -\nabla p + \nabla \left(\bar{\bar{\tau}} \right) \tag{2}$$

where τ is the stress tensor that can be calculated from Eq. (3).

$$\bar{\bar{\tau}} = \mu \left[\left(\nabla \boldsymbol{v} + \nabla \boldsymbol{v}^{T} \right) - \frac{2}{3} \nabla \cdot \boldsymbol{v} I \right] \tag{3}$$

where μ is the dynamic viscosity and I is the unit tensor while $\boldsymbol{v}^{T}$ is a transposed velocity vector.

The presented governing equations were solved together with the accompanying boundary conditions. The inlet boundary condition was set as a pressure profile varying in time using the recorded values collected during the experimental part of the research. In the same manner, pressure outflow was formulated.

The pipe deformation in the experiment is shown in Fig. 4. The contraction effect in the MB section was implemented into the simulations by reproducing the data coming from image analysis, as presented in Fig. 3 and described in the previous subsection. As it was mentioned, the temporal lumen change of the pipe was modelled

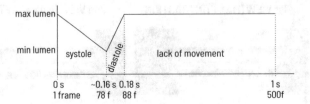

Fig. 4 Process of the tube lumen contraction

by dynamic mesh distortion and re-meshing methods. One can see that the contraction (systole) period was notably longer than releasing (diastole) period. The maximum pipe contraction occurred at the 0.156 s of the cycle. To bring the cycle closer to the heart one additional valve decreasing the speed of the release phase will be implemented in further research.

4 Results

As it was mentioned in the model description, the boundary conditions were set in the model according to the experimentally recorded pressures. In Fig. 5, the comparison of the pressures implemented in the model and the experimental data are juxtaposed. The pipe contraction and relaxation occurred during the first 0.2 s of the cycle where the pressure wave was mapped with sufficient consistency.

The pressure field estimated by the numerical model for the maximum pipe distortion is presented in Fig. 6. The whole domain is shown in black-and-white while the zoom of the MB section is shown in colours. The minimum pressure in the MB section for this time instant could be observed in the region behind the centre of the MB. The pressure drop in the MB section is lower than 1 kPa.

The velocity fields in the myocardial bridge section are presented in Fig. 7 for three time instants. The scale was unified for all presented fields. The first field represents the time instant at 0.07 s of the cycle and shows the moment a bit before the middle of the contraction period. The next field, representing 0.15 s, shows the maximum hose distortion during the cycle. For that moment both within the MB and at the same time in the whole domain the maximum velocity occurs. The last presented velocity field, for 0.3 s of the cycle, shows the flow within the hose of the default shape.

5 Conclusions

The numerical model reproducing the behavior of the flow at the dedicated test rig was developed. The test rig was built to investigate the process of the pipe distortion in in-vitro conditions mimicking the MB behavior occurring in the human body.

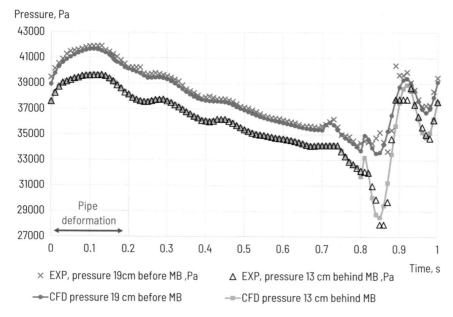

Fig. 5 Pressure introduced in the model on the base of experimental records

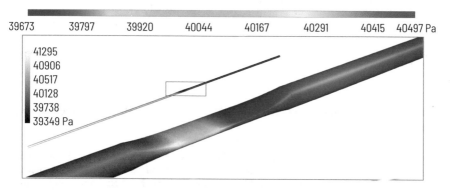

Fig. 6 Pressure fields on the MB walls in Pa: gray-scale for the whole numerical domain, color scale in the MB section

The aim of the presented research was to reproduce in the numerical model exact experiment, not to mimic real heart work.

The boundary conditions assumed in the model were set as the pressure varying in time according to experimental data recorded by pressure transducers. The varying flow was simulated under the additional load coming from the dynamic shape distortion of the pipe. The results of the model covered the velocity and pressure fields in the defined domain. The model was able to get reasonable results despite rapid pressure changes and large domain distortions. The experience gained in this

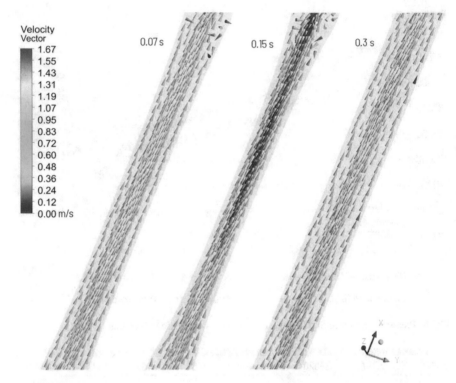

Fig. 7 Velocity fields in m/s zoomed to the MB section for three time instants: 0.07 s, 0.15 s and 0.3 s of the cycle

research will be used to simulate the behavior of the real MB using patient specific data.

Acknowledgements This research is supported by the National Science Centre (Poland) within project No. 2017/27/B/ST8/01046 and by the Silesian University of Technology within the Rector's scientific research and development grant No 08/60/RGJ20/0254. This help is gratefully acknowledged herewith.

References

1. Alegria, J.R., Herrmann, J., Holmes, D.R., Lerman, A., Rihal, C.S.: Myocardial bridging. Eur. Hear. J. **26**(12), 1159–1168 (2005). https://doi.org/10.1093/eurheartj/ehi203
2. Aygun, F., Caldir, M., Ciftci, O., Ozulku, M., Gunday, M.: Co-existence of myocardial bridge, thrombus and stenosis in the same coronary segment. J. Med. Cases **6**(6), 243–246 (2015)
3. Cranicianu, A.: Anatomische Studien über die koronarterien und experimentelle Untersuchungen über Durchgan-gigkeit. Virchows Arch. [Pathol. Anat.] **238**, 1–8 (1922)
4. Hazirolan, T., Canyigit, M., Karcaaltincaba, M., Dagoglu, M.G., Akata, D., Aytemir, K., Besim, A.: Myocardial bridging on MDCT. Am. J. Roentgenol. **188**(4), 1074–1080 (2007). https://doi.

org/10.2214/AJR.06.0417

5. Ishii, T., Ishikawa, Y., Akasaka, Y.: Myocardial bridge as a structure of "double-edged sword" for the coronary artery. Ann. Vasc. Dis. **7**(2), 99–108 (2014). https://doi.org/10.3400/avd.ra.14-00037

6. Matsuzaki, Y., Ikeda, T., Matsumoto, T., Kitagawa, T.: Experiments on steady and oscillatory flows at moderate reynolds numbers in a quasi-two-dimensional channel with a throat. J. Biomech. Eng. **120**(5), 594–601 (1998). https://doi.org/10.1115/1.2834749

7. Reyman, H.C., Disertatio de vasis cordis propriis. Medizinische Dissertation, Universität Göttingen, 1–32 (1737)

8. Wentzel, J.J., Corti, R., Fayad, Z.A., Wisdom, P., Macaluso, F., Winkelman, M.O., Fuster, V., Badimon, J.J.: Does shear stress modulate both plaque progression and regression in the thoracic aorta?: Human study using serial magnetic resonance imaging. J. Am. Coll. Cardiol. **45**(6), 846–854 (2005). https://doi.org/10.1016/j.jacc.2004.12.026

9. Yu, M., Zhou, L., Chen, T., et al.: Myocardia ischemia associated with a myocardial bridge with no significant atherosclerotic stenosis. BMC Cardiovasc. Disord. **15**, 165 (2015). https://doi.org/10.1186/s12872-015-0158-2

Numerical Model of the Aortic Valve Implanted Within Real Human Aorta

Marcin Nowak, Wojciech Adamczyk, Bartlomiej Melka, Ziemowit Ostrowski, and Ryszard Bialecki

Abstract Cardiovascular system diseases are the main cause of deaths in developed and developing countries. The main reasons are myocardial infarction, heart failure, stroke and valvular diseases. These are caused mainly by arteriosclerosis. The valvular diseases involve a significant burden for the health care system and their frequency is rising with the patient age. This work describes the tools and numerical models appropriate for modeling the blood flow through the synthetic aortic valve and demonstrates the preliminary model used by authors. The overset mesh technique was applied to capture synthetic valve movement implanted within the aortic root, the aorta arch and the main branches of cardiovascular system. As the analyzed geometry scope does not include the whole cardiovascular system, there are artificial boundaries present at the inlet and at the outlets. To capture the cardiac system influence on the pressure values at these boundaries, the lumped parameter model was implemented.

Keywords CFD · Blood flow · Aortic valve · Moving mesh

M. Nowak · W. Adamczyk · B. Melka · Z. Ostrowski (✉) · R. Bialecki
Biomedical Engineering Lab., Department of Thermal Engineering, Silesian University of Technology, Konarskiego 22, 44-100 Gliwice, Poland
e-mail: ziemowit.ostrowski@polsl.pl

M. Nowak
e-mail: marcin.nowak@polsl.pl

W. Adamczyk
e-mail: wojciech.adamczyk@polsl.pl

B. Melka
e-mail: bartlomiej.melka@polsl.pl

R. Bialecki
e-mail: ryszard.bialecki@polsl.pl

E. Piętka et al. (eds.), *Information Technology in Biomedicine*, Advances in Intelligent Systems and Computing 1186, https://doi.org/10.1007/978-3-030-49666-1_21

1   Introduction

The diseases of cardiovascular system (CVDs) are the leading cause of deaths in the world. According to the World Health Organization (WHO), CVDs caused 31% of deaths in 2015 in the world, while in Europe 45% of all diseases are the consequence of CVDs [20]. Although disability-adjusted death due to CVDs have been decreasing in most European countries over the last decade, CVDs are responsible for the death of more than 64 million in Europe (23% of all death) and 26 million death in the EU (19%) [20]. Looking on these numbers, it is clear that the problem is quite large and cannot be downplayed by the society.

The main reason for the increased cardiovascular mortality is arteriosclerosis with its consequences, such as myocardial infarction, heart failure or stroke. The most life threatening valve disease is severe aortic stenosis. The pooled prevalence of severe aortic stenosis reaches 3.4% in patients 75 year old and older [17]. In the USA alone, about 65,000 surgical aortic valve replacements are performed yearly.

This research demonstrates the development of the numerical model, based on application of the complex overset mesh technique, to model movement of the leaflets and simulate their impact on the blood flow patterns downstream the valve. A set of numerical simulations was carried out using commercial CFD ANSYS Fluent package extended by User Defined Functions (UDF) implemented into the solution procedure. The responses of blood circulatory system on modeled section of the arterial tree and aortic valve performance were captured by implementation of the lumped parameter model (LPM) into the solution procedure, based on the electrical analogy [19]. The valve leaflets were modeled as non-deformable and its movement was modeled using the angular profile based on the literature [18]. The mesh motion was simulated using the overset technique. The laminar turbulence model was applied. The impact of heart valve presence within modeled domain, especially on the calculated mass flow rates from subsequent branches, also was investigated. The blood was treated as non-Newtonian fluid—Carreau model. The set of numerical simulations was carried out using geometrical model of the 8-year-old female patient with coarctation (CoA) [2], in conjunction with the attached aortic root geometry.

The novel character of the presented work is detailed description of the overset mesh technique for modeling heart valves, and analysis of the aortic valve hemodynamics including the whole arterial tree, coupled with the lumped-parameter Windkessel model. The state of the art studies consider only ventricular aortic portion and the aortic root in the geometry scope. The future goal is to develop virtual diagnostic procedure, that can be included into the stepwise integrated approach for the assessment of aortic stenosis severity.

2 Numerical Model

Typically used approach for modeling heart leaflets movement is application of the Fluid-Structure Interaction (FSI), where the forces that act on the leaflets can be accurately retrieved form fluid simulation. Nobili et al. [15] shows the application of FSI technique for modeling in silico the dynamics of a bileaflet synthetic heart valve (BV). Amindari et al. [4] has presented methodology for aortic valve hemodynamics modeling, based on application of the commercial numerical software, ANSYS, where fluid solver—Fluent and structural solver—Mechanical were connected through the System Coupling module to enable FSI process. There are number of approaches that can be used for modeling FSI depending on the computational resources, geometry complexity and the level of the coupling. In the case of large deformation of entire structure, like heart ventricles during systole and diastole, an example is application of the arbitrary Lagrangian–Eulerian (ALE) approach [9]. The drawback of mentioned approach is the solver complexity, ill-conditioned solver and long computational time resulted from the solving of the monolithic matrix. More novel methods—Immersed Boundary Method (IBM) and Lattice Boltzmann Method (LBM) enable more stable FSI computing [21]. All mentioned approaches have one common feature, namely the computational cost is quite large and high instability.

The overset mesh technology allows to perform calculations on the overlapping meshes—the stationary background mesh and component mesh. The computation process is done on the *solve cells*. The interpolation is realized between the *donor cells* and the *receptor cells*, where the latter receive the data from the former. This method was used as well for updating the geometry and mesh due to the leaflets' movement. The computational stability and solver convergence were improved due to the avoidance of generation some low-quality cells in the gap vicinity in the case of dynamic mesh usage instead. Moreover, it enabled the hexahedron structural mesh creation and preserving during body movement in the most part of the two individual leaflet' surroundings and at the background as well. The additional advantage of the overset meshing is the limitation of the Fluent wall-clock time, because this utility is less consuming than smoothing or remeshing, and elimination of the negative cell volume error. This error will stop the solution process. Furthermore, the dynamic mesh could effect in deterioration of the cells quality, especially increased skewness parameter. Maintaining the high-quality cells, especially in the vicinity of the moving or deforming bodies, is crucial to improve accuracy and stability in the simulation.

To mimic the pulsatile blood flow, at the inlet to the computational domain (see Fig. 3) the velocity profile in function of time was prescribed using UDSs [2]. The measurement data was acquired using a cardiac-gated, 2D, respiratory compensated, phase-contrast cine sequence with through-plane velocity encoding.

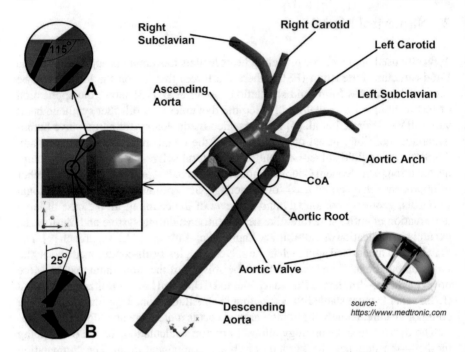

Fig. 1 Numerical geometry of the aorta with valve and subsequent branches

2.1 Geometry and Numerical Mesh

Three different regions can be distinguished at developed model, i.e. ascending and descending aorta, aortic arch with its major branches, aortic root with sinuses and the artificial valve Fig. 1. The real 8-year old female aorta model [2], used in authors earlier work [16] was used in presented work. The geometry was acquired using the Gadolinium-enhanced magnetic resonance angiography. The Geomagic Design X (3D Systems Corporation) [3] was used to convert the base surface triangulated .stl file into the format supported by computer aided design (CAD) systems. The three-dimensional (3D) geometry of the aortic root was created based on the measurement data published by [11]. Its geometry consist of three identical aortic sinuses. Furthermore, each sinus is symmetrical, so only 60° portion was modeled and then the mirror operation was realized, resulting in the complete sinus. The aortic valve geometry was created based on the user manual provided with *Medtronic® Open Pivot^{TM}* documentation [1]. The considered valve version's inside diameter is equal 16.8 mm.

The background, i.e. aortic geometry, was discretized with the hybrid mesh approach. For this purpose, this geometry was divided into 12 regions. The regions where the branches are connecting, i.e. aortic arch and the end of the brachiocephalic artery (bifurcation region), as well as the ventriculoaortic ring surrounding, were meshed with the unstructured tetrahedral elements. The final background mesh con-

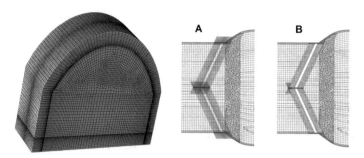

Fig. 2 Overset component mesh, cross-section through the background and components meshes, **a**—before the matching process and **b**—after matching process

sists of 1.7 mln hybrid elements. To create the quasi-structural mesh, component geometries were divided, each into 18 bodies, meshed individually, with different methods and settings. The selected methods and cell growth rates ensured the increasing cell size going from all leaflets' walls and the proper quality parameters. The final single component mesh reached 115,500 cells and its 14 bodies were discretized into structural hex type (Fig. 2).

2.2 Modeling Response of Cardiovascular System

To prescribe proper outlet boundary conditions in the limited section of the aorta, the three elements Windkessel model developed based on the electric analogy has been implemented into the solution procedure. Model constants include two resistances, i.e. proximal R_1 (simulates aortic or pulmonary resistance) and distal R_2 (peripheral resistance), as well as one compliance C which represents the compliance of the veins. The final form of the ordinary differential equation (ODE) that was used is defined as

$$\frac{dP(\tau)}{d\tau} = \left(1 + \frac{R_1}{R_2}\right)\frac{Q(\tau)}{C} + R_1\frac{dQ(\tau)}{d\tau} - \frac{P(\tau)}{R_2 C} \tag{1}$$

where P stands for pressure, Q defines the volumetric flow rate, and τ is time. The ODE (1) was integrated within subsequent steps of solution procedure using fourth-order Runge–Kutta technique with adaptive control of the integration time.

2.3 The Valve Leaflets Motion

To enable the modeling of movable rigid structures, as both valve leaflets, the valves angle time functions were taken and adapted from [14]. For each leaflet, the angle

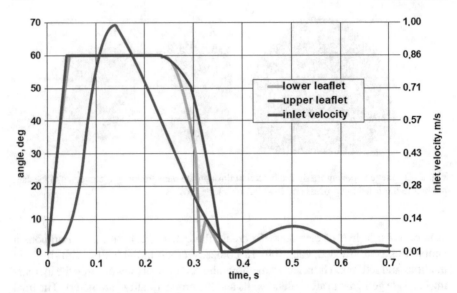

Fig. 3 Velocity inlet profile and the leaflet angle profiles; the value of 0° refers to the fully closed state

polynomial time functions $\theta(\tau)$ were created. Finally, the angular velocities were calculated as time derivatives $\omega = \frac{d\theta(\tau)}{d\tau}$, as this is the input value of the UDF macro `define_cg_motion`. The angular velocity function is formed as (2):

$$\omega(\tau) = \frac{\pi}{180°} \cdot (a_1 \cdot \tau + a_0) \tag{2}$$

where multiplier $\frac{\pi}{180°}$ is used to transform degrees into radians. The angle curves are shown in Fig. 3. The asymmetry between leaflets kinematics is caused by the 3D geometry and is stronger during closing than opening phase. The irregular aortic root geometry, with three symmetrical sinuses, also is found as the factor having an impact onto asymmetrical valve motion.

3 Results and Discussion

The pressure drop was calculated between two points located on the centerline, 3.5 mm before the valve and 3.5 mm behind, considering its opened state. Figure 4 shows the pressure drop between indicated points. The curve monotonicity is concurrent with the inlet velocity profile. The oscillations are visible during the moments when the valve is moving and are more apparent when the valve become fully closed or fully opened. The maximum value achieved about 0.8 kPa and is very close to the validated pressure drop values in [6, 13], where pressure drops are slightly above

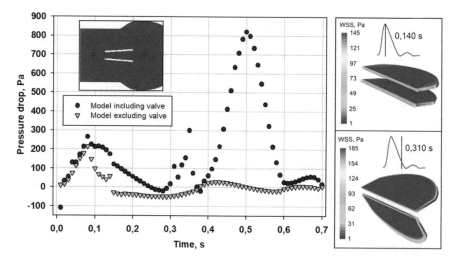

Fig. 4 Pressure drop calculated between two central points shown at the inset for two analyzed models (left); high wall shear stress values presented for two time instants (left)

0.8 kPa and 1.3 kPa, respectively. To observe the separated velocity profile influence on the pressure drop, additional calculations were performed for the case excluding the moving valve. The maximum pressure drop was 4 times lower than in the model with the valve. The conclusion was made, that the transvalvular drop oscillations are more dependent on the leaflet movement than on the inlet velocity profile (Figs. 4 and 3).

Figure 5 presents the velocity components—streamwise (x-velocity) and vertical (y-velocity). Five different time instants were considered: the moment when valve started to open (0.01 s), the opening completion (0.05 s), the maximum inflow time (0.14 s), the closing start-up (0.24 s) and closing completion (0.36 s). The x-velocities are plotted on three lines located behind the valve, in its middle cross-section. The y-velocity is plotted for the valve centerline. The bottom right picture fragment shows the line locations.

The regurgitation is undesirable and beside the reversed flow is can be observed when the valve is in the fully closed state, due to the leakage regions [7]. It reduces the net flow through the valve, however, the backflow contributes to the leaflets washout. Some degrees of this phenomenon is visible close to the sinus wall region when the valve is starting to open and when it is closing, nevertheless, considering the values presented on the scales, this phenomenon is not substantial. As the upper leaflet closing startup is slightly earlier than lower, thus in moment *0.27* s discussed effect is present only in the upper gap region. The streamwise velocity distributions remains quite similar moving away from the valve and its changes are related to local maxima stabilizing and the influence of 3D aortic geometry. When the fully opened state is achieved, the flow field is visibly divided into three quite symmetrical regions—one central and two lateral. The unsymmetrical irregular patterns at the beginning of the heart cycle are related to the stagnation of the flow and are rapidly eliminated with the increasing inflow. The greatest difference between maximum and minimum streamwise velocity values is equal 1.38 m/s and is observed just behind the valve during the peak systole phase.

The axial velocity (Fig. 5, red curve) fall behind the maximum 0.14 m/s and minimum −0.9 m/s values. When the leaflets are fully opened and stationary, the courses become highly dependent on the ascending aorta geometry curvature. Beside these moments, the vertical velocity depends almost only on the unsymmetrical leaflets motion.

A common indicator used in the assessment of the aortic valve performance is the Effective Orifice Area (EOA). This coefficient is the measure of the effective valve opening during the forward flow phase and determine how well a valve design utilize its primary orifice area. It is related to the degree how the prosthesis itself obstructs the flow. It can be calculated both experimentally and using simulation results, with equation described by Gabbay, based on the principle of energy conservation [12]:

$$EOA = \frac{Q_{RMS}}{51.6\sqrt{\Delta \bar{p}}} \tag{3}$$

where EOA—effective orifice area (cm^2), 51.6—gravitational constant, $\bar{p}$—mean systolic pressure drop (mmHg) and Q_{RMS}—root mean square of the systolic flow rate (ml/s):

$$Q_{RMS} = \sqrt{\frac{1}{n}\sum_{i=1}^{n} Q_i^2} \tag{4}$$

The valve stenosis results in low EOA values, which is related to the higher pressure loss and increased heart workload. The bileaflet type mechanical valve construction overcome the drawback of low EOA values related to former mechanical valve types—caged-ball and ball-and-cage. The EOA typically falls between the values $1.04 - 4.05$ cm^2 [7]. For the same construction type, it is proportional to the valve diameter and may vary in patients. The measured value by [5] for the St Jude Medical® bileaflet valve was equal 2.08 cm^2 and 3.23 cm^2 for size 21 mm and 25 mm, respectively. The calculated value using our simulation results considers 21 mm type (with inside diameter equal 16.8 mm) and was equal 2.99 cm^2, which indicate the appropriate prosthesis performance.

The negative pressure transients (*NPTs*), called also *surges*, are the high and rapid pressure drops [10]. NPTs could result in cavitation which can cause the leaflet structural failure and deterioration. It is observed, that the pressure values are rapidly changing especially during the time from 0.30 s to 0.31 s. This is the moment when the leaflets angular velocity is very high and in the case of the lower leaflet the closure is almost complete, to open subsequently for a while. The minimum negative pressure achieved −1 kPa. Presented results coincide with the conclusions for the cavitation bubbles presence made by [8] and suggest, that there is still the room for enhancement in the optimum mechanical valve geometry as well for the material improvement.

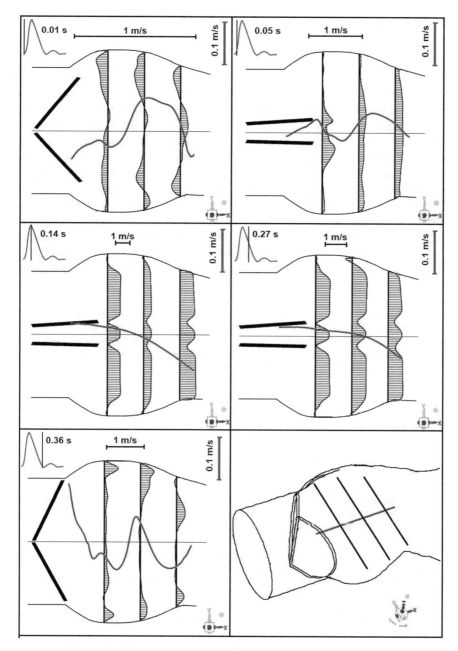

Fig. 5 Streamwise velocity profiles for three locations (x-velocity, hatched graphs) and the vertical velocity component (y-velocity, red curve)

4 Summary

We described geometry acquisition approaches and realization of the overset mesh in the case of more challenging applications, such as when very small gaps and moving domain occurs. The overset mesh proved to be a very stable, efficient and reliable mesh update strategy for the aortic valve modeling. The simulation results were validated against the measurement data available in literature and compared with additionally created model excluding the valve, showing its impact onto the velocity field, pressures and outlet mass flows. Main parameters concerning the valve performance were determined, such as the pressure drops, regurgitation flows and the effective orifice area. The results indicated the proper work of the artificial valve in the 8-year old girl's circulatory system. Some typical phenomenons for mechanical bileaflet valves are present, such as the negative pressure transients and high shear stresses that could effect in the cavitation bubbles or the blood cells lysis, accordingly. Our future goal is to develop virtual diagnostic procedure with the inhouse six degrees of freedom solver, that can be included into the stepwise integrated approach for the assessment of aortic stenosis severity.

Acknowledgements This research is supported by the National Science Centre (Poland) within projects no. 2014/13/B/ST8/04225 and 2018/29/B/ST8/01490. The research team express their grateful gratitude for the Medtronic® company, Poland, for providing mechanical properties of the valves based on user manuals. The research is also supported by the Silesian University of Technology within 08/060/RGJ18/0154 found.

References

1. Medtronic® Open Pivot: Instructions for use
2. Source of the medical data from. www.vascularmodel.com/. Accessed 03 Jan 2016
3. 3D Systems: Geomagic. www.geomagic.com/en/products/design/overview
4. Amindari, A., Saltik, L., Kirkkopru, K., Yacoub, M., Yalcin, H.: Assessment of calcified aortic valve leaflet deformations and blood flow dynamics using fluid-structure interaction modeling. Inform. Med. Unlocked **9**, 191–199 (2017)
5. Bech-Hanssen, O., Caidahl, K., Wallentin, I., Ask, P., Wranne, B.: Assessment of effective orifice area of prosthetic aortic valves with Doppler echocardiography: an in vivo and in vitro study. J. Thorac. Cardiovasc. Surg. **122**(2), 287–295 (2001)
6. Borazjani, I., Ge, L., Sotiropoulos, F.: High-resolution fluid-structure interaction simulations of flow through a bi-leaflet mechanical heart valve in an anatomic aorta. Ann. Biomed. Eng. **38**(2), 326–344 (2010)
7. Bronzino, J.: The Biomedical Engineering HandBook, 2nd edn. CRC Press LLC, Boca Raton (2000)
8. Chandran, K., Dexter, E., Aluri, S., Richenbacher, W.: Negative pressure transients with mechanical heart-valve closure. Ann. Biomed. Eng. **26**, 546–556 (1998)
9. Chnafa, C., Mendez, S., Nicoud, F.: Image-based large-eddy simulation in a realistic left heart. Comput. Fluids **94**, 173–187 (2014)
10. Fleming, K., Dugandzik, J., Lechavellier, M.: Susceptibility of Distribution Systems to Negative Pressure Transients. AwwaRF and American Water (2006)

11. Grande, K.J., Cochran, R.P., Reinhall, P.G., Kunzelma, K.S.: Stress variations in the human aortic root and valve: the role of anatomic asymmetry. Ann. Biomed. Eng. **26**(4), 534–545 (1998)
12. Gray, R.J., Chaux, A., Matloff, J.M., DeRobertis, M., Raymond, M., Stewart, M., Yoganathan, A.: Bileaflet, tilting disc and porcine aortic valve substitutes: in vivo hydrodynamic characteristics. J. Am. Coll. Cardiol. **3**(2), 321–327 (1984)
13. Kadhim, S., Nasif, M., Hussain, H.A.K., Rafat, A.W.: Computational fluid dynamics simulation of blood flow profile and shear stresses in bileaflet mechanical heart valve by using monolithic approach. Simulation **94**(2), 93–104 (2018)
14. Le, T.B., Sotiropoulos, F.: Fluid-structure interaction of an aortic heart valve prosthesis driven by an animated anatomic left ventricle. J. Comput. Phys. **244**, 41–62 (2013)
15. Nobili, M., Morbiducci, U., Ponzini, R., Gaudio, C., Balducci, A., Grigioni, M., Montevecchi, F., Redaelli, A.: Numerical simulation of the dynamics of a bileaflet prosthetic heart valve using a fluid-structure interaction approach. J. Biomech. **41**, 2539–2550 (2008)
16. Nowak, M., Melka, B., Rojczyk, M., Gracka, M., Nowak, A., Golda, A., Adamczyk, W., Isaac, B., Białecki, R., Ostrowski, Z.: The protocol for using elastic wall model in modeling blood flow within human artery. Eur. J. Mech. - B/Fluids **77**, 273–280 (2019)
17. Osnabrugge, R., Mylotte, D., Head, S., VanMieghem, N., Nkomo, V., LeReun, C., Bogers, A., Piazza, N., Kappetein, A.: Aortic stenosis in the elderly: disease prevalence and number of candidates for transcatheter aortic valve replacement: a meta-analysis and modeling study. J. Am. Coll. Cardiol. **62**(11), 1002–1012 (2013)
18. Votta, E., Le, T., Stevanella, M., Fusini, L., Caiani, E., Redaelli, A., Sotiropoulos, F.: Toward patient-specific simulations of cardiac valves: state-of- the-art and future directions **46**(2), 217–228 (2013)
19. Westerhof, N., Lankhaar, J., Westerhof, B.: The arterial windkessel. Med. Biol. Eng. Comput. **47**(2), 131–141 (2008)
20. Wilkins, E., Wilson, L., Wickramasinghe, K., Bhatnagar, P., Leal, J., Luengo-Fernandez, R., Burns, R., Rayner, M., Townsend, N.: European Cardiovascular Disease Statistics 2017 edition. European Heart Network (2017). http://www.ehnheart.org/images/CVD-statistics-report-August-2017.pdf
21. Yanhong, L.: A lattice Boltzmann model for blood flows. Appl. Math. Model. **36**(7), 2890–2899 (2012)

Establishment of an In-Silico Model for Simulation of Dehydration Process in Human Skin to Compare Output Parameter with Clinical Study

Jana Viehbeck, Alexandra Speich, Swetlana Ustinov, Dominik Böck, Michael Wiehl, and Rainer Brück

Abstract The skin is an important indicator of fluid deficiency as it contains 30% of the extracellular body water. A continuous fluid loss changes the water content of the skin and consequently its composition. With help of electromagnetic waves it is possible to analyze the hydration state of the tissue. The factors that influence the measurement of dehydration are still unknown and cannot be changed directly in humans. Therefore, an in-silico model for the controlled change of system parameters is necessary. The hydration status of the tissue can be simulated by adding a degree of dehydration to the model. The results show a tendency towards stronger reflection behavior with increasing dehydration. However, as was determined in the simulation and internal study, the reflection measurement of the electromagnetic waves has strong personal differences. A determination of the hydration status may only be considered by a temporal change of the reflection behavior.

Keywords Dehydration · Skin model · Simulation · Electromagnetic waves

1 Introduction

If there is a fluid deficit in the body, it uses its own fluid reserves to compensate. The skin has an essential role, because it saves a very large proportion of easily

J. Viehbeck (✉) · A. Speich · S. Ustinov · D. Böck · M. Wiehl
Senetics Healthcare Group GmbH & Co. KG, Ansbach, Germany
e-mail: jana.viehbeck@senetics.de

A. Speich
e-mail: alexandraspeich@web.de

S. Ustinov
e-mail: swewil@web.de

D. Böck
e-mail: dominik.boeck@senetics.de

R. Brück
University Siegen, Siegen, Germany
e-mail: Rainer.Brueck@uni-siegen.de

© The Editor(s) (if applicable) and The Author(s), under exclusive license
to Springer Nature Switzerland AG 2021
E. Pietka et al. (eds.), *Information Technology in Biomedicine*, Advances in Intelligent
Systems and Computing 1186, https://doi.org/10.1007/978-3-030-49666-1_22

accessible, extracellular water [1]. The precise factors influencing the measurement of dehydration are unknown and cannot be changed directly on humans. Therefore, an in-silico model for the controlled change of system parameters is necessary. The skin consists of several layers. Not every skin layer is equally involved in the dehydration, because they store different amounts of body fluid. The subcutaneous fat tissue, for example, contains about 20% of water [2], whereas the dermis represents the interstitial space of the body and consists most of the extracellular water [1].

2 State of Science and Development

There are currently several innovative approaches in the field of simulation of human skin models and the approaches differ according to the area of interest. The analysis of absorption and scattering behavior at wavelengths is mainly used in the medical field for the diagnosis and treatment of skin diseases [3].

The simulation of electromagnetic waves in the microwave range is currently being carried out primarily with regard to the effects of daily electromagnetic radiation, as in mobile phones or wireless network. In this area there are some solution mechanisms based on a finite difference time domain (FDTD) simulation which output is the SAR value. The Specific Absorption Rate (SAR) is a value for damage of tissue by electro-magnetic exposure. Examples of these simulation approaches are the software packages FEMLAB or SEMCAD [4]. The FDTD grid consists of rectangular cells to which specific material properties are assigned. Therefore, the knowledge of the dielectric properties (permittivity, permeability) of different human tissues is also relevant for the simulation. One problem is the frequency dependence of the parameters, which greatly limits the realistic simulation. In most cases the skin will be designed as a whole, which results in the assumption of the material parameters of Gabriel (scientist of high-frequency technology, special field: measurement of dielectric material properties of human tissue types) [4, 5].

The use of microwave antennas to analyze the hydration state has only recently become known. Therefore, there are no established simulation approaches in this regard. For the analysis of the dehydration behavior of the skin, two issues have to be considered. On the one hand, the more detailed modeling of the human skin and the definition of the associated dielectric material properties are necessary [6, 7]. The problem of detailed modeling has already been worked on and published [6]. On the other hand, it is relevant to know about the recognition of water distribution and regulation in humans and their skin during dehydration. This problem has been experimentally processed in a clinical study [8].

The combination of a detailed skin layer model including the dehydration of different skin layers has not yet been investigated.

3 Materials and Methods

3.1 Modelling and Meshing

In order to obtain a simulated solution that is as accurate as possible, the following two questions have to be considered [9]:

- How detailed is the model?
- Is the meshsize small enough?

The electromagnetic simulation is divided into three sections—Preprocessing, Processing and Postprocessing. The preprocessing includes modeling, parameter assignment, and meshing of these structures. Processing is only the simulation of the propagation of electromagnetic waves in the medium. In the postprocessing, the evaluation and visualization of the simulation results takes place.

For the simulation, a skin model with the dimensions of (50×50) mm^2 and a depth of >100 mm is designed. The measuring range is between 2.5 and 3.5 GHz with an excitation frequency of 3 GHz. The FDTD data structure stores all parameters, boundary conditions and termination criteria. For the simulation box, in which the model is located, absorbing boundary conditions are applied. To simulate the sinusoidal oscillation of the network analyzer, a Gaussian excitation is used. The meshing has to be as coarse as possible and as fine as necessary. In practice, a cell size of $\lambda/15$ or $\lambda/20$ is selected, and λ is the material specific wavelength (Table 1).

A simplified nine-layered model was modeled [6, 7]. The dielectric material properties of the individual layers are only partially available.

Table 1 Permittivity and electrical conductivity of the various skin layers of the multilayer model [5]

No.	Layer	Relative permittivity [–]	Electrical conductivity [S/m]
1	Stratum corneum	50.742	2.7292
2	Epidermis	N/A	N/A
3	Capillary	N/A	N/A
4	Dermis	N/A	N/A
5	Upper blood vessels	N/A	N/A
6	Subcutis	5.224	0.1300
7	Muscle	52.058	2.1421
8	Cortical bone	11.066	0.5062
9	Spongy bone	17.943	1.0062

N/A: There are no specific values available in literature

Table 2 Water and cell content of certain tissue layers

Layer	Water content [%]	Cell content [%]
Epidermis	60	40
Capillary system	60	40
Dermis	70	30
Upper blood vessels	70	30

The permittivity of the layers 2–5 are calculated by determining the total permittivity of the various constituent layers. The calculation is based on the cell and water content of the different layers.

For the liquid parts, the experimentally determined "body fluid" dielectric properties are used (see Table 2). The dry cell content of the layers largely consists of proteins. Pure protein has a relative permittivity of approximately 2 [–] at a frequency of 3.2 GHz. The dielectric loss factor is 0.1 (compare to Table 3) [10]. The total permittivity is calculated very simply as follows [11]:

$$\epsilon_{R_{total}} [-] = (WC_{tissue} \cdot \epsilon_{R_{Bodyfluid}}) + (PC_{tissue} \cdot \epsilon_{R_{Protein}}) \tag{1}$$

with WC = Water Content from 0.0 to 1.0; PC = Protein Content from 0.0 to 1.0.

Attached, the dielectric properties of the tissue layers used are shown at a frequency of 3 GHz.

Table 3 Dielectric material properties at a frequency of 3 GHz

No.	Layer	Relative permittivity [–]	Electrical conductivity [S/m]
2	Epidermis	41.490	2.0505
3	Capillary	41.490	2.0505
4	Dermis	48.072	2.3098
5	Upper blood vessels	48.072	2.3098
	Body fluid[a]	67.817	2.9559
	Pure proteins[b]	2.000	0.0334

[a]Not calculated, the dielectric material properties comes from literature [5]
[b]Not calculated, the dielectric material properties comes from literature [10]

The base of the simulation is the calculation of Maxwell equations using the FDTD solution method. The evaluation and visualization of the simulation results is done by calculating the Reflection Frequency behavior of the antenna. The diagram represents the percentage reflection frequency:

$$\% f_{ref}[\%] = \frac{f_{ref}[GHz]}{f_{trans}[GHz]} \cdot 100[\%] \tag{2}$$

with f_{trans}: Defined input parameter in preprocessing; f_{ref}: Calculated via simulation of the reflection behavior of electromagnetic waves with Maxwell equations using FDTD solution method $\% f_{ref}$: Percentage reflection frequency of the transmitted frequency. From 0 to 100%.

3.2 Modelling of the Dehydration Model

The body uses its stored fluid reserves at the beginning of dehydration in order to keep the circulation stable. The skin—mainly the dermis—is one of its largest water reservoirs. Depending on the degree of dehydration, the percentage of water in the individual skin layers changes as a result. In the simulation, up to 15% water is removed from the layers "epidermis", "capillaries", "dermis" and "lower vascular network". A fluid withdrawal of more than 15% water is related to the death of the patient, therefore the percentage withdrawal of more than 15% is not considered in the simulation (Table 4).

The effects are shown in the layer-specific relative permittivities, and consequently in the total permittivity of the layered model.

Table 4 Simplified water content and protein content of the tissue layers at dehydration level of 15% [11]

No.	Layer	Water content [%] at 15% dehydration:	Cell content [%]
2	Epidermis	45	55
3	Capillary	45	55
4	Dermis	55	45
5	Upper blood vessels	55	45

4 Results

4.1 Dehydration of Skin via In-Silico Simulation

With the aid of the developed application program for the simulation of electromagnetic waves, the reflection behavior in the euhydrated and dehydrated state can
be simulated. In the multi-layered simulation approach, a reflection frequency of
2.228 GHz is simulated at an excitation frequency of 3 GHz. This corresponds to
74.3% of the excitation frequency. The result is shown in Fig. 1 with a degree of
dehydration of 0%. Various dehydration levels between (0–15)% were simulated.
The detection of the dehydration state of (0–5)% is urgently needed for the daily
use in the context of the nursing area. Therefore, simulations were performed in
the range of (0–5)% with 1% intervals. As can be seen from the simulation results,
the reflection frequency increases with the degree of dehydration. The percentage
increase in the reflection frequency is small and amounts to several megahertz. The
change in the percent reflection frequency per degree of dehydration is up to 0.2%.
Larger dehydration levels of, for example 5%, can be clearly seen from the simulation
results [11].

   As a result of the simulation, an increase of the reflection frequency with increasing
degree of dehydration can be shown.

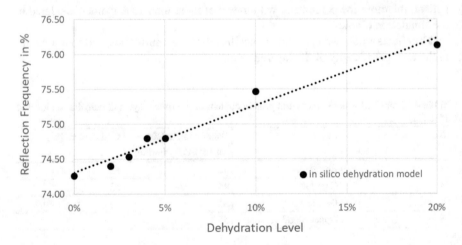

Fig. 1 Reflection frequency of the dehydrated in-silico model. There is some increase while dehydration [11]

4.2 Comparison of the Reflection Behavior with Different Skin Models

For the comparison of the reflection behavior of the in-silico model, a technical and a biological skin model were established within the scope of two bachelor theses [12, 13]. The technical skin model consists of the base materials gelatin and water. The biological skin models are porcine ex-vivo models. To compare the reflection behavior of the in-silico model while dehydration, the other skin models were dehydrated. The models were applied with a dehydration status of (1–10)%.

If the reflection behavior of the skin models during dehydration is compared, it can be determined that the reflection frequency tends to increase with increasing dehydration.

In addition the reflection behavior of the in-silico model can be compared to real human dehydration evaluation. There is a clinical evaluation of an innovative electromagnetic waves sensor by a dehydration study of 9 participants. The new sensor detected the reflection frequency of participants forearm while dehydration of (0–5)%. The results show an increase of the reflection frequency while ongoing dehydration. With a constant transmitted frequency and an increase of reflection frequency, there is identified an increase of the related percentage reflection frequency [8].

5 Discussion

5.1 Restrictions of the Simulation

Capillaries and the Upper Blood Vessels are anchored as a layer at specific locations, but not included in the respective tissue type. Capillaries are modeled as a "tissue layer". In reality, there is a combination of tissue and blood in a complex variation. The different layers have been assumed to be planar planes, but this does not correspond to reality [11]. The stratum corneum is the outermost skin layer of the human– also called cornea. For the simulation, the dielectric properties of cornea were used. In this context, cornea is specifically the cornea of the eye, this layer contains more fluid than the cornea of the remaining body regions. In reality, the dielectric properties would be slightly lower. Unfortunately there are no literature values available for the stratum corneum.

The penetration depth into the tissue at an excitation frequency of 3 GHz is almost 2 cm. This fact also requires the inclusion of muscle and bone besides the various skin components. Although the different layer thicknesses were determined by a literature search, they are very specific according to locality and person and therefore in reality, they differ very strongly [7, 14, 15]. The reason for this is the deviations of the different participants among themselves as well as the deviations of the measuring position.

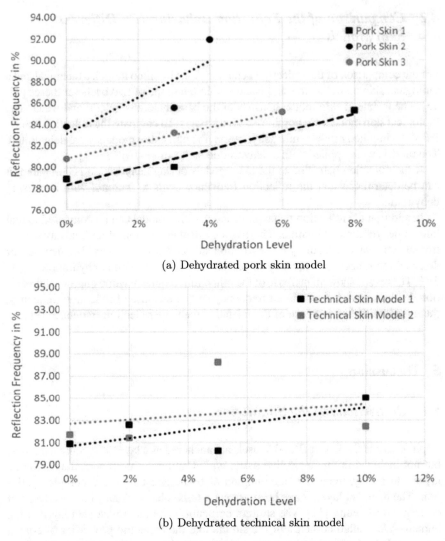

(a) Dehydrated pork skin model

(b) Dehydrated technical skin model

Fig. 2 a Reflection frequency of the dehydrated porcine skin models. There is an increase of reflection frequency while dehydration [13]. **b** Reflection Frequency of the dehydrated technical skin models. There is an increase of reflection frequency while dehydration [12]

For the layers "epidermis", "capillaries", "dermis" and "Upper Blood Vessels" no dielectric material properties are known. Therefore, permittivity and electrical conductivity were determined by a very trivial approximation method. The respective layers were classified into their respective dry matter and liquid content for the determination of their dielectric material properties. Since the dry mass of human skin consists of protein to a large extent, the dielectric material properties of protein were used for this purpose. However, the dry mass still contains lipids, ions and other inorganic constituents [14], which were neglected in this simulation but which may affect the relative permittivity. The water content of the different skin layers was compared in several models, however this differs greatly depending on the model [7, 16].

The in-silico model is a simplified simulation model of the dehydration process in human skin. To make this model more specific, the electromagnetic properties of the different skin layers has to be measured or calculated. For this simulation, the focus was to get knowledge about the trend of the percentage reflection frequency while dehydration. An increase in the reflection frequency tends to be recognizable as the degree of dehydration increases. However, the percentage increase is very small. It has been argued that the difference of the person has more influence on the reflection behavior than the change of the permittivity by dehydration. Because of this, it is confirmed here that a statement about the degree of hydration can only be made by analyzing the temporal change of the reflection behavior of a person.

The results confirm the theory that an analysis of the degree of dehydration of the skin by means of electromagnetic waves is possible due to a change in the dielectric properties upon dehydration. However, this method only includes the dehydration of the skin and provides no information about the total body water and other water reservoirs of the body [11].

5.2 Comparison with Other Skin Models

The presented skin models show an increase of the reflection frequency with progressing dehydration. This knowledge was also confirmed in a clinical study [8].

With small water changes of $\pm 1\%$, the determination of the reflection frequency in the microwave range is currently not suitable, because the differences are not always clearly recognizable. For larger water changes $> \pm 5\%$, this approach provides clearer results.

6 Outlook

The results show that it is possible to measure the loss of water in the skin using electromagnetic waves. During dehydration, there is less fluid in the skin, which can be detected by means of electromagnetic waves via the reflection behavior of the skin layers. Materials with less liquid content have a lower permittivity and consequently a higher reflection frequency. This knowledge is confirmed by the in-silico model. This simulation coincide with the results of a clinical study, in which patients were purposefully dehydrated for 3 days. The evaluation was conducted using a microwave sensor. The reflection frequency was increased subsequently [8].

If the dielectric material parameters of tissue layers can be noticed, it is possible to describe the simulation in more detail and to illustrate the relationship between water loss in the skin and the reflection frequency more specifically [11].

In order to be able to reliably detect water loss in the tissue even in smaller ranges ±1%, additional sensors need to be used.

Acknowledgements This publication is a review of 3 thesis papers [11–13]. We would like to thank Swetlana Ustinov (B. Eng.) and Katja Müller (M. Sc.) for the establishment of the biological skin models by as well Alexandra Speich (B. Eng.) for the establishment of technical skin models. This Research was made possible by the international project NexGen (Next Generation of Body Monitoring), funded by the Federal Ministry of Education and Research (BMBF Germany).

References

1. Rieger, H., Schoop, W.: Herausgeber. Klinische Angiologie, Berlin (1998) (in German). https://doi.org/10.1007/978-3-662-08104-4
2. Schmidt, R.F., Lang, F., Heckmann, M.: Herausgeber. Physiologie des Menschen: mit Pathophysiologie: mit Online-Repetitorium. Sonderausgabe der 31. Auflage. Springer, Berlin (2017). https://doi.org/10.1007/978-3-642-01651-6(in German)
3. Rüdlinger, R., Gnädinger, M.: Licht in der Dermatologie. Swiss Med Forum **11**(34) (in German). https://doi.org/10.4414/smf.2011.07590
4. Lazhar, B., Mohammed, D., Redouane, T.: Numerical modeling of electromagnetic interaction between a radio frequency sources and the human body. In: 2015 4th International Conference on Electrical Engineering (ICEE), pp. S. 1–6 (2015). https://doi.org/10.1109/INTEE.2015.7416711
5. Italian National Research Council. Dielectric Properties of Body Tissues: HTML clients [Internet]. An Internet resource for the calculation of the Dielectric Properties of Body Tissues
6. Huclova, S., Erni, D., Fröhlich, J.: Modelling and validation of dielectric properties of human skin in the MHz region focusing on skin layer morphology and material composition. J. Phys. D: Appl. Phys. **45**(2), 025301 (2011). https://doi.org/10.1088/0022-3727/45/2/025301
7. Querleux, B.: Computational Biophysics of the Skin. Pan Stanford Publishing, Singapore (2014)
8. Viehbeck, J., Wiehl, M., Sening, W., Brück, R.: Untersuchung der Mikrowellenfrequenz und des Return Loss einer neuen Sensortechnologie zur Detektion des Hydratationsstatus. VDE-Verlag, Berlin (2019). (in German)
9. Weiland, T., Timm, M., Munteanu, I.: A practical guide to 3-D simulation. IEEE Microw. Mag. **9**, 62–75 (2009). https://doi.org/10.1109/MMM.2008.929772
10. Klauenberg, B.J., et al.: Radio Frequency Radiation Dosimetry and Its Relationship to the Biological Effects of Electromagnetic Fields. Springer, Dordrecht (2000)
11. Viehbeck, J.: Entwicklung eines in-silico Hautmodells durch die Simulation von elektromagnetischen Wellen im Nahfeld zur Analyse des Hydratationszustandes von Gewebe [Master Thesis]. OTH Regensburg, Regensburg (2017). (in German)
12. Speich, A.: Entwicklung eines Hautmodells zur Dehydratationsanalyse [Bachelor Thesis]. Hochschule Ansbach, Ansbach (2018). (in German)
13. Ustinov, S.: Etablierung von ex-vivo Hautmodellen zur Analyse eines Hydratationssensors [Bachelor Thesis]. Hochschule Ansbach, Ansbach (2018). (in German)
14. Groenendaal, W., von Basum, G., Schmidt, K.A., Hilbers, P.A.J., van Riel, N.A.W.: Quantifying the composition of human skin for glucose sensor development. J. Diabetes Sci. Technol. **4**(5), 1032–1040 (2010). https://doi.org/10.1177/193229681000400502

15. Magnenat-Thalmann, N., et al.: A computational skin model: fold and wrinkle formation. IEEE Trans Inf Technol Biomed. Dezember **6**(4), 317–23 (2002). https://doi.org/10.1109/titb.2002.806097

16. Wang, R.K., Tuchin, V.V.: Advanced Biophotonics: Tissue Optical Sectioning [Internet]. CRC Press (2016). https://doi.org/10.1201/b15256

SAR Evaluation in Human Head Models with Cochlear Implant Near PIFA Antenna Inside a Railway Vehicle

Mariana Benova, Jana Mydlova, Zuzana Psenakova, and Maros Smondrk

Abstract The simulation and analysis of electromagnetic field (EMF) distribution inside a railway vehicle are studied with special emphasis on their distribution in the human head model with a cochlear implant in case of two persons close to each other. Research was carried out using modelling of EMFs based on the Finite Integration Method. Simulations were performed and analyzed in cases where passengers were exposed to long-term radiofrequency field stemming from the use of mobile phones during railway transport. Results were evaluated based on the specific absorption rate (SAR)—the measure of electromagnetic energy absorption in the body. Dual band (900/1800 MHz) PIFA antennas were designed and employed as the radio frequency source. Two passenger head models (namely SAM models and homogenous head phantom models) include a cochlear implant. Results have shown that the calculated maximum values of the SAR in railway vehicle are higher than values obtained in simulation in open space and additionally, the obtained values are higher than those established within the European maximum SAR limit. In that environment they are comparable for both of used human head models.

Keywords Electromagnetic field · Specific absorption rate · Cochlear implant · PIFA antenna · Railway vehicle

M. Benova (✉) · J. Mydlova · Z. Psenakova · M. Smondrk
Faculty of Electrical Engineering and Information Technology, University of Zilina, Zilina, Slovakia
e-mail: mariana.benova@fel.uniza.sk

J. Mydlova
e-mail: jana.mydlova@fel.uniza.sk

Z. Psenakova
e-mail: psenakova@fel.uniza.sk

M. Smondrk
e-mail: maros.smondrk@fel.uniza.sk

© The Editor(s) (if applicable) and The Author(s), under exclusive license to Springer Nature Switzerland AG 2021
E. Piętka et al. (eds.), *Information Technology in Biomedicine*, Advances in Intelligent Systems and Computing 1186, https://doi.org/10.1007/978-3-030-49666-1_23

289

1   Introduction

The increase of mobile phone (MP) usage and their possible impact on health is a significant worldwide topic due to electromagnetic radiation. Use of those high frequency (HF) sources of electromagnetic fields (EMF) near people with active implantable device (ID) may cause disturbing interference with device or a body tissue thermal effect around implant [1]. One of those ID is cochlear implant (CI) which replace the function of damaged inner ear or cochlea. The communication via mobile phone is also common for people with CI. As research shows [2], approximately 60% use a mobile phone daily, especially to make calls to people whose voice they know. MP as a source of EMF may cause undesired interactions with the CI such as growling or creaking the processor depending on the mobile phone type. Additionally, due to metallic part inside the human head there is different distribution of EMF. Thus, it is necessary to respect exposure limits and eliminate risk to lowest possible levels. These principles are related to the MP's antenna power output, varying between 0.25–3 W, based on different factors. Identification of possible adverse effects in addition to the performance monitoring and other factors, such as the penetration depth of the radiation, exposure limits and biological effects relies on the good knowledge of EMF theory. Moreover, previous research has shown that the use of numerical modeling can be highly effective [3, 4]. Electromagnetic interference is caused by both electric and magnetic components of EMF in audio and ultrahigh frequencies [5]. The International Commission on Non-Ionizing Radiation Protection sets exposure limits of the EMF fields for the human safety purposes [6]. The specific absorption rate (SAR) limits for wireless communication devices were established based on the purpose of the wireless device and generally consider an open space, e.g. a home or an office environment. However, the situation is more complicated when these wireless devices are used in more complex environments, for example automobile applications [7–9] or railway vehicles; the chassis of which are in the form of cubical metallic blocks with irregular boundaries [10].

The aim of this article is to simulate and analyze EMF distribution for SAR calculation inside a human head model with cochlear implant in the case of two persons close to each other, while one person is using the mobile phone within the railway vehicle. Two passenger head models (namely SAM models and homogenous head phantom models) encompass a cochlear implant, and the dielectric properties of the tissue layers are set according to the evaluated frequency band. We also analyze the influence of distance between the mobile phone and head of the human phantom, and the distance between two passengers.

Table 1 The specification of railway vehicle materials and components

	Type of material	μ_r [–]	ε_r [–]	γ [S/m]	ρ [kg/m^3]
Window, door	Lead glass	1	6	1×10^6	4200
Vehicle construction	Steel 1008	1	9.64	4.86	8.28
Seats	Lead	0.999	1	4.8×10^6	11340
Inside walls	Wood	1	1.9	0.31	500

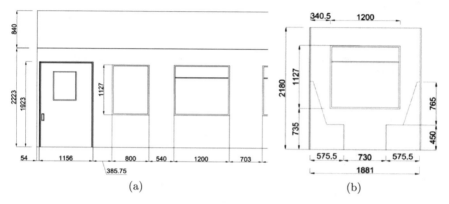

Fig. 1 Railway vehicle geometrical layout **a** outside; **b** inside sideview of the one section

2 Numerical Models and Methods

2.1 Model of Railway Vehicle

We suppose typical railway vehicle type Bmz with 3+3 arrangement. This type of compartment coach with 11 sections is widely used in the long-distance railway traffic. There are 22 pcs of triple sets in total. Specification of materials and individual components of railway vehicle are summarized in Table 1, where μ_r is the relative permeability, ε_r is the relative permittivity, γ is the electrical conductivity and ρ is specific density of the railway vehicle materials. The total railway vehicle size is $26100 \times 2824 \times 3062$ mm (length $\times$ width$\times$ height). For our simulation we selected only one section with six sets (Fig. 1).

2.2 Cochlear Implant and Human Head Models

A cochlear implant (CI) is a prosthetic replacement for the inner ear and is only appropriate for people who receive minimal or no benefit from conventional hearing

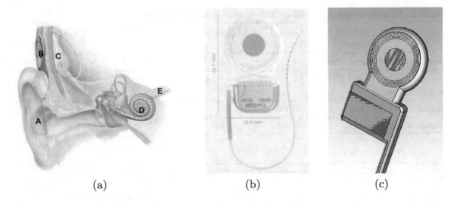

(a) (b) (c)

Fig. 2 A cochlear implant **a** in the ear area, where A is the sound processor, B is a coil, C is an outside implant and D is an inner implant [12], **b** picture of real CI made by MED-EL [13], **c** a numerical model of CI [14]

Table 2 The specification of cochlear implant materials and components

Part of CI model	Assigned material	μ_r [–]	ε_r [–]	γ [S/m]	ρ [kg/m^3]
Implant over cover	Silicone elastomers	1	2.9	5.3×10^{-4}	1124
Implant case	Titanium alloy	1	1	5.9×10^5	4700
Coil	Gold	1	1	4.561×10^7	19320
Magnet	Titanium alloy	1	1	5.9×10^5	4700

aids. Part of the device is surgically implanted in the skull behind the ear and miniscule wires are inserted into the cochlea. The other part of the device is external and consists of a microphone, a speech processor, and connecting cables [11]. Proper localization and placement of the CI is important when creating a simulation model (Fig. 2). CI uses an external microphone and sound processor that is generally worn behind the ear. A transmitter sends radio-frequency signals to a surgically implanted electronic chip, the receiver and stimulator unit, which stimulates the auditory nerve with electrodes that have been threaded through the cochlea [10].

For the purpose of our simulations, we constructed the cochlear implant based on the real-life counterpart shown in Fig. 2a. This model represents the shape and size of commonly implanted CI made by MED EL [14]. Dielectric parameters thereof are listed in Table 2.

Most manufacturers and testing laboratories are currently focusing on using homogeneous, fluid-filled human heads for mobile phone testing. Human head phantoms, both SAM model with hand [14] and homogeneous simplified body model [15], have been developed to help estimate SAR from mobile phones. Measurement accuracy when utilizing homogeneous head designs is highly dependent on the proper selection of the dielectric properties of tissues. Their properties have to be set according

Table 3 The dielectric, magnetic and material properties of SAM model [14] and human body model (SHB) [15]

Model	ε_r [–] 900 MHz	γ [S/m] 900 MHz	ε_r [–] 1800 MHz	γ [S/m] 1800 MHz
SAM model	41.5	0.97	40	1.4
SHB - outer layer	3.5	1.6×10^{-3}	3.5	1.6×10^{-3}
SHB - inner layer of head	41.5	0.97	40	1.4
SHB - inner layer of body	55	1.05	53.3	1.52

to the evaluated frequency band. Likewise, SAR results are only valid when proper material properties are used according to the evaluated frequency band.

Specific Anthropomorphic Mannequin (SAM) like a model of human head was used for calculation of SAR, as it is specified in standard EN50361. The head is modelled by a liquid (inside part of head) covered a shell (outside part of head) which represents the average material properties of these two significant parts of human head. The dielectric properties were evaluated for proposed source frequency 900 and 1800 MHz [14]. A standardized hand model with the dielectric properties given in the Table 3 was considered in the simulations. Those dielectric parameters were taken from the standard [16]. The simulations carried out confirmed that the hand model should be considered in simulations for more accurate results to determine the impact of a mobile phone to a person with implanted CI.

The simplified human body (SHB) model contains a sphere (head) and several blocks (chest, legs, hands) and is modelled as a two-layer structure. The body is situated in sitting position with a total height of 1310 mm. The outer layer has a thickness of 2 mm and has frequency independent parameters. The inner layout is represented by homogeneous structure with dielectric parameters shown in Table 3— for both considered frequencies and in accordance with the IEEE 1528–2013 [6], and EN 62209—1:2016 standards [17]. However, due to simplification, both the head and the body have different dielectric parameters when directly compared related to real human body tissues. The cochlear implant is situated in the right part of human models

2.3 Source of High Frequency Field Exposure

A dual-band (900 MHz–0.5 Watts output power, 1800 MHz–1 Watt output power) PIFA antenna was designed and used as source of the high frequency electromagnetic field—mimicking the mobile phone (Fig. 3a) with their radiation pattern (Fig. 3b). We chose a two-band design with a U-shaped slot. The dual-band antenna covers both commonly used frequency bands and S11 parameters are approximately –15 dB

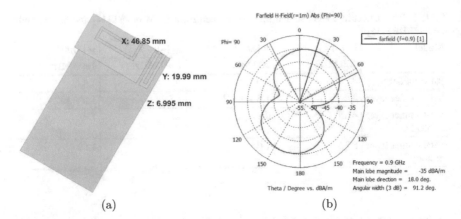

(a)   (b)

Fig. 3 a Design of dual-band PIFA antenna for 900 and 1800 MHz, and **b** Radiation pattern for two-band PIFA antenna

for 900 MHz and −12 dB for 1800 MHz. This ratio describes how well the antenna input impedance is matched to the reference impedance.

2.4 Numerical Modelling

This study is based on electromagnetic modelling using the Finite Integration Technique (FIT) implemented within CST Microwave Studio. The FIT-based time-domain solver was applied on hexahedral mesh. The problem addressed in this study deals with the calculation of the electric field distribution E. Subsequently, the spatial-averaged SAR W/kg in 10 g of tissue was calculated utilizing the algorithm described in the IEEE C95.3-2002 standard given by the following equation:

$$\text{SAR}(\mathbf{r}) = \frac{1}{V} \int_{element} \frac{\gamma(\mathbf{r}) \, |\mathbf{E}(\mathbf{r})|^2}{\rho_m(\mathbf{r})} d\mathbf{r}^3 \tag{1}$$

where |E| is the maximal value of electric field intensity [V/m] in the tissue, γ is the electrical conductivity [S/m] of the tissue, ρ_m is the mass density of the tissue [kg/m³] and **r** [m] is the position within the tissue, [18], To estimate SAR value in human tissue at certain depth, the intensity of electric field or the electric field strength **E** must be known. Distribution of the **E** is defined as follows:

$$\nabla \times \mu_r^{-1} (\nabla \times \mathbf{E}) - k_0^2 \left(\varepsilon_r - j \frac{\gamma}{\omega \varepsilon_0} \right) \mathbf{E} = 0 \tag{2}$$

where k_0 is the wave vector in free space [m⁻¹], ∇ represents the rotation vector operator, ε_r is the relative permittivity, ε_0 is the vacuum permittivity [F/m], μ_r is the

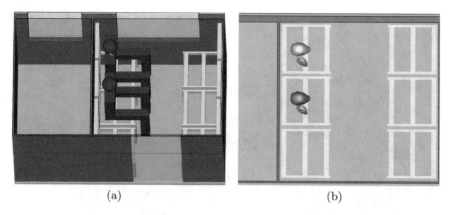

(a)   (b)

Fig. 4 The situation of the overall numerical model with **a** two simplified human body models or **b** two human SAM models placed in railway vehicle

relative permeability and ω is the angular wave frequency [rad/s], [19]. This absorbed power per tissue mass (SAR) averaged over the whole body or arbitrary 10 g tissue mass element is a well-established dosimetry quantity. As per IEEE C95.3-2002, the limiting values of the mentioned quantity are 0.08 W/kg for whole body averaged SAR and 2 W/kg for locally averaged SAR in general population.

The aim of this study was to obtain the spatial distribution of the electric field within the head tissue for both passengers when they are exposed to a near electromagnetic field generated by a mobile phone placed on the right side of the one person head. We used two types of human head models. Figure 4 shows two situations which were simulated—two human head SAM models with one electromagnetic source and two human simplified body models placed near each other, again with one electromagnetic source for two mobile telecommunication bands.

3   Results and Discussion

Spatial electric field distribution within the two types of human head models with CI was calculated for both mobile telecommunication bands (900 and 1800 MHz) and different distances between the head surface and mobile phone for human model with CI. The results were processed in order to compute the spatial-averaged SAR (10 g) as well as the peak spatial-averaged SAR (10 g) distribution considering specific dielectric parameters of the body and head tissue. In our simulation scenarios, we consider two distances (17 and 22 mm) between the PIFA antenna and the head surface. The reason was that we want to know direct influence of EMF in the secure distance if it could cause not regularly function of CI and influence of EMF to another passenger (B) sitting close to first passenger (A) on the right too. The distance between them is about 37 cm. Fig. 5 shows the spatial-averaged SAR distribution for 900 MHz

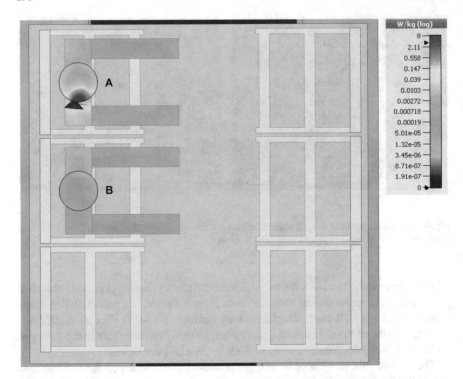

Fig. 5 The representative example of the spatial-averaged SAR distribution for one exposure scenario of two human body models (model A containing implanted CI model) in perspective view for 17 mm distance between the PIFA antenna and the head surface in case of 900 MHz carrier frequency

carrier frequency when considering the 17 mm distance between the PIFA antenna (mobile phone) and head surface for simplified human body (SHB) models. Figure 6 shows the spatial-averaged SAR distribution for both carrier frequency in the same scenario for two SAM models. For comparison purposes, the same simulations were performed in free space—that is, the human body models were out of railway vehicle.

The simulation results of the peak spatial averaged SAR (10 g) values for 17 and 22 mm distances between head surface and PIFA antenna, carrier source frequency (900 and 1800 MHz) and type of human head model (SHB and SAM) for two passengers (A and B) inside the railway vehicle or in the free space are placed in the Table 4.

Based on the results of the peak spatial averaged SAR (10 g) for passenger A prolonged exposure to mobile phones for 900 MHz (e.g. longer calls) in enclosed spaces could be potentially dangerous for the human body, given that all obtained SAR values exceed the European maximum SAR limit of 2 W/kg. From this point of view the optimal distance between the mobile phone and the cochlear implant is about 25 mm. In this case we obtained the peak spatial-averaged SAR values about 1.965 W/kg. Additionally, in each case the maximal SAR values inside the head

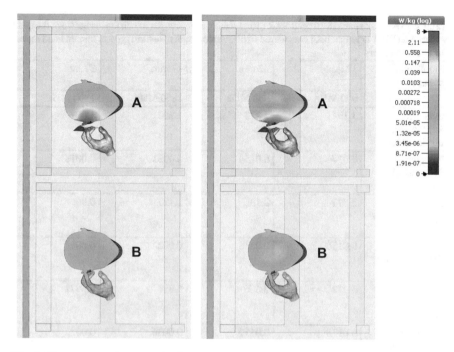

Fig. 6 The representative example of the spatial-averaged SAR distribution for one exposure scenario of two SAM models (model A containing implanted CI model) in perspective view for 17 mm distance between the PIFA antenna and the head surface in case of **a** 900 MHz carrier frequency, **b** 1800 MHz carrier frequency

were localized about 2 mm from the surface of head, oriented directly towards the CI. This could pose a potential threat for the CI users due to inhibition of perceived sound levels. Our simulation results show that passenger B sitting close to the person with active mobile phone is out of danger from this source since to very small SAR 10 g values. On the other hand, when we compare the previously mentioned simulation results with simulations performed in the open space, the SAR values are about 10% higher than in the open space scenario. It means that the greatest power dissipation occurs while sending messages in places with weak signal - implying inverse relationship, e.g. the weaker the signal, the greater the transmitted power as is especially evident in places with steel walls, cars, trains, etc. However, it should be noted that all results were obtained using the simplified model of railway vehicle and model of the human body, and possibly other sources of EM fields were not taken into the consideration. Using the standard IEEE Std 1528-2013 we can obtain uncertainty in SAR correction for deviations in dielectric and material properties. Our results have shown that the mean power uncertainty 2.7% for the spatial-averaged SAR (10 g) with $\pm 20\%$ maximal change in permittivity ε or conductivity γ.

Table 4 The peak spatial averaged SAR (10 g) results according to the distances between the head surface and PIFA antenna, both considered EMF source frequencies and type of human head model for two passengers

Simulation scenario	17 mm	22 mm	17 mm	22 mm
	900 MHz	900 MHz	1800 MHz	1800 MHz
Passenger A: SHB model inside vehicle	3.191	2.373	1.252	1.067
Passenger B: SHB model inside vehicle	0.0174	0.0153	0.0031	0.0018
Passenger A: SHB model free space	2.872	2.136	1.127	0.96
Passenger B: SHB model free space	0.0156	0.0138	0.0028	0.0012
Passenger A: SAM model inside vehicle	3.272	2.666	0.897	0.8571
Passenger B: SAM model inside vehicle	0.0178	0.0157	0.0036	0.0022
Passenger A: SAM model free space	3.01	2.452	0.8253	0.789
Passenger B: SAM model free space	0.016	0.0144	0.0033	0.002

4 Conclusion

Previous research has shown that the metallic implants may change the distribution of the electric field strength inside living tissue. Metallic implants may thus modify absorption of EMF energy around them by means of the scattering of the incident EM wave. It is very important to highlight potential risks stemming from use of CI in specific situations. One such situation can arise when a person is sitting in a railway vehicle and operates a mobile phone with additional person in the proximity. Our simulation results have shown that the calculated peak spatial-averaged SAR values are about 1.6/1.2 times higher for 900 MHz exposure and 17/22 mm distance between the head surface and PIFA antenna than the recommended maximum values established by the European SAR limit. Our simulation results have shown the passenger B sitting close to person with active mobile phone is out of danger from this source due to the small SAR 10 g values. Inside a railway vehicle they are comparable for both of used models of human head (simplified human body (SHB) models and SAM models). By comparing this simulation results with simulations performed in the open space, we have found that the SAR values are about 10% higher than simulations performed in the open space. It means, the greatest power dissipation occurs while sending messages in places with weak signal—implying inverse relationship, e.g. the weaker the signal, the greater the transmitted power as is especially evident in places with steel walls, cars, trains, etc.

Acknowledgements This work was supported project ITMS: 26210120021, cofounded from EU sources and European Regional Development Found.

References

1. Psenakova, Z., Hudecova, J.: Influence of Electromagnetic Fields by Electronic Implants in Medicine. Elektronika ir Elektrotechnika **7**, 37–40 (2009)
2. Need to read – all about CI. http://ci-a.at/. Accessed 05 Jan 2019
3. Vidal, N., Lopez-Villegas, J.M.: Changes in electromagnetic field absorption in the presence of subcutaneous implanted devices: Minimizing increases in absorption. IEEE Trans. Electromag. Compatib. **52**(3), 545–555 (2010)
4. Campi, T., Cruciani, S., Santis, V.D., Feliziani, M.: EMF safety and thermal aspects in a pacemaker equipped with a wireless power transfer system working at low frequency. IEEE Trans. Microw. Theory Tech. (2016)
5. Levitt, H.: The nature of electromagnetic interference. J. Am. Acad. Audiolo. **12**(6), 322–326 (2001)
6. EN 62209-1:2006. Human exposure to radio frequency fields from hand-held and bodymounted wireless communication devices – Human models, instrumentation, and procedures – Part 1: Procedure to determine the SAR for hand-held devices used in close proximity of the ear (frequency range of 300 MHz to 3GHz), (2006)
7. Chan, K.H., Leung, S.W., Siu, Y.M.: Specific absorption rate evaluation for people using wireless communication device in vehicle. In: 2010 IEEE International Symposium on Electromagnetic Compatibility, Fort Lauderale, vol. 5711364. Florida, USA (2010)
8. Salah, I.Y., Khalil, A.: High resolution numerical modelling of in-vehicle mobile cars. Int. J. Electromag. Appl. **5**(1), 66–72 (2015)
9. Gombarska, D.; Smetana, M.; Janousek, L.: High-frequency electromagnetic field measurement inside personal vehicle within urban environment In: MEASUREMENT 2019: Proceedings of the 12th International Conference (2019)
10. Psenakova, Z., Mydlova, J., Benova, M.: Investigation of SAR (Specific absorbtion rate) in different head models placed in shielded space. In: 2019 20th International Conference on Computational Problems of Electrical Engineering (CPEE), pp. 1–3. IEEE (2019)
11. Niparko, J.K.: Cochlear Implants: Principles & Practices. Lippincott Williams & Wilkins (2009)
12. Cochlear implants. Accessed 05 Jan 2019. https://www.westchesterhearingcenter.com/services/hearing-solutions/cochlear-implants/cochlear-implants-img4/, http://www.patedu.com/englisha/topic/cochlear-implants
13. Synchrony®System In Sync with Natural Hearing. Accessed 12 Dec 2018. https://s3.medel.com/pdf/24318CE_r5_1-synchronySystemFS-WEB.pdf
14. Mydlova, J., Benova, M., Psenáková, Z., Smondrk, M.: Evaluation of specific absorption rate in SAM head phantom with cochlear implant with and without hand model near PIFA antenna. In: Advances in Intelligent Systems and Computing. Springer Nature, Switzerland AG (2019). ISBN 978-3-030-23761-5

15. Mydlova, J., Benova, M, Stefancova, V., Pitlova, E.: Assessment of SAR in human body model with the cochlear implant inside a railway vehicle. Proceedings of the 13th International Scientific Conference on Sustainable Modern and Safe Transport Transportation Research Procedia (2019)
16. Dielectric properties of body tissues in the frequency range 10 Hz – 100 GHz. http://niremf. ifac.cnr.it/tissprop/#appl
17. IEEE 1528–2013 Standard: IEEE Recommended Practice for Determining the Peak Spatial-Average SAR in the Human Head from Wireless Com. Devices: Measurement Techniques
18. EN 62209-1:2016 Measurement procedure for the assessment of specific absorption rate of human BS exposure to radio frequency fields from hand-held and body-mounted wireless communication devices. Devices used next to the ear (Freq. range of 300 MHz to 6 GHz)
19. Golio, M.: The RF and Microwave Handbook, 2nd edn., vol 3. CRC Press, Boca Raton (2008)

Medical Data Analysis

Methods Supporting the Understanding of Structural Information by Blind People and Selected Aspects of Their Evaluation

Michał Maćkowski, Katarzyna Rojewska, Mariusz Dzieciątko, Katarzyna Bielecka, Mateusz Bas, and Dominik Spinczyk

Abstract The perception of structural information in mathematical formulas and charts is a challenge for the blind. The article presents the method of designing information system supporting the understanding of structural information by blind people. The article presents the 5 stages of the presented methodology: general principles of design, methods enabling data mining, content layout design, tools supporting the presentation of content and method for assessing user satisfaction. The results section presents evaluations of the described stages taken from the literature and own results based on a research group of 15 blind people. User satisfaction was examined for two thematic modules of developed by the authors of the platform for self-learning mathematics by the blind: algebra and mathematical analysis modules. From among 5 assessment categories proposed at the evaluation stage: presentation of information, gradation of difficulty, ease of decision making, ease of use of the user interface, simplicity of the user interface, the biggest differences in the assessment

M. Maćkowski
Faculty of Automatic Control, Electronic and Computer Science, Silesian University of Technology, 16 Akademicka, 44-100 Gliwice, Poland
e-mail: michal.mackowski@polsl.pl

K. Rojewska
Clinical Hospital No. 1 in Zabrze, Department of Pediatrics, School of Medicine with the Division of Dentistry in Zabrze, Medical University of Silesia in Katowice, 15-18 3th Maja, 41-800 Zabrze, Poland

M. Dzieciątko
SAS Institute Sp z o.o. Polska, ul.Gdańska 27/31, 01-633 Warszawa, Poland
e-mail: mariusz.dzieciatko@sas.com

K. Bielecka · M. Bas · D. Spinczyk (✉)
Faculty of Biomedical Engineering, Silesian University of Technology, 40 Roosevelta, 41-800 Zabrze, Poland
e-mail: dominik.spinczyk@polsl.pl

K. Bielecka
e-mail: katabie861@student.polsl.pl

M. Bas
e-mail: mateusz.bas@polsl.pl

E. Piętka et al. (eds.), *Information Technology in Biomedicine*, Advances in Intelligent Systems and Computing 1186, https://doi.org/10.1007/978-3-030-49666-1_24

of the two modules were observed in the categories of information presentation and user interface simplicity.

Keywords Perception of structural information · Blind people · Alternative methods of presenting structured information

1 Introduction

Blind people experience a number of difficulties in learning technical subjects, including the interpretation of structural information contained in materials containing mathematical formulas and graphs. The presented problem is the current topic of research and implementation. The increased interest of the largest corporations dealing with data presentation (SAS® Graphics Accelerator tool from SAS Institute) [1] proves the great importance of this issue. Moreover, Berkley University in cooperation with Elsevier developed the methodology of data mining in the form of charts adapted to the needs of the blind people [2].

The purpose of the work is to review the stages that occur during the creation of a tool supporting the understanding of structural information by the blind and the visually impaired. As part of the work, a methodology will also be developed that allows the authors to assess the satisfaction of mathematical content adapted for the blind. Such issue will be verified on a selected research group.

2 Materials and Methods

Based on the literature review, several stages were distinguished in the production cycle of the tool supporting the understanding of structural information by the visually impaired and blind:

1. General principles of design
2. Methods enabling data mining
3. Content layout design
4. Tools supporting the presentation of content
5. Method for assessing user satisfaction

2.1 General Principles of Design

We can distinguish general rules for creating charts for the blind or visually impaired persons. The information collected is summarised in the Table 1.

Table 1 General rules for creating charts for the blind [3]

Rule	Description
Content	– presentation not only of the chart description but also of any interactions or relationships on the chart,
	– graduation of difficulties and complexity of information. Adapting the level of knowledge and skills to the blind person. When designing touch graphics, the age and experience of the reader should be taken into account,
	– identification of trends, increasing and decreasing functions,
	– cohesion and the unequivocal nature of the information. Presenting information in a clear and concise manner. Omission of irrelevant information,
	– ensuring that blind people can make decisions
Location	– selection the appropriate scale,
	– a margin of at least 10,0 mm across the whole side,
	– avoid clutter, too close to each other or similar elements that are difficult to distinguish. Transparency should be ensured by providing gaps between adjacent textures or where lines intersect other lines or textures. A gap is not required only when the contrast is clear
Appearance	– designing objects in the most meaningful way for the user. This is not an accurate representation,
	– a single graphic should contain no more than five different area textures, five different line styles, and five different types of point symbols,
	– omission of decoration and decorative effects

2.2 Methods Enabling Data Mining

Elsevier making charts accessible for people with visual impairments. A collaboration between Elsevier and Highcharts created one version of the chart available to everyone (Fig. 1). A screen reader translates hidden chart detail information. Obtained improved system of descriptive markers for graphs. Description of the chart structure, giving information about the chart type, axis and long description of what can be found on the chart. Described also interactions and relationships in the chart. Currently it gives the possibility to understand dynamic graphs and obtain the information you need independently [2].

2.3 Content Layout Design

Google supports various accessibility plugins for visually impaired users such as Extension Accessibility Developer Tools, High Contrast, ChromeVox [6]. Presentation of content so that elements become more accessible and usable. This can be done by:

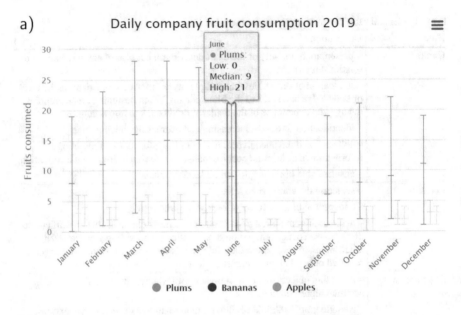

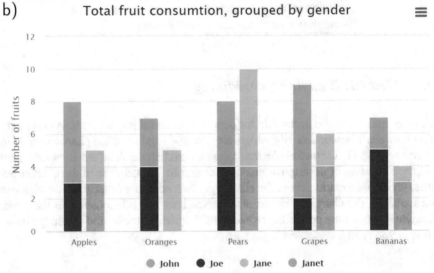

Fig. 1 Accessible chart (**a**) and chart for people without visual impairments (**b**) [4]

- enlarging the text size,
- customizing color contrasts (Fig. 2),
- using screen readers,
- subtitles or captions on videos,
- alternative image text to describe images (Fig. 3).

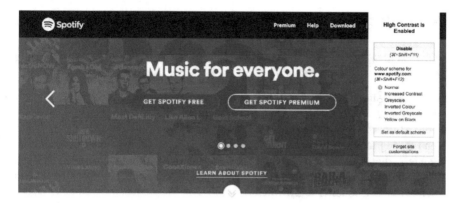

Fig. 2 Example of customizing color contrasts of a web page [6]

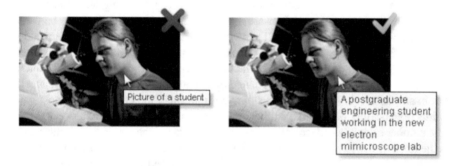

Fig. 3 Example of alternative text usage on an image [6]

Several authors from the article entitled "Web Accessibility for Visually Impaired People: Requirements and Design Issues" organized three workshops with various stakeholders. A set of requirements devised from the workshops guided the process of building a middleware prototype. A prototype of middleware that allows content to be adjusted by displaying and transforming content in a more accessible way adapted to user preferences and alternative representations of content using voice narrators and other sounds. The aim is to provide personalised visual adaptations for different levels of disability and to increase the accessibility of web content. This is based on combining the original page with the middleware version, where it removes from the original version e.g. unimportant images, leaves only what is related to the content. The relevant content is transformed into a clickable form. By pointing the cursor on a paragraph, the paragraph is highlighted in yellow. Text with a larger font is displayed and moves from left to right and is read by the screen reader [7].

2.4 Tools Supporting the Presentation of Content

SAS Graphics Accelerator is a browser extension, which provides for the chart (Fig. 4):

- text descriptions such as chart type, title, X and Y axis labels, and more,
- tabular data. It is possible to export data to a CSV file,
- sonication, which allows the user to see graphics with rising tones for higher values and falling tones for lower values. Sounds are played through the left speaker at the left edge of the object and then played to the right within the sonified data set. The sounds that are played can be speed-dependent or controlled with the keys to select the next tones (Fig. 5).

SAS Studio enables visually impaired students to complete video courses with a screen reader, magnifying glass, or braille monitor. The SAS support page offers several sample SAS Graphics Accelerator enabled chart types, among other things heat maps. Sonification and Heat Maps are used to understand the relationship between two continuous variables (Fig. 6). The two variables are represented on the x and y axes. Typically, an independent variable is represented on the x-axis, and a dependent variable is represented on the y-axis. The heat map divides the Cartesian plane into a grid. The colour of each cell is represented by the number of given points in that cell. For example, a cell with zero points may be light blue, the cell with the most data points may be dark blue, and the other cells have an intermediate tint between them. The number of points in each cell represents the values of the z-axis, where the z-axis is the third dimension. The z-axis is the height of the textures in the touch graphics. The sound presentation of the Z-axis will be represented by a specific sound. The sound pitch represents the number of given points in the corresponding cell [1].

2.5 Method for Assessing User Satisfaction

Based on the literature review and previous authors' work, a methodology was prepared to assess the satisfaction of mathematical content adapted for the blind. For this purpose, an evaluation questionnaire was prepared (in cooperation with a psychologist), where each participant had to answer the following questions:

1. Is the information presented clearly and comprehensibly?
2. Is the principle of gradation of difficulty maintained?
3. Does the mathematics learning platform allow the user to make conclusions and make decisions?
4. Is the interface of the math learning platform simple and orderly?
5. Does the interface of math learning platform lack of decorative details?

Each of the above questions could be answered by the user in the following way: I totally disagree (1 point), I rather disagree (2 points), I have no opinion (3 points), I rather agree (4 points), I totally agree (5 points).

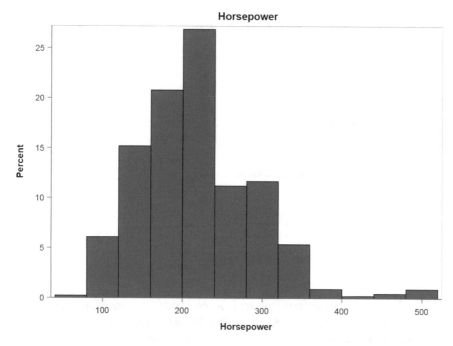

Fig. 4 Example of graph for the SAS graphics accelerator [5]

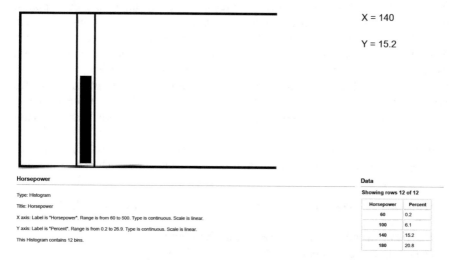

Fig. 5 Example of SAS sonification view for histogram from Fig. 4 [5]

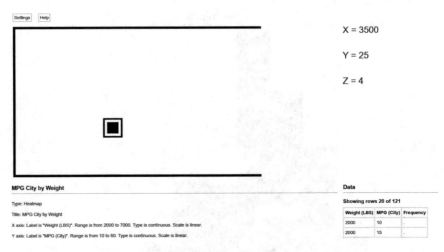

Fig. 6 Example of SAS sonification and heat map [5]

Based on the methodology prepared in the above way, mathematical content adapted to the needs of the blind was evaluated. In the previous works of the authors, a platform for learning mathematics by blind people was presented [8, 9]. In the developed platform, in order to present effectively the structural information contained in the math formulas, a set of rules was prepared to create alternative descriptions, containing additional information not only about the symbols appearing in the formula but also about its structure. The developed set of exercises from a given area is available in the form of an internet portal, which a blind user can use to learn using a computer and an installed screen reader program. Moreover, the platform was developed in Polish language, mainly because Polish language was native for all participants, which provided them with maximum comfort. The users were equipped with a computer with the Internet access and a screen reader Non Visual Desktop (NVD).

The selected research group consisted of 15 students. Each person was blind or visually impaired. Psychological consultation allowed the authors to adopt the following inclusion criteria:

- The group includes persons whose degree of visual impairment or blindness was significant.
- The vision disability was acquired during their lives.
- The group was consistent with the duration of disability,
- People in the group did not have any other disabilities.

The research group assessed alternative content for two branches of mathematics: algebra and mathematical analysis (exercises related to solving Riemann integrals by parts or substitution). After solving 5 exercises from algebra and then mathematical analysis, each participant assessed the platform based on a previously prepared questionnaire. Answering all questions was possible in nominate scale with grades form 1 to 5 with step size equals one. Then the sum of points obtained by a particular participant was divided by the maximum number of points possible to obtain and expressed in percent scale. Finally, the average value for each question in the survey was calculated from all the answers given by the participants.

3   Results

The Results section presents the results obtained from the literature for those stages for which evaluation results were found: methods enabling data mining and designing the content layout, as well as self-obtained results in the section on user satisfaction evaluation.

3.1   *Evaluation of the Enabling Data Mining Stage*

Highcharts has been tested on a blind person since birth. According to Lucy Greco, this method allows the user to interact with the chart, to understand all relations on it. The advantage is that it is not only a description of the chart. Lucy said it gives you the possibility to understand dynamic charts, to obtain independent information. There is no need for a volunteer or an assistant who has to be paid for. Independent reading and interpretation of the charts gives a blind person the opportunity to analyse the data at a suitable time and date. The risk with the help of a sighted person is that the person who provides you with information has his or her own interpretation of the chart, and this is not desirable. This takes away the possibility of forming one's own opinions from a blind person [2].

3.2   *Evaluation of the Content Layout Design Stage*

A prototype of middleware was tested by 4 people from the Terrassa School of Optics and Optometry of Universitat Politecnica de Catalunya. The participants were between 28 and 70 years with different types of disabilities, years of low vision and internet usage per day. They used Window Eyes screen reader. They received an email containing two links and an instruction manual. The first link contained the middleware and the second included the evaluation survey. The evaluation process consisted of three steps:

– familiarization with the middleware interface and its functions,
– randomly assign a user to a particular web page to find specific information,
– answering questions. The questions concerned demographic data, experience with technology, type and level of visual impairment. The second category of questions

were questions used to evaluate whether a person was able to find the required information on a particular website. The third category of questions was based on using the Likert scale and open-ended questions to evaluate the usefulness of middleware [7].

The authors of the article summarized the results and recorded them in a table (Table 2).

3.3   *Evaluation of the Assessing User Satisfaction Stage*

Based on the collected research results presented in Table 3, it can be easily noticed a variety of test results for the assessment of mathematical content adaptation for the blind referring to algebra and analysis. The greatest discrepancy can be seen in two categories regarding the assessment: whether the information is presented clearly and comprehensively and whether the interface is simple and orderly. All research participants stated that despite the developed alternative description of mathematical expressions, some of the information provided is difficult to understand, especially when solving more advanced exercises. What is more, in the case of solving integrals, drop-down lists with sample answers appeared at particular stages of exercise solving, whose handling caused some problems for blind users.

4   Discussion and Conclusions

In addition to cognitive barriers, learning mathematics by the blind is also difficult for psychological reasons. Literature studies show low self-confidence and negative feelings associated with learning [10]. Tools supporting the learning of mathematics by the blind, such as the proposed platform or the Daisy Book Standard extended by the ability to read mathematical formulas [11] are not very common. In this you can see the reasons for the small number of people participating in the tests of other tools developed.

According to the literature review, the particular phases of developing tools for the blind people have not been subjected to "mass" testing. This analysis has shown that such research should be carried out in the future, in particular those focusing on the evaluation of tools that adapt charts for the visually impaired. Thanks to the developed methodology a quantitative assessment of the adaptation of mathematical content to the needs of the blind is possible. Based on the research, it can be concluded that this method can also be used to assess the understanding of the charts by the blind. In the future, it is planned to use sentiment analysis methods to evaluate user satisfaction [12].

The development of tools supporting the learning of mathematics by blind people and their evaluation methodologies in order to be effective in the future must go

Table 2 Prototype evaluation result [7]

Participants	Middleware feature/adaptation technique							WCAG 2.0 compliance
	Image filtering	Image resizing	Text transformation	Contrast	Content filter	Voice narrator	Amplifying lens	
A	2	2	6	3	2	2	6	Yes
B	2	2	6	1	5	6	6	Yes
C	6	3	6	3	6	3	6	No
D	6	3	6	2	6	2	6	No
Mean	4	2.5	6	2.25	4.75	3.25	6	–

Table 3 Assessment of user satisfaction results (normalized numerical values)

	Algebra	Mathematical analysis
The information is presented clearly and comprehensibly	84.7	68.0
The principle of grading of difficulty has been maintained	76.0	78.7
It allows the user to make conclusions and make decisions	82.7	89.3
The interface is simple and orderly	84.0	70.4
The interface does not include decorative details	84.0	85.3

hand with a social campaign promoting proactive attitudes. In addition, facilitation allowing for further use of acquired mathematical skills in career development (e.g. support for university studies) will increase personal motivation to learn mathematics by the blind people.

Acknowledgements The research was conducted thanks to funding from the project 2019/03/X/ ST6/01093, National Science Centre, Poland.

References

1. Reviewing charts and graphs with SAS accessibility. https://www.afb.org/aw/19/7/15075. Accessed 10 Nov 2019
2. Making charts accessible for people with visual impairments. https://www.elsevier.com/ connect/making-charts-accessible-for-people-with-visual-impairments. Accessed 21 Oct. 2019
3. The Braille Authority of North America: Guidelines and Standards for Tactile Graphics (2010)
4. Highcharts - manufacturer's website. https://www.highcharts.com/demo. Accessed 25 Oct 2019
5. SAS PRODUCTS & SOLUTIONS - manufacturer's website. http://support.sas.com/software/ products/graphics-accelerator/samples/index.html. Accessed 10 Nov 2019
6. Accessibility basics: designing for visual impairment. https://webdesign.tutsplus.com/articles/ accessibility-basics-designing-for-visual-impairment--cms-27634. Accessed 20 Nov 2019
7. Kurti, A., Raufi, B., Astals, D., Ferati, M., Vogel, B.: Web Accessibility for Visually Impaired People Requirements and Design Issues. Published by Springer International Publishing, Switzerland (2016)
8. Maćkowski, M., Brzoza, P., Spinczyk, D.: Tutoring math platform accessible for visually impaired people. Comput. Biol. Med. **95**, 298–306 (2018). https://doi.org/10.1016/j. compbiomed.2017.06.003
9. Maćkowski, M., Brzoza, P., Żabka, M., Spinczyk, D.: Multimedia platform for mathematics' interactive learning accessible to blind people. Multimedia Tools Appl. **77**(5), 6191–6208 (2018). https://doi.org/10.1007/s11042-017-4526-z
10. Spinczyk, D., Maćkowski, M., Kempa, W., Rojewska, K.: Factors influencing the process of learning mathematics among visually impaired and blind people. Comput. Biol. Med. **104**, 1–9 (2019). https://doi.org/10.1016/j.compbiomed.2018.10.025
11. Brzoza, P., Spinczyk, D.: Conference: multimedia browser for Internet Online Daisy books. In: 10th International Conference on Computers Helping People with Special Needs Location: Linz, AUSTRIA Date: JUL 11-13, 2006 Book Series: Lecture Notes In Computer Science, vol. 4061, 1087-1093 (2006)

12. Maćkowski, M., Rojewska, K., Dzieciątko, M., Spinczyk, D.: Initial motivation as a factor predicting the progress of learning mathematics for the blind. In: Pietka, E., Badura, P., Kawa, J., Wieclawek, W. (eds) Information Technology in Biomedicine. Advances in Intelligent Systems and Computing, vol 1011. Springer, Cham (2019)

Videoplethysmographic Measurements of Pulse Wave Velocity and Pulse Transit Time

Anna Pająk and Piotr Augustyniak

Abstract Oxygen-rich blood has different absorption properties than de-oxygenated one. For that reason during the heartbeat there are slight changes in colour of human skin which are invisible to an eye but detectable for the colour video camera after applying motion picture processing algorithms. Therefore, one of the new methods for touchless pulse rate measurements is videoplethysmography (VPG). With VPG techniques the blood pulse in human can be recorded in a seamless and unobtrusive way, in some applications even without subject's knowledge. Most authors are focusing on detection of the heart rate as representative to physical load and stress. In this paper we are estimating pulse wave velocity (PWV) and pulse transit time (PTT) from video footage of the skin. PWV is directly related to the stiffness of a blood vessels, so can be used to detect certain diseases early.

Keywords Videoplethysmography · Pulse wave velocity · Pulse transit time · Video signal processing

1 Introduction

Videoplethysmographic (VPG) measurement is attractive due to the possibility of contactless measurement and the use of commercially available, customer-grade video cameras. The most common place for examinations is the face, because it is uncovered most of the time, the subcutaneous artery network is dense, and the results are most reliable. In pilot research reported in this paper, a two-point VPG measurement was carried on the arm. This part of body is easily accessible and contains arterial vessels suitable for pulse detection.

A. Pająk (✉) · P. Augustyniak
AGH University of Science and Technology, Krakow, Poland
e-mail: Anna.Pajak@fis.agh.edu.pl

P. Augustyniak
e-mail: august@agh.edu.pl

E. Piętka et al. (eds.), *Information Technology in Biomedicine*, Advances in Intelligent
Systems and Computing 1186, https://doi.org/10.1007/978-3-030-49666-1_25

317

Pulse wave velocity (PWV) and its reciprocal—pulse transit time (PTT) are relatively new markers of cardiovascular risk. The relationship between them can be described by formula (1).

$$PWV = \frac{L}{PTT},\tag{1}$$

where L—the distance between proximal and distal sites of artery.

Both markers are associated with flexibility of blood vessels and can be used to determine the changes in stiffness of their wall tissue. The arterials in the arm are long enough to notice a delay in pulse wave (called transit time) between the marked areas. Owing to this fact we can estimate pulse wave velocity.

The PWV (or PTT) measurement is usually made with precise evaluation of blood wave delay between two points. In case of regional PWV analysis, the pulse wave is captured on vessels of different thickness and flexibility, while the local PWV measurement assesses the wave delay along a single calibre artery. In this paper we present results of the latter method.

2 Related Work

The origins of PTT measuring can be traced back to 1959, when Weltman et al. designed a computer which, by measuring the ECG, pulse signal and knowing the length of measured artery, determined the PTT value. After the research it was concluded that PTT value decreases with increasing stiffness of blood vessels. This stiffness increases with aging, inadequate diet, smoking, etc. [1].

Most studies are focused on the evaluation of regional pulse waves. However, the local pulse wave is also being studied, although reported in few papers only. In the work of P. M. Nabeel et al. [2] local pulse wave velocity values were estimated using single-source based PPG method. Pulse of people aged 28 ± 4 years were measured. The values of $2.30 \pm 0.17 \, \mathrm{m\,s^{-1}}$ (BMI = $26.76 \, \mathrm{kg\,m^{-2}}$) and $2.80 \pm 0.23 \, \mathrm{m\,s^{-1}}$ (BMI = $30.96 \, \mathrm{kg\,m^{-2}}$) were obtained in people aged about 24 years. The respondents had a BMI of 26–$30 \, \mathrm{kg\,m^{-2}}$, so they were overweight.

Pereira et al. in their article [3] included studies in which 16 patients aged 55 ± 7 years were measured using MRI method. Estimated pulse rate was measured in the aorta. The obtained results oscillated around the mean value of $5.65 \pm 0.75 \, \mathrm{m\,s^{-1}}$.

There are many non-invasive methods for pulse and PWV measuring. Currently, research is focused on videoplethysmography (VPG) as a cheap and contactless method. Usually the visible light is employed, although to obtain reliable results, adequate lighting and minimalizing patient movements are necessary. In order to perform the test both visible and infrared video cameras are used. There is also a possibility of measurements in infrared or thermal spectra, where the dependence of the temperature change on the moment of heart evolution is studied [4]. The most frequently surveyed region is the face. In Ming-Zher Poh et al. studies, the ROI was selected so as to cover 60% of the surface area from the central part of detected face.

If no face was found or more faces were detected, the coordinates closest to previous frame were used. The signal from every pixel was divided into three channels (red, green and blue), and then the variability of the intensity of every colour in time was analized. The strongest variability and the highest SNR showed the green component. After applying appropriate filtration and amplification it was possible to determine the pulse rate. Reliability of the method is studied in [5]. The author used the YUV color model which was recommended as not requiring the use of independent or principal component analysis.

The VPG is a fast method and it has several prospective applications e.g. in emergency medicine, where the patient's life parameters should be determined quickly. In the paper by Ming-Zer Poh et al. the measurement results differed from the reference by 3 to 5 bpm what was found sufficiently accurate as heart rate approximation [6].

There is a method similar to VPG and is called imaging photoplethysmography (iPPG). Anton M. Unkafov in his research as a ROI region selected the whole face and facial region below eyes (definitely better results were obtained from the whole face). In order to increase the SNR, pixels without pulse rate information (e.g. hair or shaded areas) were removed from the ROI area. Then the remaining pixels were detrended and filtered with a moving average or a band-pass filter. The pulse rate was approximated using the interbeat interval (IBI) or maximal power spectra density (PSD) method [7].

Przybyło et al. wrote in their paper [8] about the importance of lightning selection. The worst results were obtained for infrared light and dim daylight. For both types of illumination SNR was negative, while for fluorescent artificial light and incandescent light bulb SNR was above zero. In paper [9] Mędrala and Augustyniak concluded that the temperature of lightning has influence on the quality of pulse rate estimation. The best results were obtained for warm lightning (colour temperature of 2700 K).

The other significant thing which has compelling meaning in estimate pulse rate is the skin tone. Królak in her paper [10] measured 12 people of different ethnicity and proved that different colour of skin has other light absorption properties.

3   Methods

3.1   Study Conditions

With the use of RGB camera it is possible to record and analyze the changes in tone of the skin for three different colours: red, green and blue. The measurement was carried out on the arm. There arteries are not winding, so approximating the length of artery to the distance between two measurement points selected on the skin is quite accurate.

To conduct the study we used a RGB camera (connected to a computer), a program for dividing the recorded colour image into three components (red, green and blue)

Fig. 1 The measuring system

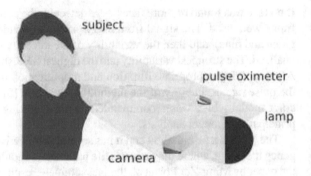

and a program to analyze the data. The number of frames per second recorded by camera was 16 fps.

The examination was performed with three subjects: a white woman at the age of 23 (Woman) and two white men at the age of 23 (Man 1) and 24 (Man 2). The left arm of the subject was lying on a table at heart level. The footage of examined body part was recorded for about twenty seconds. During filming, the subject was asked not to make any movements in order to avoid the formation of motion artifacts. This procedure was designed to prevent the formation of motion artifacts. The arrangement of measuring system is shown in Fig. 1. The distance between the arm and the camera was 25 cm. The distance between the camera and the lamp was 30 cm.

The measurement was made in constant conditions. To achieve such conditions there was used artificial lightning (brightness and intensity of natural light varies depending on the time of day and year and on the place of Earth). The place, where measurements took place, was illuminated with a warm light bulb of 806 lm and the colour temperature of 2700 K.

As a reference measurement of the pulse rate we used a pulse oximeter applied to the index finger. During the study, the values of pulse rate were read from the device and then the average value from the obtained data was taken for analysis.

3.2 Image and Signal Processing

In the resulting image, two regions were selected, where the colour changes in each colour channel were measured. During this examination the following sites were selected: elbow bend area and inguinal bend area. The region of interest (ROI) size was 64×64 pixels.

As in examinations of Ming Zher Poh [6], Unfakov [7] and Mędrala [9], colours of each of the selected fragments of the image were divided into three components. This manoeuvre was performed for each frame of the film, resulting in changes in individual colours over time.

In next step, we calculated the mean value for every component from each image of the video sequence inside both ROIs. In result we obtained a one-dimensional vector for every colour.

The data from all components has been centred in order to better illustrate the obtained results. For this purpose, the formula (2) was used.

$$D(n) = d(n) - \frac{\Sigma_{i=1}^{M}(d_i - \overline{d})}{M},$$
(2)

where $D(n)$—value after centering, $d(n)$—value obtained in examination, $\overline{d}$—mean value of obtained data, M—number of all individual measurements.

After centring, the data was whitened. The goal of whitening is to remove the underlying correlation in the data and preparing it for further analysis.

Then we used the independent component analysis (ICA) algorithm. ICA is a case of blind source separation. During recording the video, the camera's sensors can receive mixed signals from each channel and additional common fluctuations and noise (e.g. small movements, changes in lightning). Therefore, the dependence of the amplitude of each channel (red, green and blue) on time was determined as $x_r(t)$, $x_g(t)$, $x_b(t)$ and subjected to ICA algorithm. Assuming that the three statistically independent sought sources (determined as $s_r(t)$, $s_g(t)$, $s_b(t)$) are a linear combination of signals from each channel, the Eq. (3) is true.

$$\overrightarrow{x}(t) = \mathbf{M} \cdot \overrightarrow{s}(t),$$
(3)

where: $\overrightarrow{x}(t)$—column vector of channels $[x_r(t), x_g(t), x_b(t)]$, $\overrightarrow{s}(t)$—column vector of sources $[s_r(t), s_g(t), s_b(t)]$, $\mathbf{M}$—square (3×3) matrix of the mixture coefficients.

Using the ICA algorithm, it is necessary to find such a mixing matrix $\mathbf{M}$ that its inversion, called the separating matrix $\mathbf{N}$. Then:

$$\widehat{s}(t) = \mathbf{N}\overrightarrow{x},$$
(4)

where: $\widehat{s}(t)$—estimate of the vector $\overrightarrow{s}$ which contains the independent sought sources.

Afterwards the $s_r(t)$, $s_g(t)$, $s_b(t)$ was filtered with a fourth order Butterworth low-pass filter with a cutoff frequency of 4 Hz. Thanks to it the high frequency noise were deleted.

Then the graphs with these changes were analysed. As the ICA returns components in random order, we have to select one of them for further analysis. To maximize the signal-to-noise ratio we analyzed the variability of values in a frame sequence and used the component where the variability index was the highest. It was found in the relation to the moment of heartbeat for second component, therefore only this component was further analyzed. The Fig. 2 shows the intensity dependence for each component on time. The change of intensity is most visible and regular for second component.

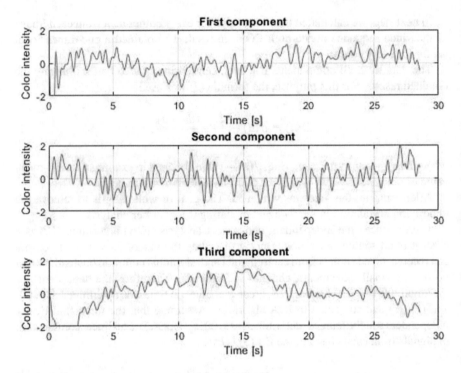

Fig. 2 Dependence of colour intensity of each independent components on time

After overlapping two graphs of the most varying signal a program was searching for a value of time delay that would yield best match of pulse waves from two ROIs. Peaks were detected by a custom-written MATLAB script and then the delay between peaks was determined in a ROI placed further from the heart (elbow fold) from a ROI placed closer to the heart (inguinal region). The path the pulse travelled was the distance between the centers of both ROIs. After using formula (5), successive values of the local pulse wave velocity were saved in the file. The absolute value in the denominator was used to eliminate negative speeds for reverse naming of ROIs.

$$v_i = \frac{f_s \cdot d}{100 \cdot |x_{i1} - x_{i2}|},$$ (5)

where v_i—pulse wave velocity [m s^{-1}], f_s—sampling frequency (16 fps), d—the distance between the centers of the designated image fragments [cm], x_{i1}—peak time in the i-th frame for the first ROI (green channel), x_{i2}—peak time in the i-th frame for the second ROI (green channel).

Then the calculated blood pressure rates were averaged and the standard deviation of each result was determined.

4   Experimental Evaluation of the Method

4.1   Results of Measurement Accuracy

A pulse oximeter applied to the index finger was used as a reference measurement device. Through the different absorption properties of oxygen-rich and non-oxygenated blood, it measures the heart rate and the saturation (oxidation) of blood. The signal measured by the pulse oximeter can be divided into two components: constant and pulsating. Thanks to the pulsating component it is possible to determine the heart rate. Table 1 shows pulse rate obtained with the VPG measurements and the pulse oximeter readouts. Heart rate estimates were taken from the elbow bend area, due to more stable lighting.

Maximum error of the estimated heart rate was 6 bpm. The average error of this value was 4 bpm (6.24%).

4.2   Results of Local Pulse Wave Velocity

As the regions of interest have been selected at a certain distance (20 cm) on the arm, there is a possibility to observe the delay of the pulse wave (i.e. the transit time) related to the build-up of vascular deformation. Thanks to the relationship (1) we can determine PWV value. Figure 3 shows the results obtained for the woman and the men parameters.

Using formula (5) the rate of local pulse wave propagation in the brachial artery was calculated. The results are presented in Table 2.

Table 1   Accuracy of heart rate estimation

Person	Pulse oximeter (bpm)	VPG (bpm)	Error of estimation (%)
Woman	68	62	8.82
Man 1	59	55	6.78
Man 2	64	62	3.13

Table 2   Local pulse wave velocities and its standard deviations

Person	Pulse wave velocity ($m s^{-1}$)	Standard deviation ($m s^{-1}$)
Woman	1.54	0.92
Man 1	2.27	0.99
Man 2	1.48	0.98

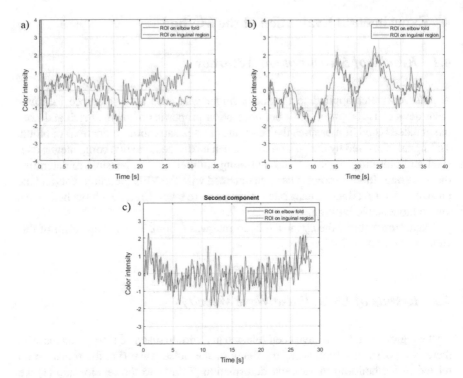

Fig. 3 Dependence of selected independent component intensity of each ROI on time for Woman (**a**), Man 1 (**b**) and Man 2 (**c**)

5 Discussion

Mędrala and Augustyniak in their paper [9] came to the conclusion that the VPG measurement of heart rate does not have to be limited to the face only. Their hypothesis is confirmed by the research reported in the current paper, where the heart rate was determined on the arm of the examined person. The estimated pulse rate from the arm does not have a perfect correlation with the measurement obtained from the reference pulse oximeter but it is sufficiently accurate to detect incorrect pulse. The maximal difference was 6 bpm. Results on pulse rate reported in [5] are far better (1.85–2.67 bpm) due to more reliable measurement from the human face. Nevertheless this author findings that scene changes and subject motion affect the measurement reliability are consistent with ours.

The estimated local pulse wave velocity were: $1.54 \pm 0.92\,\mathrm{m\,s^{-1}}$, $2.27 \pm 0.99\,\mathrm{m\,s^{-1}}$ and $1.48 \pm 0.98\,\mathrm{m\,s^{-1}}$. The results obtained by P. M. Nabeel et al. [2] $(2.3 \pm 0.17\,\mathrm{m\,s^{-1}}$ and $2.8 \pm 0.23\,\mathrm{m\,s^{-1}})$ are slightly higher than ones from current article. The difference is due to other BMI ranges. In both experiments the people were in similar age but in [2] the examined persons were overweight (BMI of 26–

$30\,\mathrm{kg\,m^{-2}}$) and in this measurement the subjects were within normal range range (BMI of 19–$25\,\mathrm{kg\,m^{-2}}$).

In Pereira's research [3] the results of ultrasound measuring oscillated between $5.65 \pm 0.75\,\mathrm{m\,s^{-1}}$. This is much higher than results obtained in current research. The reason for this difference is: (1) higher age of subjects and (2) different place for measurements. The expected PWV value in people at age 55 is much higher than PWV of people at age 25 due to higher blood vessels stiffness.

On the basis of the above comparisons, it can be concluded that the data received in current experiment are realistic. This gives hope for further development of the VPG method in local and regional PWV measurements.

The value of the local heart rate in our article was determined by the recording from an RGB camera. In case of [2] measurements, the measurements were made in the infrared range. Cameras recording images in the visible light range are much easier to access than cameras with the possibility of infrared recording, which proves that our algorithm can be used more widely. The studies mentioned in the Pereira [3] article were carried out using MRI method. To conduct an MRI examination, one must be qualified and experienced. This results in a significant reduction in the number of people who can take measurements. The equipment used for this test is expensive and not commonly available. There is no such limitation in our method.

The main problem during the measurements was the question of lightning. The right choice of light source is a key issue on VPG examinations [9]. Care should also be taken to ensure that there is no shading on the parts of the body that are measured, which could cause the results to be distorted. The problem could be hairy skin on the arms in men too. The subject should stay in motionless in order to minimise interference and noise caused by movements. Unfortunately, this factor cannot be completely eliminated, therefore motion compensation algorithms would be highly welcome.

The perfect matching of colour change time series from two recording zones can only be expected for pulse wave delays equal to a multiple of camera frame interval (i.e. the inverse of frame rate). The resulting quantization of the delay value increases when the distance of measurement zones shortens. On the other hand lengthening of the distance may be not possible along a single calibre artery for anatomical reasons. Increasing the camera frame rate may be the most straightforward method for reducing the delay quantization error, but it is impractical due to costs of high speed cameras and augmented requirements about lighting. The alternative way to be further investigated is application of mathematical methods to calculate the cross-correlation of the pulse waveforms with time shift of a fraction of frame interval.

The aim for next tests is to carry out examinations with more people to verify the accuracy and correctness of local pulse wave velocity marking. Care must be taken to ensure that measurements are reproducible and as little as possible dependent on environmental conditions. We would try to use YUV colour mode in pulse wave velocity analysis. The relationship between RGB and YUV colour is linear, as suggested by Rumiński in [5], so we will test the effectiveness of other colour spaces in case of unsatisfactory results.

The VPG measurements have several prospective applications in different areas of life surveillance because of their non-contact sensing capabilities and fairy cheap instrumentation. It is possible to automatically detect and follow the region of interest, which would avoid disturbance caused by movements.

Acknowledgements Research supported by the AGH University of Science and Technology in year 2020 from the subvention granted by the Polish Ministry of Science and Higher Education; grant no.: 16.16.120.773.

References

1. Molisz, A., Faściszewska, M., Wożakowska-Kapłon, B., Siebert, J.: Pulse wave velocity – reference range and usage. Folia Cardiologica, tom 10, nr 4, strony 268–274 (2015)
2. Nabeel, P.M., Jayaraj, J., Mohanasankar, S.: Single-source PPG based local pulse wave velocity measurement: a potential cuffless blood pressure estimation technique. Institute of Physics and Engineering in Medicine (2017)
3. Pereira, T., Correia, C., Cardoso, J.: Novel methods for pulse wave velocity measurement. J. Med. Biol. Eng. **35**, 555–565 (2015)
4. Li, J.: Pulse Wave Velocity Techniques. Springer Nature Switzerland AG (2019)
5. Rumiński, J.: Reliability of pulse measurements in videoplethysmography. Metrol. Meas. Syst. **23**(3), 359–371 (2016)
6. Poh, M.-Z., McDuff, D.J., Picard, R.W.: Non-contact, automated cardiac pulse measurements using video imaging and blind source separation. Opt. Express **18**(10) (2010)
7. Unfakov, A.M.: Pulse rate estimation using imaging photoplethysmography: generic framework and comparison of methods on a publicly available dataset. Biomed. Phys. Eng. Express **4** (2018)
8. Przybyło, J., Kańtoch, E., Jabłoński, M., Augustyniak, P.: Distant measurement of plethysmographic signal in various lightning conditions using configurable frame-rate camera. Metrol. Meas. Syst. **23**(4), 579–592 (2016)
9. Mędrala, R., Augustyniak, P.: Taking Videoplethysmographic Measurements at Alternative Parts of the Body – Pilot Study, PCBBE (2019)
10. Królak, A.: Influence of Skin Tone on Efficiency of Vision-Based Heart Rate Estimation. Springer International Publishing AG (2018)

Biomechanical Methods of Validating Animations

Filip Wróbel, Dominik Szajerman, and Adam Wojciechowski

Abstract Skeletal animation being one of the most distinct technics in real-time computer graphic is constantly evolving, since the time it was first implemented. New features, methods of synthesis and processing are being actively worked on and shipped in commercial titles. One missing aspect of this subbranch of rendering is proper automatic validation for humanoid movements. In response to that niche a study was prepared. It consisted of typical industry standard animation environment, used state-of-the-art animations resources and run with repeatable results in controlled environment. On these bases motion data for selected animated joints were measured and stored. Collected test data was analyzed against biomechanical constraints of human body. With conclusion of promising results, further research and possible applications were proposed.

Keywords Animation validation · Biomechanics in animation · Biomechanically correct animation

1 Introduction

Animating humans in graphical applications and video games is matter constantly being improved and worked on. This is a part of wider research aimed at making the movement of humanoid characters in games more reliable [3]. Over the years performance growth allowed for more complex, fluent and detail animations leading to better reception of animation by users. Additionally spare computing capabilities

F. Wróbel · D. Szajerman (✉) · A. Wojciechowski
Institute of Information Technology, Lodz University of Technology, Łódź, Poland
e-mail: dominik.szajerman@p.lodz.pl
URL: http://it.p.lodz.pl/

F. Wróbel
e-mail: filip.wrobel@dokt.p.lodz.pl

A. Wojciechowski
e-mail: adam.wojciechowski@p.lodz.pl

© The Editor(s) (if applicable) and The Author(s), under exclusive license
to Springer Nature Switzerland AG 2021
E. Piętka et al. (eds.), *Information Technology in Biomedicine*, Advances in Intelligent
Systems and Computing 1186, https://doi.org/10.1007/978-3-030-49666-1_26

327

allowed for more processing of the animation both pre and mid simulation. This enabled such features like inverse kinematics, run-time animation blending or procedural animations. All of these feature (and many more) had created more fluent and attractive experience for the users. It is worth remembering that even though they are the final judges of the animation quality it is not their task to find error and flaws.

During the process of creating animations it is always the creators call when quality and believability is sufficient and whether all issues are resolved. It is present both in process of creating them by hand and recording them with motion capture equipment. Knowing that human perception is varied and subjective there is constant need for creating universal tool for verifying animations. Knowing the problem of validation and question was stated "How can animation quality and correctness be automatically and equally verified?".

2   Related Work

Problem of missing true validation method was known for the entire history of skeletal animation, and so there were many attempts at tackling the issue. When creating new ways to blend animations or synthesize new ones researchers often come up new ideas as to how measure accuracy and quality of newly synthesized motions. Another common place for grading animations and verifying their parameters are researchers conducted in order to filter noise or correct small imperfections of motion capture software [10].

One of the less complex methods for validating animations: perceptual studies. In these participants are tasked with watching animations and grading them respectively. This method was used in study [4] where researchers using Laban Movement model procedurally animated character with emotions accordingly to OCEAN personality model. This kind of animation appraisal is highly subjective, non sensitive to details and prone to changes of the test group. On the other side of the spectrum there were attempts at correcting and validating animation when comparing animation data from motion capture to kinematic calculations. Paper [11] proposed correction of motion capture data with the use of aforementioned method basing its data on biomechanical model. Similarly to the first one, study [2] referred to test group opinion. It took on problem of visualizing animations for easier recognition during perceptual studies. Paper proposed method of displaying animations as movement trails, but concluded that even though result were above average recognition rate they were worse compared to traditional representation (playing animation). Different approach to validating final animation is presented in paper [7]. In this one motion data is captured on two different motion capture hardware. One of which is inferior and often presents lacking tracking data. Final assessment of processed animation if comparison between reference animation (captured on superior hardware), flaw animation and corrected flaw animation.

Above papers were focusing on bringing innovation to the field of animation synthesis and animation processing [1]. What this paper would like to propose are means of validating animation correctness for human skeletal animation. Additionally proposed method can be applied without any prior processing to any animation of human skeleton. Finally proposed approach is based on biomechanical data for human joints with goal of robustness in mind.

3 Methodology

3.1 Test Environment

Fulfilling goal of created such method requires preparation of a test that validates the ability to verify animation integrity and believability with the use of biomechanical data about human skeleton. For this for happen test environment was created—framework able to calculate animations according to industry skeletal animation standard, render resulting animation and record every frame of the animation. Animation processing and rendering implementation was consulted with resource [6]. For convenience of the testing and independence from computing performance, ability to run and record animation headless was added. For test runs were chosen three modes of run-time animation processing for animation testing:

1. No processing and single animation rendering, as most basic one displaying source material (no blending).
2. Animation blending showcasing how mixing animations changes their characteristics (blending pair of animations).
3. Animation blending based on barycentric coordinates displaying case of most common locomotion case (three animation blend).

Then source material was chosen out of industry standard animation material recorded in motion capture studio and fine tuned by hand of experienced animators. Said animations were created as a part of research and development project [12]. Animations were recorded using Vicon Motion Capture System. It consisted of 10 cameras capturing at 120 Hz. Captured animations were saved with local joint rotation data and re-sampled down to match video game standard. Selected animations are depicting human character standing idle, walking in 8 directions and expressing emotional gestures. Emotional gestures were vivid, predefined animations used to broadcast information about agent emotional state. Blending them with locomotion allows for easy introduction artifacts to the resulting animations. Above allowed for testing on industry and state of the art level of animation source material. Animations were then formed into trial runs. All trial runs with their descriptions were placed in Table 1.

Table 1 Simulation run names and their descriptions

Run name (Test name)	Description
Idle	Idle animation of man standing
Walk	Animation of walking man
Anger gesture	Animation of man threatening with his fist
Anger blend	Idle and anger run blended together
Locomotion	Standard locomotion blendspace with 8 directional movement animations and 9th animation of idle man standing; simulation of full turnaround of movement direction; meaning simulation of walking in every direction on traversal plane

For the matter of biomechanics skeletal joint with best equivalents in human skeleton were selected. There were chosen three joints for in-depth analysis: **Knee joint**, **Hip joint**, and **Wrist joint**.

First two joints are important for locomotion animations, but with different aspects of movement. Third joint was hand joint, which is often important for gestures and can easily stand-out behaving unnaturally. Additionally based on [5] joint were selected with respect to Degrees of Freedom and having them be varied between each other. Knee joint being hinge joint allows only one axis of freedom (One degree of freedom). Hip being "ball-and-socket" joint allows for three degrees of freedom. Finally wrist being "candyloid" joint is limited to two degrees of freedom.

For these joints data about limitations of their natural behaviour was extracted. Joint ROMs (Range of Motions) and maximum angular velocities were selected as basic verification criteria. Joint ROMs were sourced from [5] (for knee and hip) and [13] (for wrist). Collectively limitations of said joints, motion names and axes were presented in Table 2. Cells with name "–" are desired to be constant. All these limitations are result of biomechanical restrictions of human joint. It is worth noting that local virtual joints and their axes of movement were matched for later comparison.

All measures in this study and source material refer to neutral rotation as starting position. All given data about biomechanical constraints rely on initial joint alignment. When collecting joint rotation data results were compensated accordingly.

Finally maximum angular velocities were extracted from study [8]. These parameters were collected and presented in Table 3 and were addressed as ROAV (Range of Angular Velocity). There values were measured in sport environment and allow for some tolerance when analyzing animations aiming for realism.

Table 2 Ranges of Motion for Biomechanical constrain for knee, hip and wrist joints. Values are expressed in degrees. Cells marked with "–" represent degrees of freedom that are biomechanicaly constraint and should not take part in animation. Motion names are consisted with [5]

Joint name	Parameter name	Axes					
	Simulation axis	−X	+X	−Y	+Y	−Z	+Z
Knee	Biomechanical movement	–	–	–	–	Flection	Extension
	Biomechanical constraints [degrees]	0	0	0	0	−120	0
Hip	Biomechanical movement	Internal rotation	External rotation	Abduction	Adduction	Extension	Flexion
	Biomechanical constraints [degrees]	−51.7	52.3	−37.8	20.1	−20.9	135.1
Wrist	Biomechanical movement	–	–	Adduction	Abduction	Extension	Flection
	Biomechanical constraints [degrees]	0	0	−33.7	25.3	−78.5	78.9

Table 3 Ranges of Angular Velocities for Biomechanical constrains

Joint	Knee		Hip		Wrist	
Simulation axis	(−Z)	(+Z)	(−Z)	(+Z)	(−Z)	(+Z)
Biomechanical movement	Flection	Extension	Extension	Flexion	Extension	Flection
Biomechanical constraints [degrees per second]	−1266.24	1833.46	−956.84	779.22	−2881.98	3019.49

3.2 Research Method

Having both biomechanical limitations of skeleton and real simulation data it was possible to determine which keyframes and animations were incorrect from biomechanical standpoint. Dissecting collected data it was possible to read different flaws in animation, based on particular series of data. Initially bare ROMs compared to reference biomechanical ROMs clarify whether animation is displaying any unnatural movement. Then ROAV provides information if animation is exceeding another limitation of human capabilities: joint rotation velocity. Lastly most basic verification mostly based on ROMs is validation of degrees of freedom. This is related directly to human joint structure and comes from the fact that not every joint in human body allows for rotation in every degree of freedom.

These three methods allow to determine invalidation of animation but do not provide enough data for direct correction. From now on biomechanical analysis of animation evolves into statistical analysis of biomechanical data.

3.3 Conducting Tests

With prepared environment and selected animations simulation runs were ready to be conducted. First and second animation scenarios were run for double the time of longest animation in particular test. That way it was possible to test full length of animation and its looping characteristics. For the locomotion test run: it was possible to simulate and record every possible blend of directional movement shown to the played in typical locomotion animation in video game environment. All of test were run with native speed of animation, with sixty sample per second update frequency, fixed time-step and in headless mode. Given these parameters result animation parameters were run independent, which was later confirmed by statistical check and random frame comparison (comparison of a few consecutive runs).

With prepared environment, selected animations and chosen focus points tests were conducted. Motion data for these was collected and stored.

From the collected simulation records data series were extracted for the joints of interest. Then for every joint and animation set Range of Motion and Range of Angular Velocity were calculated. Tables 4, 5 and 6 contain ranges of movement respectively for Knee, Hip and Wrist joints. ROAV were placed Table 3. These four tables hold values for appraising animations against biomechanical restrictions of average human (biomechanical data source from: [5, 9, 13]). For every measured ROM, test run and selected joints six measures were calculated. Firstly there is "ROM magnitude" which is just the size of the ROM. Secondly there is value marked as "out of Range magnitude" which tells how many degrees out of measured ROM are outside of biological constraints. Thirdly there is "longest distance from ROM" which describes the distance to the furthest point from biomechanical constraints. Last three are mean, standard deviation and median values of the recorded rotations.

Additionally Angular Velocities for main axis of movement for selected joints were calculated and presented their ROAVs in Table 7. For convenience measured ROAVs were presented with repeated Biomechanical constraints.

3.4 Data Analysis

For every joint analysis can be started with checking "longest distance from ROM" and "out of Range magnitude". First of the two informs if there is even a single excess in animation ROM and how significant it was. Second from the pair specifies scale of

Table 4 Ranges of Motion and additional parameters measured during simulation runs for knee joint. Additional parameters were described Sect. 3.3

Run name	Simulation axis name	(-X)	(+X)	(-Y)	(+Y)		(-Z)	(+Z)	
							Flection	Extension	
Idle	Biomechanical movement name	–	–	–	–		Flection	Extension	
	Biomechanical constraints [degrees]	0.00	0.00	0.00	0.00	0.00	-120.00	0.00	120.00
	ROM	7.06	8.17	-1.64	-1.02		-9.41	-7.67	
	ROM magnitude		1.11			0.63			1.74
	out of Range magnitude		1.11			0.63			0.00
	longest distance from ROM		8.17			1.64			0.00
	mean		7.60			-1.24			-8.54
	sd		0.29			0.17			0.55
	median		7.53			-1.23			-8.42
Walk	ROM	-2.03	-0.41	-11.02	1.74		-76.01	0.18	
	ROM magnitude		1.62			12.76			76.19
	out of Range magnitude		1.62			12.76			0.18
	longest distance from ROM		2.03			11.02			0.18
	mean		-1.09			-3.17			-26.96
	sd		0.41			4.11			23.58
	median		-0.97			-1.65			-18.38

(continued)

Table 4 (continued)

	Simulation axis name	(−X)	(+X)		(−Y)	(+Y)		(−Z)	(+Z)	
Anger gesture	ROM	−20.13	7.08		−6.15	−0.87		−18.36	−8.73	
	ROM magnitude			27.21			5.28			9.63
	out of Range magnitude			27.21			5.28			0.00
	longest distance from ROM			20.13			6.15			0.00
	mean			−11.83			−4.30			−12.23
	sd			8.35			1.72			2.68
	median			−14.97			−5.18			−11.85
Anger blend	ROM	−6.50	7.58		−3.68	−0.95		−14.00	−8.24	
	range magnitude			14.08			2.73			5.77
	out of Range magnitude			14.08			2.73			0.00
	longest distance from ROM range			7.58			3.68			0.00
	mean			−2.19			−2.63			−10.55
	sd			4.13			0.80			1.37
	median			−3.78			−3.06			−10.21
Locomotion	ROM	1.41	5.62		−4.04	1.00		−47.50	−3.59	
	ROM magnitude			4.21			5.04			43.91
	out of Range magnitude			4.21			5.04			0.00
	longest distance from ROM			5.62			4.04			0.00
	mean			3.42			−1.35			−20.53
	sd			0.80			0.99			10.13
	median			3.30			−1.24			−18.54

Table 5 Ranges of Motion and additional parameters measured during simulation runs for hip joint. Additional parameters were described Sect. 3.3

Run name	Simulation axis name	(−X)	(+X)		(−Y)	(+Y)		(−Z)	(+Z)	
	Biomechanical movement name	Internal rotation	External rotation		Abduction	Adduction		Extension	Flexion	
	Biomechanical constraints [degrees]	−51.70	52.30	104.00	−37.80	20.10	57.90	−20.90	135.10	156.00
Idle	ROM	8.86	9.74		−3.05	−1.74		6.34	8.05	
	ROM magnitude			0.88			1.31			1.71
	out of Range magnitude			0.00			0.00			0.00
	longest distance from ROM			0.00			0.00			0.00
	mean			9.37			−2.29			7.16
	sd			0.22			0.32			0.38
	median			9.42			−2.33			7.17
Walk	ROM	3.24	10.48		−3.84	3.00		−22.72	33.74	
	ROM magnitude			7.25			6.83			56.46
	out of Range magnitude			0.00			0.00			1.82
	longest distance from ROM			0.00			0.00			1.82
	mean			6.57			−0.39			10.27
	sd			1.66			1.95			18.87
	median			6.21			−0.69			13.59

(continued)

Table 5 (continued)

	Simulation axis name	(−X)	(+X)		(−Y)	(+Y)		(−Z)	(+Z)	
Anger gesture	ROM	8.63	19.14		−13.67	−0.73		4.01	20.92	
	ROM magnitude			10.52			12.94			16.90
	out of Range magnitude			0.00			0.00			0.00
	longest distance from ROM			0.00			0.00			0.00
	mean			14.75			−9.06			9.98
	sd			4.38			3.65			5.95
	median			16.86			−11.27			6.58
Anger blend	ROM	8.87	14.36		−8.19	−1.30		5.27	14.35	
	range magnitude			5.49			6.89			9.08
	out of Range magnitude			0.00			0.00			0.00
	longest distance from ROM range			0.00			0.00			0.00
	mean			12.09			−5.71			8.69
	sd			2.12			1.82			2.90
	median			13.15			−6.69			7.12
Locomotion	ROM	1.65	13.40		−12.89	9.84		−6.27	22.30	
	ROM magnitude			11.75			22.72			28.56
	out of Range magnitude			0.00			0.00			0.00
	longest distance from ROM			0.00			0.00			0.00
	mean			8.01			−0.61			9.37
	sd			2.18			4.40			6.26
	median			8.03			−0.65			10.19

Table 6 Ranges of Motion and additional parameters measured during simulation runs for wrist joint. Additional parameters were described Sect. 3.3

Run name	Simulation axis name	(−X)	(+X)	(−Y)	(+Y)	(−Z)	(+Z)
	Biomechanical movement name	—	—	Adduction	Abduction	Extension	Flection
	Biomechanical constraints [degrees]	0.00	0.00	−33.70	25.30 (59.00)	−78.50	78.90 (157.40)
Idle	ROM	−35.14	−33.22	−14.38	−12.85	5.55	7.06
	ROM magnitude	1.92				1.53	1.51
	out of Range magnitude	1.92				0.00	0.00
	longest distance from ROM	35.14				0.00	0.00
	mean	−34.16		−13.70			
	sd	0.45		0.36			
	median	−34.22		−13.70			
Walk	ROM	−32.28	−15.92	−12.69	0.01	−10.64	−7.81
	ROM magnitude	16.35				12.71	2.83
	out of Range magnitude	16.35				0.00	0.00
	longest distance from ROM	32.28				0.00	0.00
	mean	−23.97				−5.17	−9.22
	sd	5.42				3.80	0.88
	median	−23.25				−5.59	−9.25

(continued)

Table 6 (continued)

	Simulation axis name	(−X)	(+X)		(−Y)	(+Y)		(−Z)	(+Z)	
Anger gesture	ROM	−37.79	−32.00		−6.74	8.75		−10.01	−4.08	
	ROM magnitude			5.78			15.49			5.93
	out of Range magnitude			5.78			0.00			0.00
	longest distance from ROM			37.79			0.00			0.00
	mean			−34.52			−3.48			−5.87
	sd			1.75			3.18			1.90
	median			−34.90			−3.75			−5.07
Anger blend	ROM	−35.73	−32.37		−10.48	−2.18		−2.22	1.41	
	range magnitude			3.37			8.30			3.63
	out of Range magnitude			3.37			0.00			0.00
	longest distance from ROM range			35.73			0.00			0.00
	mean			−34.06			−8.61			0.18
	sd			0.87			1.55			0.95
	median			−34.19			−8.76			0.52
Locomotion	ROM	−33.97	−22.00		−13.87	−7.12		−3.67	2.59	
	ROM magnitude			11.97			6.75			6.26
	out of Range magnitude			11.97			0.00			0.00
	longest distance from ROM			33.97			0.00			0.00
	mean			−27.66			−10.24			−1.19
	sd			2.51			1.32			1.28
	median			−27.48			−10.11			−1.40

Table 7 Ranges of Angular Velocities for Biomechanical constrains and ROAVs measured during simulation for Knee, Hip and Wrist joint. All values are in [degrees/s]

Joint	Knee		Hip		Wrist	
Simulation axis name	(−Z)	(+Z)	(−Z)	(+Z)	(−Z)	(+Z)
Biomechanical movement name	Flection	Extension	Extension	Flexion	Extension	Flection
Biomechanical constraints	−1266.24	1833.46	−956.84	779.22	−2881.98	3019.49
Idle animation	−12.42	11.29	−5.37	7.53	−14.40	7.80
Walk animation	−507.57	871.66	−232.73	250.61	−33.44	16.27
Anger gesture animation	−55.22	71.96	−101.43	112.72	−38.24	36.99
Anger blend	−70.83	95.22	−128.62	145.54	−62.49	57.25
Locomotion	−1014.81	971.39	−337.45	267.70	−53.54	39.85

the excess and combined with pure ROM magnitude can determine if proportion of undesirable movements to feasible ones. Additionally comparing values of "longest distance from ROM" with SD (standard deviation) can present whether issues are related more with initial pose setup or following movements. Finally mean and median values narrow where the weight of the animation lies and with relatively low SD where what is most popular neighborhood of rotation values.

It is also worth coming back to validation with the use of Range Of Angular Velocities, any of them exceeding the reference values for skeleton, can be marked as flawed and examined closer.

4 Results and Discussion

The largest values of "out of Range magnitude" and "longest distance from ROM" are both largest for rotation in X axis of knee joint in test run "anger animation" (Table 4). It is important to note that this joint is not supposed to rotate in this axis. This movement can be marked as a mistake during animation or motion capture process. With such high standard deviation for an axis that should remain close to still incorrect movement can be expected. Whole range of unwanted movement in simulation run can be observed (Fig. 1). For final confirmation animation was rendered twice side-by-side with frozen frames on the Fig. 2. It is worth noting that x rotation for joint knee means rotation in traversal plane. With that in mind it can be observed that right knee expresses unnatural looking twist marked with the pink frame. With the last one there are four appraisal methods that align with their verdict each consecutive one giving more insight into about source of the flaw. Last part is visual validation which is always final but too subjective and fuzzy scale to measure beyond sanity validation.

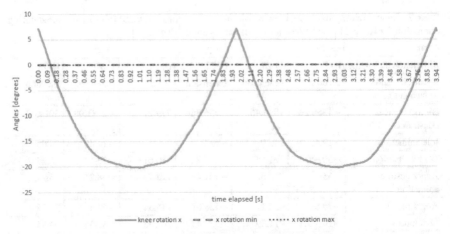

Fig. 1 Rotation in axis X for knee in simulation run anger gesture

Fig. 2 Render of animation "anger gesture" side-by-side in first frame of the animation (left) and halfway through the animation (right)

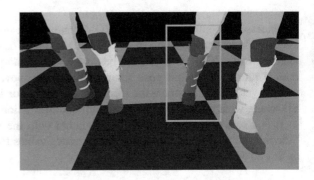

Moving onto second example set of movements this paper goes through simple yet satisfying study of hip motions. In Table 5 it is quick to determine that test run "walk" has both the largest values of "longest distance to ROM" and "out of Range magnitude". With such diminishing difference this excess can be accounted as negligible. Figure 3 presents hip movement in z axis which despite having largest standard deviation for the overwhelming part it is withing biological limits.

There was check for large values of "longest distance to ROM" and "out of Range magnitude" in data from measuring wrist joint in the test run (Table 6). This joint is middle ground between first and second presented joints in terms of degrees of freedom. Looking at the data for this joint it can be noticed that for axes in which joint can rotate, the biomechanical constraints are easily met. Nevertheless looking at the third axis large excesses can be noticed in ROM.

Values for "exceed factor" being ratio of "longest distance from ROM" to "out of range magnitude" were calculated. "Exceed factor" determines which animation run has the most focused and most biomechanically incorrect data. Results were collected in the in Table 8. Based on the calculated score "idle" and "anger blend" runs

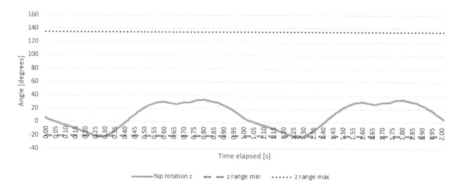

Fig. 3 Rotation in axis Z for hip in simulation run "walk"

Table 8 Results for calculating exceed factor for wrist joint (in degrees)

Run name	Out of Range magnitude	Longest distance from ROM	Exceed factor
Idle	1.92	35.14	18.29
Walk	16.35	32.28	1.97
Anger gesture	5.78	37.79	6.53
Anger blend	3.37	35.73	10.61
Locomotion	11.97	33.97	2.84

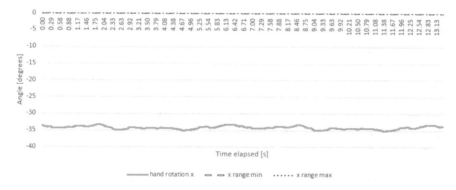

Fig. 4 Rotation in axis X for wrist in simulation run "idle"

were assume as the most flawed. For them values of rotation over the cycle of the animations were plotted resulting in charts Figs. 4 and 5. On both of these it is possible to notice small variation in values but relatively big offset from biomechanical constraint. This could mean that animations were most likely created with correct approach but mistake was made in the stage of rigging or mapping animations. For reference partial render of the two aforementioned animations was included with third animation "walk" as a comparison (Fig. 6).

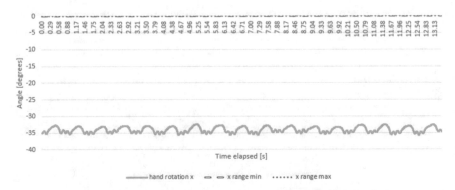

Fig. 5 Rotation in axis X for wrist in simulation run "anger blend"

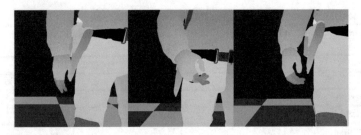

Fig. 6 Partial renders of first frame of three animations: "idle", "anger gesture" and "walk". Respectively from left to right

5   Conclusions

In search of finding a proper way to validate animations biomechanical aspect of human skeleton was approached. Data about possible joint degrees of freedom were collected and mapped local joint rotations to biomechanical descriptions of joint movements. Biomechanical data was then collected processed to match layout of the collected test data. With the use of reference ROM (biomechanical constraints for human skeleton) additional measured for every tested joint and additional measure in form of "Exceed factor" were calculated. Reasoning based on these preparations allowed this paper to statistically distinct flaw animations from biomechanically feasible ones. With more work to be done on this topic it is planed to prepare automated system for validating correctness of animations and suggesting potential origins of discovered flaws.

References

1. Bartniak, A., Guzek, K., Napieralski, P.: 3D animation of plant development using L-systems. In: XV International Conference – SMC (2013)
2. Carreno-Medrano, P., Gibet, S., Marteau, P.F.: Perceptual validation for the generation of expressive movements from end-effector trajectories. ACM Trans. Interact. Intell. Syst. **8**(3), 1–26 (2018). https://doi.org/10.1145/3150976
3. Daszuta, M., Wróbel, F., Rynkiewicz, F., Szajerman, D., Napieralski, P.: Affective pathfinding in video games. J. Appl. Comput. Sci. **26**(2), 23–29 (2018)
4. Durupinar, F., Kapadia, M., Deutsch, S., Neff, M., Badler, N.I.: PERFORM: perceptual approach for adding ocean personality to human motion using laban movement analysis. ACM ToG **36**(4), 1 (2016). https://doi.org/10.1145/3072959.2983620
5. Faisal, A.I., Majumder, S., Mondal, T., Cowan, D., Naseh, S., Deen, M.J.: Monitoring methods of human body joints: state-of-the-art and research challenges. Sensors **19**(11), 2629 (2019). https://doi.org/10.3390/s19112629
6. Gregory, J.: Game Engine Architecture. Taylor & Francis Ltd. (2009)
7. Holden, D., Saito, J., Komura, T., Joyce, T.: Learning motion manifolds with convolutional autoencoders. In: SIGGRAPH ASIA 2015 Technical Briefs on - SA '15. ACM Press (2015). https://doi.org/10.1145/2820903.2820918
8. Jessop, D.M., Pain, M.T.: Maximum velocities in flexion and extension actions for sport. J. Hum. Kinet. **50**(1), 37–44 (2016)
9. Moromizato, K., Kimura, R., Fukase, H., Yamaguchi, K., Ishida, H.: Whole-body patterns of the range of joint motion in young adults: masculine type and feminine type. J. Physiol. Anthropol. **35**(1), (2016)
10. Pszczoła, P., Bednarski, R.: Creating character animation with optical motion capture system. In: Wojciechowski, A., Napieralski, P. (eds.) CGI (2016)
11. Seemann, W., Stelzner, G., Simonidis, C.: Correction of motion capture data with respect to kinematic data consistency for inverse dynamic analysis. ASMEDC (2005). https://doi.org/10.1115/detc2005-84964
12. Teyon: R&D Project: From Robots to Humans no. POIR.01.02.00-00-0133/16 (2016)
13. Than, T., San, A., Myint, T.: Biokinetic study of the wrist joint. Int. J. Collab. Res. Intern. Med. Public Health **4** (2012)

One 'Stop Smoking' to Take Away, Please! A Preliminary Evaluation of an AAT Mobile App

Tanja Joan Eiler, Tobias Forneberg, Armin Grünewald, Alla Machulska, Tim Klucken, Katharina Jahn, Björn Niehaves, Carl Friedrich Gethmann, and Rainer Brück

Abstract In recent years, the approach-avoidance task (AAT) has proven to be a successful therapeutic procedure in the treatment of addictions. So far, the AAT has been used in combination with a joystick on a desktop computer, and our transfer into virtual reality (VR) already shows promising results. However, both approaches are bound to a specific location. For this reason, we are developing a mobile application that can be used regardless of time and place, whenever an affected person feels

---

Eiler and Forneberg contributed equally to this research.

T. J. Eiler (✉) · T. Forneberg · A. Grünewald · R. Brück
Medical Informatics and Microsystems Engineering, University of Siegen, 57076 Siegen, Germany
e-mail: tanja.eiler@uni-siegen.de
URL: http://www.uni-siegen.de/lwf/professuren/mim/

T. Forneberg
e-mail: tf@t-forneberg.de

A. Grünewald
e-mail: armin.gruenewald@uni-siegen.de

R. Brück
e-mail: rainer.brueck@uni-siegen.de

A. Machulska · T. Klucken
Department of Clinical Psychology, University of Siegen, 57076 Siegen, Germany
e-mail: alla.machulska@uni-siegen.de

T. Klucken
e-mail: tim.klucken@psychologie.uni-siegen.de

K. Jahn · B. Niehaves
Department of Information Systems, University of Siegen, 57076 Siegen, Germany
e-mail: katharina.jahn@uni-siegen.de

B. Niehaves
e-mail: bjoern.niehaves@uni-siegen.de

C. F. Gethmann
Research College FoKoS, University of Siegen, 57076 Siegen, Germany
e-mail: carl.gethmann@uni-siegen.de

© The Editor(s) (if applicable) and The Author(s), under exclusive license to Springer Nature Switzerland AG 2021
E. Piętka et al. (eds.), *Information Technology in Biomedicine*, Advances in Intelligent Systems and Computing 1186, https://doi.org/10.1007/978-3-030-49666-1_27

the need for it. Therefore, we conducted a feasibility study with thirty people who evaluated three interaction variants as well as the usability of the application. Based on these results, the app will be optimized in order to carry out a large-scale randomized controlled trial which will evaluate the effectiveness of the app compared to the desktop and VR AAT.

Keywords Addiction · Approach-avoidance task · AAT · Approach bias · Cognitive bias · Cognitive bias modification · CBM · Dual process model · Mobile applications · Smoking · Therapy · Usability

1   Introduction and Motivation

According to estimates by the Federal Ministry of Health, the number of deaths caused by the effects of tobacco consumption in Germany amounts to about 120.000 people a year, of which about 3.300 are caused by passive smoking. Furthermore, the use of these legal drugs leads to considerable costs, that have to be paid by society as a whole. It is estimated that the macroeconomic damage caused by tobacco consumption in Germany is around 79.1 billion euros per year [4].

The Global Burden Of Disease study from 2015 shows that the number of smokers in Germany relative to the total population in the same year was 19.4% for women and 25.2% for men. With these age-standardized values, Germany is in the middle of the international rankings. The relative number of smokers in Germany, as in most countries, has been declining steadily for many years. However, this decline is rather small, averaging less than one percentage point per year [18].

Due to these health and economic consequences, it is reasonable to carry out further research in the field of substance dependence therapy. Although there are already various therapeutic offers, these are not being used by all people who are actively interested in combating their dependency. Possible reasons for this are limited availability and the corresponding long waiting times, or long travel distances. The social stigmatization associated with the use of such therapies can also be a factor.

Our research focuses on these areas and aims to improve access to therapeutic measures using modern digital technologies. Specifically, a virtual reality application [5–7, 14] and a smartphone application are being developed, each of which will implement the approach-avoidance task (AAT) [19, 20], a promising psychotherapeutic procedure. It is hoped that the conversion into an Android smartphone application, which is the subject of this publication, will lower the inhibition threshold for potential therapy participants by facilitating integration into daily life and reducing the risk of social stigmatization. In addition, it is seen as an opportunity to make the AAT procedure available to the general public, independent of time and place.

2 Theoretical Background

2.1 Dual Process Model of Addiction

An important model for understanding the AAT procedure is the "Dual Process Model of Addiction" [9]. According to this model, there are two different mental processes that determine what behavior results from a certain input in the form of perceived stimuli. The first of these processes is the reflective process, which is controlled and conscious. This includes, for example, deliberate considerations or stored knowledge about how harmful or useful the consumption of a substance is. The second process is the impulsive process, which is subconscious and automated. It influences attention and the approach to a stimulus without the person concerned becoming aware of it. For example, a stimulus associated with smoking, such as the sight of an ashtray or the smell of a cigarette, increases the craving of a dependent person and can unconsciously lead to automatic approach actions and subsequent consumption of cigarettes.

The increase in dependency is accompanied by an increase in the influence of impulsive processes on the behavior, at the expense of reflective processes. Associated with this are systematic tendencies to perceive, remember, think and judge deviated from a rational standard. In the case of dependency, such cognitive distortions are responsible for its retention and amplification [21].

Most established methods of addiction cessation try to achieve success by influencing the reflective processes, for example by informing the patients by a therapist about the negative consequences of their addiction. In contrast, procedures that address the impulsive processes by modifying the cognitive bias, like the AAT, attempt to restore the balance between the two processes, in favor of the reflective processes [15].

2.2 Approach-Avoidance Task

From a therapeutic point of view, the approach-avoidance task (AAT) procedure was used by Rinck and Becker [19] to test whether negative tendencies towards different stimuli can be determined without having to ask explicit questions about these tendencies. Disadvantages of explicit interviews, such as the influence of social desirability of certain answers, should be avoided this way. The procedure works in such a way that the participants are presented with a series of stimuli in the form of photos on a screen, and are required to take one action per photo. The action is either a pulling or a pushing movement of a joystick, the former accompanied by an enlargement and the latter by a reduction of the displayed image size to simulate an approaching or avoiding movement. A distinction is made between a direct variant in which the action to be performed is derived directly from the image content ("Push all images with a cigarette"), and an indirect variant in which a feature not directly related to the image content, such as the border color or the image orientation, is decisive for the action to be performed ("Push all images with a red border").

In addition, the reaction times (RTs) of the test persons are recorded for each stimulus. The RTs measured by Rinck and Becker were on average shorter if the so-called compatibility effect, i.e. the correspondence between the tendency caused by the image and the positive or negative reaction carried out, was high. In concrete terms, this means that the RTs for avoiding reactions to spider images were on average faster the more pronounced the negative tendency of a person to spiders was.

With the measured RTs, the AAT method makes it possible to determine two special forms of the cognitive bias, the approach bias and the avoidance bias. For this purpose, the median of the RTs for pulling movements is subtracted from the median of the RTs for pushing movements for each stimulus type (e.g. cigarettes vs. toothbrushes) [12, 19]. A positive value represents an approach bias, which is associated with an automatic approach to these stimuli, and a negative value indicates an avoidance bias, which causes an automatic avoidance. After their study, the researchers hypothesized that the procedure could also be used therapeutically in the sense of cognitive bias modification (CBM, see [15]).

This effect has already been proven in numerous studies (for an overview see [10]). In these trials, the participants had to push all addiction-related images, and pull all neutral or positive images. This allows to modify the impulsive processes and thus prevent automatic approximations after a successful AAT training.

These studies have also shown that there are some important prerequisites that have to be followed during AAT training. For successful retraining of automated (re-)actions, the movements performed during AAT training have to be fast, simple and intuitive. Accordingly, no chains of action are allowed. In addition, there should be no external or internal distraction factors during training, since the users need to concentrate completely on the task. Correspondingly, the distinguishing feature of the stimuli should also not be too dominant and distracting, otherwise the stimuli themselves cannot be recognized fast enough. This indicates that the distinguishing feature as well as the stimuli must be distinctive and immediately recognizable.

3   Related Work

In recent years, several attempts have already been made to transfer the AAT procedure into a mobile application. In 2015, an app was tested with 56 participants. The gesture used to control this app represented a movement of the device away from the user or towards the user. Participants had to pull faces with happy, or push faces with angry facial expressions [8]. The recorded data were compared with those of a conventional, joystick-controlled AAT procedure. The researcher's expectation that happy faces would be pulled faster than angry faces would be pushed away was only confirmed by the mobile AAT variant. Therefore, no correlation could be found between the two methods.

In 2017, the same app was used again in another study [2]. This time, however, images of different appetizing food and neutral non-food-related objects were used. The hypothesis that food should have a higher approach bias than neutral objects was confirmed. However, no significantly different bias could be found in the foods classified as differently appetizing.

Another app was evaluated in 2018 [1]. This app was mainly developed with modern web technologies, which allows it to be used on almost any mobile device with different operating systems, as the application is executed in the browser of the respective device. A wipe gesture was used for interactions, because the work is based on the findings of a meta-analysis from 2014 [17], which came to the conclusion that the movement of the arm itself does not seem to be the decisive factor for the impression of approach or avoidance. Instead, the zooming linked to a gesture is the important factor. A feasibility study with ten participants was carried out in which RTs to computer-game-related stimuli were recorded. The hypothesis that people who regularly play such games would show a higher approach bias towards these stimuli than people who do not play such games could not be clearly confirmed by the data obtained.

There are only a few works where a bias modification was attempted using a smartphone-based AAT. One study, which tried to reduce the amount of chocolate consumed by the participants, was published in 2018 [16]. A wipe gesture was used for interaction. However, the study did not reveal any clear differences in bias or post-eating behavior compared to a placebo control group and an inactive control group.

4 Design and Implementation

4.1 Requirement Analysis

In the preliminary stages of development, requirements were identified. First of all, the main features and requirements of the AAT procedure described in Sect. 2.2 must be implemented (zooming, no distracting features, etc.). Further requirements are described below:

4.1.1 Interaction Methods

It should be possible to select one of the following three input methods, which can be executed in a simple and fast manner, therefore fulfilling an important AAT requirement:

– pinch-to-zoom: By moving two fingers closer or farther apart, the displayed image is enlarged or reduced (Fig. 1, left).

Fig. 1 The three interaction methods of the mobile AAT application. From left to right: "pinch-to-zoom", "whole arm movement", and "tilting the device"

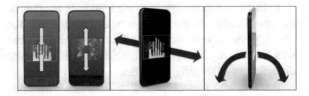

– whole arm movement: An arm movement that moves the mobile device closer to the user initiates an enlargement of the displayed image, and vice versa (Fig. 1, center).
– tilting the device: A tilt of the device that corresponds to pulling a joystick toward the user enlarges the displayed image, and vice versa (Fig. 1, right).

4.1.2 Settings

In order to offer many customization possibilities for studies with the developed app, it should have different settings to modify the sessions. In addition to the input methods, the following settings should be adjustable:

– the number of pictures per round, and the number of rounds per session
– per round, the ratio of images to be reduced to images to be enlarged
– the timeout between the display of two images
– whether a short message is displayed after each image (e.g. required RT), or whether a dialog must be confirmed before the next stimulus
– whether (and if so, which) instructions should be displayed before the start of a session

In addition, by activating and configuring a colored frame or an image rotation for each of the image categories, it can be determined whether the direct or indirect AAT procedure will be used.

4.1.3 Inclusion of Additional Images

According to their study, Kong and his colleagues have hypothesized that the personal relevance of the images shown is of great importance for therapeutic success [11]. This hypothesis can be further investigated using a function that allows the integration of self-made photos into the mobile AAT app.

4.1.4 Acquisition and Export of Data

During the use of the application the session data should be recorded and stored. Broken down into a single action, this includes the RTs, the file name of the image,

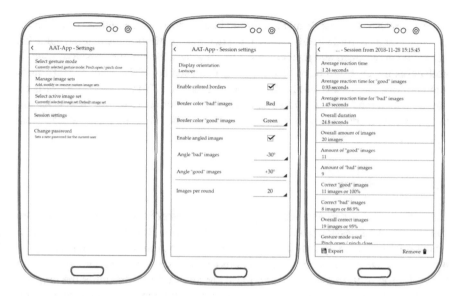

Fig. 2 Concept wireframes of the mobile AAT application. From left to right: General settings, session settings, and stored data of one session

and whether the reaction was a PUSH or PULL movement. In addition, the settings, user ID, the device used, and a timestamp have to be recorded. Furthermore, it should be possible to export the data in the .csv file format.

4.1.5 Screen Layout and Menu Structuring

In order to get initial ideas on how to implement the requirements, wireframes were created. In this way, a first impression of the user interface required by the app could be gained. Figure 2 shows some of these wireframes.

4.2 Implementation and User Interface

This section focuses on the presentation of central components of the app and their implementation, divided into login screen and the main screen.

4.2.1 Login Screen

The first screen a user sees after installing the app is the login screen, which has two fields for entering a username and a password, as well as two buttons for login or creating a new user account. While the former checks whether the entered combination of name and password already exists, the latter checks whether the entered name has not yet been assigned and then creates it in combination with the password used. In both cases the user will be redirected to the main screen. If the login or registration attempt fails, the reason will be displayed in a message. The entered passwords are hashed with a randomly generated salt and a hash function. Only this hash value and the salt value, from which the original password cannot be restored, are stored in the database.

4.2.2 Main Screen

The main screen serves as a starting point for all further functions of the app. Users can start an AAT session from here via the start button. Below is the results button, which opens an activity that displays, deletes and exports the RTs and settings of already executed sessions. Further functions can be accessed via a menu in the action bar at the top of the screen. In detail these are an info icon, that takes the user to a page with information about the app, and the possibility to log out and navigate back to the login screen.

If an account has admin authorization, a gear symbol is displayed in the action bar, which can be used to open the settings interface. This allows study leaders to change or check the general and session settings. Study participants will not be able to do so, thus avoiding any falsification of the results. Instead, these accounts are shown an "Import settings" function. When this is selected, a dialog box appears in which an URL can be entered. Behind this URL a file can be placed, which is downloaded and imported. The study instructors only have to provide a file with the currently relevant settings for download and instruct the participants to import it by entering the corresponding URL on their device.

5 Experimental Setup and Results

5.1 Study Design

A total of thirty people (fourteen females and sixteen males; mean age: 36.3 years, range: 21–65; fifteen smokers) took part in the feasibility study. Before starting the experiment, participants were given a verbal introduction. Subsequently, they were asked to download and install the developed app on their device via a download link. Their first task was to create a user account and conduct a training with the default settings. Participants were now asked to log out and log back in with an admin account. After a hint to the additional gear icon, they were asked to make some changes in the "settings" menu. They should set the control mode to "whole arm movement" and start another training. After completing this second run, they were prompted to save the current settings as a file on their device. The participants were then instructed to use an URL to import a file that reverted to the default settings. A third training should then be performed using the "tilting the device" control mode.

Next, participants were asked to import some pictures from their own devices into a new picture set and then start a training session with this set. Another feature to be evaluated by the test persons was the editing of the displayed instruction text. Finally, they were asked to use the "results" button to review the recordings of the sessions they had completed and to store the data to a .csv file using the export function.

Afterwards, questionnaires were filled out to evaluate the individual interaction variants as well as some general aspects, such as the performance, the usability, or the design of the app. The questionnaire used consisted of two pages. On the first page information on age, sex and smoking behavior was collected. In addition, the participants were asked to indicate which Android smartphone they own and which OS version is installed on it. On the second page, an evaluation of the app was given, which is based on the "Mobile App Rating Scale" [3]. It is divided into a total of 16 statements. For each of these statements, a value between one and five should be assigned, where one stood for "very bad" and five for "very good".

5.2 Observations During Execution

The verbal explanation given was well followed by all participants. The registration of a new user and the first training run in "pinch-to-zoom" mode worked without complications on all devices. The participants were also able to understand the task given in the instruction text, although most of them needed an explanation for the interaction variants "tilting the device" and "whole arm movement". The following login with the admin account and the modification of some settings were made without difficulties as well.

Especially while training in the "whole arm movement" mode, the participants felt that the task was partly unclear and additional explanations were necessary to ensure correct reactions. This was mainly because the movements in this mode had to be performed quite energetic in order to be registered.

The export of settings ran mostly without problems, but some participants did not have a file management app installed. In these cases, an attempt was made to export the file using one of the other apps offered by the OS, which did not always work, due to the fact that these only accepted certain file formats. The subsequent import of settings via an URL worked well.

The third training run, which was carried out with the "tilting the device" control mode, ran smoothly on all devices on which this mode was available. There was no geomagnetic sensor on five devices. The import of own pictures, and the display of the collected RTs ran without problems. In most cases, the export of the RTs also went without complications. On the smartphones without a file management app, the .csv file could be sent via e-mail.

Fig. 3 Smoke-related
approach bias values for
each interaction variant

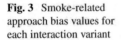

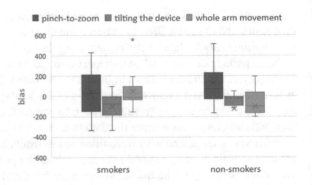

5.3   Evaluation of Reaction Times

While the usability of the app was the main focus, a first evaluation of the RTs was
carried out. For each person and each control mode completed by this person, a bias
value for smoke-related stimuli was calculated. The result of this summary is shown
in Fig. 3.

If one compares the different control modes with each other, it becomes apparent
that the bias values differ significantly from each other. In particular, it is noticeable
that the bias values of the "pinch-to-zoom" mode (smokers: M = 34, SD = 235; non-
smokers: M = 74, SD = 234) are on average significantly more positive than the bias
values of the "tilting the device" (smokers: M = −78, SD = 113; non-smokers: M
= −22, SD = 263) and "whole arm movement" (smokers: M = −8, SD = 165; non-
smokers: M = −100, SD = 183) control modes. This indicates that the participants
took on average longer to zoom-in (PULL) than to zoom-out (PUSH) in this mode.
A possible explanation for this could be that the execution of a zoom-in movement
takes longer than the execution of a zoom-out movement, for example because of
the initial hand position or better trained motor processes of zoom-out movements.
Another hypothesis is that the zoom-out movement is associated with a gripping
movement, as the fingers perform a movement similar to picking up a cigarette,
which would reverse the meaning of the performed action.

The anticipated result that smokers have a higher positive and less negative bias
value than non-smokers could not be achieved with all modes in this pilot study.
Only in the control mode "whole arm movement" smokers have a higher positive
and less negative bias than non-smokers. To confirm this effect, another study with
more participants and a longer time frame must be conducted.

5.4   Evaluation of the Questionnaires

The results of the questionnaire evaluation can be interpreted as positive. 12 out of
16 questions scored a mean value between 4 and 5 points. This also includes the

question about the "tilting the device" mode, which was rated with an average of 4.42 points. The "pinch-to-zoom" mode was rated at 3.8 points, the "whole arm movement" mode received the worst score with 3 points. The function for importing images (4.21 points) and the settings menu (4.47 points) were rated positively. The instruction text, performance of the app, menu navigation, layout, and the appearance of the app were rated with an average of more than 4 points. Almost all users could imagine using the app in combination with a therapy (4.2 points), most would also use it independently without accompanying therapy (3.87 points). The evaluation of the data on the devices used shows that almost all participants used modern smartphones that have not been on the market for more than four years.

6 Conclusion and Future Work

In summary, it can be stated that porting the AAT procedure to mobile devices in the form of an Android app is technically possible. The developed app could be executed on all test devices and, depending on the sensor equipment of the device used, always provided at least two of the three implemented control modes. Although the "whole arm movement" is still to be optimized, the performance was good on all devices, and there were no delays or crashes. All setting options required, such as the adjustment of a distinguishing feature (rotation angle, colored border), or the number of pictures shown, were successfully implemented. A configuration of these settings for study purposes is possible using the export and import functions. The functionality to import own images was also implemented. These can be managed in image sets and linked with PUSH or PULL actions.

Furthermore, the evaluation has shown that it is possible to record all RTs, whereby the time points for recordings of the "tilting the device" control mode should be improved. In addition, the accuracy of time recording and its consistency have not yet been evaluated in the use of different devices. Especially in "pinch-to-zoom" mode, the uncertainty of possibly large differences between different devices is a problem that must be solved before valid measurements can be made. In general, it can be said that the heterogeneity of the installed hardware of different devices poses a problem for the measurement of RTs and the determination of the approach bias. If it turns out that the latencies are too different, it may be necessary to limit the usable devices for a valid measurement. Alternatively, the measurement could be limited to the most reliable control mode. In addition to the small number of participants, it should be remembered that all test persons used the app for the first time and were not instructed to concentrate fully on the training and fast execution of the movements.

Nevertheless, the developed app can be further improved and then used for additional studies in which not the exact bias determination, but the therapeutic effect in the sense of a cognitive bias modification is paramount. In that case, parallel bias measurements would still have to be carried out using the desktop AAT method.

After further studies and finalizing the application, a large-scale randomized controlled trial will be carried out to determine whether the training with it is as effective as the desktop or VR AAT procedures [13]. Due to the very large target group and the possibility to integrate the training into the everyday life of the users, for example by using push notifications, the mobile AAT has a great therapeutic potential. If the results are positive, the application will be incorporated to the portfolio of a regional clinic. Furthermore, it will be discussed whether the mobile application is going to be made available to the general public free of charge. In addition, further variations of the application will be investigated. These are for instance a combination of the procedure with gamification elements, direct AAT in comparison to indirect AAT, or a port of the VR scenario to mobile devices.

References

1. Busch, C.: Implicit behavioral tendencies: porting the Approach-Avoidance Task to a mobile device (unpublished bachelor thesis) (2018)
2. Cring, C.: Approach and avoidance tendencies: using smartphones to study behavioral responses and food desires (2017). https://openaccess.leidenuniv.nl/bitstream/handle/1887/53247/Cring,%20Christina-s1899589-MA%20ThesisECP-2017.pdf
3. Cummings, E., Langrial, S., Su, W.C., Stoyanov, S.R., Hides, L., Kavanagh, D.J., Zelenko, O., Tjondronegoro, D., Mani, M.: Mobile app rating scale: a new tool for assessing the quality of health mobile apps. JMIR mHealth uHealth 3(1) (2015). https://doi.org/10.2196/mhealth.3422
4. Donath, C.: Drogen- und Suchtbericht 2018 (2018). https://www.drogenbeauftragte.de/fileadmin/dateien-dba/Drogenbeauftragte/Drogen_und_Suchtbericht/pdf/DSB-2018.pdf. (in German)
5. Eiler, T.J., Grünewald, A., Brück, R.: Fighting substance dependency combining AAT therapy and virtual reality with game design elements. In: Proceedings of 14th International Joint Conference on Computer Vision, Imaging and Computer Graphics Theory and Applications, pp. 28–37. SCITEPRESS - Science and Technology Publications (2019). https://doi.org/10.5220/0007362100280037
6. Eiler, T.J., Grünewald, A., Machulska, A., Klucken, T., Jahn, K., Niehaves, B., Gethmann, C.F., Brück, R.: A preliminary evaluation of transferring the approach avoidance task into virtual reality. In: Pietka, E. et al. (eds.) Information Technology in Biomedicine, Advances in Intelligent Systems and Computing, vol. 1011, pp. 151–163. Springer International Publishing, Cham (2019). https://doi.org/10.1007/978-3-030-23762-2_14
7. Eiler, T.J., Grünewald, A., Wahl, M., Brück, R.: AAT meets virtual reality. In: Cláudio, A.P., Bouatouch, K., Chessa, M., Paljic, A., Kerren, A., Hurter, C., Tremeau, A., Farinella, G.M. (eds.) Computer Vision, Imaging and Computer Graphics Theory and Applications, Communications in Computer and Information Science, vol. 1182, pp. 153–176. Springer International Publishing, Cham (2020). https://doi.org/10.1007/978-3-030-41590-7_7
8. Hilmar, Z.: The mobile approach-avoidance task (2015). https://doi.org/10.13140/RG.2.1.1088.3287
9. Hofmann, W., Friese, M., Strack, F.: Impulse and self-control from a dual-systems perspective. Perspect. Psychol. Sci. 4(2), 162–176 (2009). https://doi.org/10.1111/j.1745-6924.2009.01116.x
10. Kakoschke, N., Kemps, E., Tiggemann, M.: Approach bias modification training and consumption: a review of the literature. Addict. Behav. 64, 21–28 (2017). https://doi.org/10.1016/j.addbeh.2016.08.007
11. Kong, G., Larsen, H., Cavallo, D.A., Becker, D., Cousijn, J., Salemink, E., Collot D'Escury-Koenigs, A.L., Morean, M.E., Wiers, R.W., Krishnan-Sarin, S.: Re-training automatic action

tendencies to approach cigarettes among adolescent smokers: a pilot study. Am. J. Drug Alcohol Abuse **41**(5), 425–432 (2015). https://doi.org/10.3109/00952990.2015.1049492

12. Machulska, A., Zlomuzica, A., Rinck, M., Assion, H.J., Margraf, J.: Approach bias modification in inpatient psychiatric smokers. J. Psychiatr. Res. **76**, 44–51 (2016). https://doi.org/10.1016/j.jpsychires.2015.11.015

13. Machulska, A., Kleinke, K., Eiler, T.J., Grünewald, A., Brück, R., Jahn, K., Niehaves, B., Gethmann, C.F., Klucken, T.: Retraining automatic action tendencies for smoking using mobile phone-based approach-avoidance bias training: a study protocol for a randomized controlled study. Trials **20**(1), 720 (2019). https://doi.org/10.1186/s13063-019-3835-0

14. Machulska, A., Eiler, T.J., Grünewald, A., Brück, R., Jahn, K., Niehaves, B., Ullrich, H., Klucken, T.: Promoting smoking abstinence in smokers willing to quit smoking through virtual reality-approach bias retraining: a study protocol for a randomized controlled trial. Trials **21**(1), 583 (2020). https://doi.org/10.1186/s13063-020-4098-5

15. MacLeod, C., Mathews, A.: Cognitive bias modification approaches to anxiety. Annu. Rev. Clin. Psychol. **8**, 189–217 (2012). https://doi.org/10.1146/annurev-clinpsy-032511-143052

16. Meule, A., Richard, A., Dinic, R., Blechert, J.: Effects of a smartphone-based approach-avoidance intervention on chocolate craving and consumption: randomized controlled trial. JMIR mHealth uHealth **7**(11), e12,298 (2019). https://doi.org/10.2196/12298

17. Phaf, R.H., Mohr, S.E., Rotteveel, M., Wicherts, J.M.: Approach, avoidance, and affect: a meta-analysis of approach-avoidance tendencies in manual reaction time tasks. Front. Psychol. **5**, 378 (2014). https://doi.org/10.3389/fpsyg.2014.00378

18. Reitsma, M.B., Fullman, N., Ng, M., Salama, J.S., Abajobir, A., Abate, K.H., Abbafati, C., Abera, S.F., Abraham, B., Abyu, G.Y.: Smoking prevalence and attributable disease burden in 195 countries and territories, 1990–2015: a systematic analysis from the Global Burden of Disease Study 2015. LANCET **389**(10082), 1885–1906 (2017). https://doi.org/10.1016/S0140-6736(17)30819-X

19. Rinck, M., Becker, E.S.: Approach and avoidance in fear of spiders. J. Behav. Ther. Exp. Psychiatry **38**(2), 105–120 (2007). https://doi.org/10.1016/j.jbtep.2006.10.001

20. Solarz, A.K.: Latency of instrumental responses as a function of compatibility with the meaning of eliciting verbal signs. J. Exp. Psychol. **59**(4), 239–245 (1960). https://doi.org/10.1037/h0047274

21. Wiers, C.E., Kühn, S., Javadi, A.H., Korucuoglu, O., Wiers, R.W., Walter, H., Gallinat, J., Bermpohl, F.: Automatic approach bias towards smoking cues is present in smokers but not in ex-smokers. Psychopharmacology **229**(1), 187–197 (2013). https://doi.org/10.1007/s00213-013-3098-5

The Classifier Algorithm for Recognition of Basic Driving Scenarios

Rafał Doniec, Szymon Sieciński, Natalia Piaseczna,
Katarzyna Mocny-Pachońska, Marta Lang, and Jacek Szymczyk

Abstract This paper concerns three common but not recognizable driving practices based on sequences of signals from accelerometers, gyroscopes and electroocu-lograms obtained using state-of-the-art smart eyeglasses. As a result we obtained recordings from twenty volunteers with a set of flagged data assigned to specific actions taken while driving a car during driving lessons. Proposed method achieved a high level of accuracy based on data from smart eyeglasses, predicting appropriate activity classes in approximately 85% of cases without prior knowledge.

Keywords Smart glasses · Driving · Pattern recognition · Wearable devices

R. Doniec · S. Sieciński (✉) · N. Piaseczna · M. Lang · J. Szymczyk
Department of Biosensors and Processing of Biomedical Signals, Faculty of Biomedical
Engineering, Silesian University of Technology, Roosevelta 40, 41-800 Zabrze, Poland
e-mail: szymon.siecinski@polsl.pl

R. Doniec
e-mail: rafal.doniec@polsl.pl

N. Piaseczna
e-mail: natalia.piaseczna@polsl.pl

M. Lang
e-mail: marta.wadas@gmail.com

J. Szymczyk
e-mail: jacek.szymczyk@polsl.pl

K. Mocny-Pachońska
Department of Conservative Dentistry with Endodontics, School of Medicine with
the Division of Dentistry, Medical University of Silesia in Katowice, Plac Akademicki 17,
41-902 Bytom, Poland
e-mail: kpachonska@sum.edu.pl

E. Piętka et al. (eds.), *Information Technology in Biomedicine*, Advances in Intelligent
Systems and Computing 1186, https://doi.org/10.1007/978-3-030-49666-1_28

1 Introduction

Recognition of activity is not a new field; it can be stated unequivocally that categories of activity recognition have already been created [6, 9, 15]. Particularly well described are those primarily related to our basic needs and everyday life: breathing, eating, sleeping, walking [1, 3, 4], and so on. In this paper, we define a sequence of such basic activities as a scenario.

In addition to vital signals, each person can be characterized by his or her cognitive abilities. Cognition, a term that describes mental processes, typically reasoning, consciousness, perception, knowledge, intuition and judgment, is a vital feature of a driver [10]. Using this well-established convention, we decided to analyze activities accompanying the common task of car driving.

The purpose of the study was to recognize the discrete scenarios that take place during a driving session. This task involved the need to acquire a sufficient amount of data using JINS MEME ES_R glasses [7, 8] and analyzing the data in order to extract the scenarios. Based on the accuracy of activity recognition, we concentrated on four scenarios related to driving a car described further in this paper.

2 Materials and Methods

2.1 Technology Used

We used the JINS MEME ES_R (JINS) smart glasses to acquire the data. The device contains the three-point electrooculography and six-axis inertial measurement unit (IMU) with an accelerometer and a gyroscope [17]. The JINS MEME is a micromechanical patented technology [11] thanks to which we can register and detect:

- blink occurrence, its speed and strength,
- vertical and horizontal eye movement,
- head movements.

Technological advances and the availability of various mobile devices allow us the unprecedented opportunity to continuously record sensor data [2].

2.2 Experiments

The experiment was carried out in accordance with the recommendations of the Ethics Committee of Medical University of Silesia (The resolution KNW/ 0022/ KB1/ 18 from 16 October 2018).

The experiment was conducted on 20 volunteers of which ten were experienced drivers with a minimum of ten years' driving experience (age between 40 and

Fig. 1 Experiment setup. The driver (left) is wearing JINS glasses connected to the computer (foreground) while recording the signals

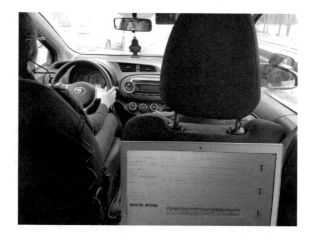

68 years), and ten were students who attended a driving school (age between 18 and 46 years). We gave each driver the same set of defined tasks to perform while wearing the JINS glasses and acquired sensor data to the computer during the drive. The sensor data were linked to the tasks by the same person who observed the driver from the rear seat. The tests were conducted under real road conditions in accordance with the Chap. 4 of the Act on Vehilcle Drivers [18]. Before the experiments we obtained the permit issued by the Provincial Police Department in Katowice. The cognitive aspects of driving lessons were assessed by tracking head, eye and eyelid movements as the indicators of driver's performance reduction and concentration due to fatigue or stress.

Driving tests were performed on a route of 28.7 km which was followed by all the participants and the average journey took approximately 75 min. To ensure the comfort of drivers during the test, experienced drivers drove their own vehicles and learner drivers drove the same car under a supervision of a driving instructor. The car for learner drivers was properly marked and adapted for driving lessons (see Fig. 1).

The following basic driving scenarios were isolated based on the data acquired with the JINS glasses and observing the drivers in action:

1. driving through a roundabout (turning right, driving straight ahead and turning left);
2. driving through a crossroads (turning right, driving straight ahead and turning left);
3. parking (parallel, perpendicular, slant).

In addition, compound scenarios included:

- journey through a motorway,
- drive straight ahead in city traffic,
- passage of a section straight ahead outside of urban area,
- drive straight ahead in residential traffic.

It should be added that experienced drivers generally completed the route faster than learner drivers, regardless of road conditions.

2.3 Classifier

Classification of activities and scenarios was based on the designation of Best Fit Sequences (BFSs) from a sequence of flagged activities visible in data acquired using the JINS glasses. Best Fit Sequence approach is based on the codebook approach described in papers [9, 13–15]. Best Fit Sequence (BFS) is the most frequent sequence of signals associated with flagged activities.

The flagged activities are further separated by a time window for a given width and result from a series of sub-sequences of time-shifted windows. Best Fit Sequence Dictionary (BFSD) is constructed from a set of BFSs as a part of training phase, as shown in Fig. 2. The first step in constructing a BFSD is to find the most suitable BFSs. The length of each BFS equals the length of sub-sequenced data sets from the classifier training data set, which matches the time window width w. A time window is moved from the beginning to the end of the analyzed set of data (see Fig. 2).

We used two different ways of moving the time window—sliding and overlapping. Sliding is when moving step equals the time window width w. If moving step is smaller than w—we define it as overlapping. Choosing an appropriate w and window movement parameter i affect the classifier accuracy; dense sampling of sub-sequences lead to higher accuracy than using more scarce sampling [5]. We changed not only the width of time windows ($w \in \{8, 16, 32, 64, 128\}$ samples, where sampling frequency is 100 Hz), but also the way that the windows were chosen (in sequence or randomly).

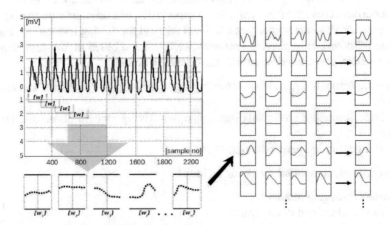

Fig. 2 BFSD construction. Image derived from [15]

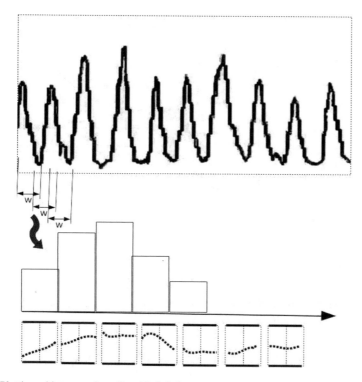

Fig. 3 Plotting a histogram from Best Fit Sub-Sequences

The second classification step grouped all extracted sub-sequences into N different clusters. The distance between the two sub-sequences is measured as the Euclidean distance. Because k-means clustering depends on randomly chosen centroids, it takes tens to hundreds of iterations in order to select the best result. Based on the best grouping result, a BFSD consisting of N BFSs is thus obtained, with each centroid representing one BFS. The optimal number of BFSs (N) must be determined experimentally.

After grouping sub-sequences into clusters, each cluster center becomes a BFS. Each sub-sequence is then assigned in a given sequence to the most similar BFS. Then we extract the histogram representing the frequency of each BFS (see Fig. 3).

After assembling our BFSs into a BFSD, we used half of the labelled data set to train the activity classifier related to driving, based on sequential, multidimensional data from sensors that corresponded to measurements of three quantities (measured by the 3-axis accelerometer, 3-axis gyroscope and four-channel EOG). It should be noted that the BFSD may contain more base vectors (x, y, z) than the input data dimension (Fig. 4). Excessive completeness reduces sensitivity to noise, while the use of sparse coding may help achieving optimal BFSD structure and capturing the optimal order of data patterns [12].

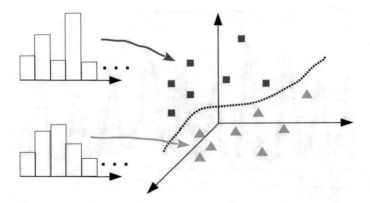

Fig. 4 BFS assignment

3 Results

We calculated the entropy from each window. The common formula for the entropy of random variable x into set of values $x_1, x_2, \ldots, x_n$ is:

$$H(X) = \sum_{i=1}^{n} p(x_i) \log_r \frac{1}{p(x_i)} = -\sum_{i=1}^{n} p(x_i) \log_r p(x_i) \tag{1}$$

$$\lim_{p \to 0^+} p \log(p) = 0 \tag{2}$$

where $r = 2$ according to the theory of information and entropy unit is a bit.

The data presented includes several features: high probabilities (p) and low entropy (H) in each activity class. The desired situation is low entropy which indicates that the probability in one activity class is significantly higher than in other classes.

In the first experiment in which seven activities were analyzed, experiments were carried out on the data from the driving school. The data were divided into seven classes:

- driving on a highway,
- parking in front,
- parallel parking,
- slope parking,
- driving around a roundabout,
- driving in city traffic,
- driving in residential traffic.

The main goal was to recognize the activity by classifier trained on the raw data. Unfortunately, the results were not very promising—the maximum that we managed to achieve was 62% of activities that were classified correctly, even before averaging the results of two runs (2-fold cross-validation). Therefore, in the next experiment, only 4 classes of activity were used:

- driving on the motorway,
- parking,
- urban traffic,
- traffic in the neighborhood,

to which the collected data were assigned and we managed to achieve much better results, with the best average probability value (i.e. percentage of correctly classified activities) from two runs being 85%.

In summary, we are able to recognize four activities related to driving a car with a sufficiently high probability.

4 Conclusions

Comparing our investigations to research (including literature review and related works), it should be noted that we operated on a similar number of subjects within each experimental group. The differences were in the number of signals taken from sensors and monitoring devices. We relied only on signals from the accelerometer, EOG electrodes and gyroscope furnished in the JINS glasses. The experimental results presented in this article show that the BFSD approach can be successfully used to diagnose activities related to driving a car. In the case of data from JINS glasses only, the proposed method achieved a high level of accuracy in results, predicting appropriate activity classes in approximately 85% of cases without prior knowledge. Moreover, a test based on entropy BFSs turned out to be an easy-to-use analytical tool to acquire time window characteristics for a given class of activities. These can be used to build a knowledge based on cognitive activities related to driving a car. Currently, there is an insufficient number of studies and research about the characteristics of particular classes of cognitive activity in this area.

Future work will concentrate on the implementation and contribute to the development and decoding of more complex activities related to driving a car, e.g. mobile phone calls, avoiding road obstacles or responding to traffic incidents. The results may be implemented in determining individual driver's traits, such as diabetes, narcolepsy and vision defects. This approach may help improve the learning outcomes in driver training and examination centers by the arbitrary evaluation of person's ability to drive a car.

References

1. Bao, L., Intille, S.S.: Activity recognition from user-annotated acceleration data. In: Pervasive Computing, Lecture Notes in Computer Science, Berlin, Heidelberg, vol. 3001, pp. 1–17 (2014). https://doi.org/10.1007/978-3-540-24646-6_1
2. Bulling, A., Blanke, U., Schiele,. B.: A tutorial on human activity recognition using body-worn inertial sensors. ACM Comput. Surv. **46**(3), Article 33 (2014). https://doi.org/10.1145/2499621
3. Chen, L., Hoey, J., Nugent, C.D., Cook, D.J., Yu, Z.: Sensor-based activity recognition. IEEE Trans. Syst. Man Cybern. Part C (Appl. Rev.) **42**(6), 790–808 (2012). https://doi.org/10.1109/TSMCC.2012.2198883
4. Cook, D.J., Krishnan, N.C.: Activity learning: discovering, recognizing, and predicting human behavior from sensor data. John Wiley & Sons, Hoboken (2015)
5. Grzegorzek, M.: Sensor data understanding. Logos Verlag Berlin GmbH, Berlin (2017)
6. Ishimaru, S., Kunze, K., Uema, Y., Kise, K., Inami, M., Tanaka, K.: Smarter eyewear: using commercial EOG glasses for activity recognition. In: Proceedings of the 2014 ACM International Joint Conference on Pervasive and Ubiquitous Computing: Adjunct Publication, UbiComp '14 Adjunct, pp. 239–242. ACM, New York, NY, USA. https://doi.org/10.1016/0022-2836(81)90087-5
7. Ishimaru, S., Kunze, K., Tanaka, K., Uema, Y., Kise, K., Inami, M.: Smart eyewear for interaction and activity recognition. In: Proceedings of the 33rd Annual ACM Conference Extended Abstracts on Human Factors in Computing Systems, CHI EA '15, pp. 307–310. ACM, New York, NY, USA (2015). https://doi.org/10.1145/2702613.2725449
8. Kanoh, S., Ichi-nohe, S., Shioya, S., Inoue, K., Kawashima, R.: Development of an eyewear to measure eye and body movements. In: 2015 37th Annual International Conference of the IEEE Engineering in Medicine and Biology Society (EMBC), pp. 2267–2270 (2015). https://doi.org/10.1109/EMBC.2015.7318844
9. Łagodzinński, P., Shirahama, K., Grzegorzek, M.: BFSD-based electrooculography data analysis towards cognitive activity recognition. Comput. Biol. Med. **95**, 277–287. https://doi.org/10.1016/j.compbiomed.2017.10.026
10. Mitas, A.W., Ryguła, A., Pyciński, B., Bugdol, M.D., Konior, W.: Driver biomedical support system. In: Piętka, E., Kawa, J. (eds) Information Technologies in Biomedicine. Lecture Notes in Computer Science, vol. 7339, pp. 277–285. Springer, Berlin, Heidelberg (2020). https://doi.org/10.1007/978-3-642-31196-3_27
11. Petersen, K.E.: Micromechanical membrane switches on silicon. IBM J. Re. Dev. **23**, 376–385 (1979). https://doi.org/10.1147/rd.234.0376
12. Raina, R., Battle, A., Lee, H., Packer, B., Ng, A.Y.: Self-taught learning: transfer learning from unlabeled data. In: Proceedings of the 24th International Conference on Machine Learning, ACM, pp. 759–766 (2007). https://doi.org/10.1145/1273496.1273592
13. Shirahama, K., Köping, L., Grzegorzek, M.: Codebook approach for sensor-based human activity recognition. In: Proceedings of the 2016 ACM International Joint Conference on Pervasive and Ubiquitous Computing: Adjunct (UbiComp '16). Association for Computing Machinery, New York, NY, USA, pp. 197–200 (2016). https://doi.org/10.1145/2968219.2971416
14. Shirahama, K., Grzegorzek, M.: Emotion recognition based on physiological sensor data using codebook approach. In: Piętka E., Badura P., Kawa J., Wieclawek W. (eds) Information Technologies in Medicine. ITiB 2016. Advances in Intelligent Systems and Computing, vol. 472, pp. 27–39. Springer, Cham (2016). https://doi.org/10.1007/978-3-319-39904-1_3
15. Shirahama, K., Grzegorzek, M.: On the generality of codebook approach for sensor-based human activity recognition. Electronics **6**, 44 (2017). https://doi.org/10.3390/electronics6020044

16. https://jins-meme.com/en/products/es/ (Accessed 9 Jan. 2020)
17. https://jins-meme.com/en/researchers/specifications/ (Accessed 13 Feb. 2020)
18. Act of 5 January 2011 on Vehicle Drivers (Dz. U. 2011 Nr 30 poz. 151) http://prawo.sejm.gov.pl/isap.nsf/DocDetails.xsp?id=WDU20110300151

Monitoring Temperature-Related Hazards Using Mobile Devices and a Thermal Camera

Mariusz Marzec

Abstract The paper proposes an algorithm that allows for automatic detection of thermal hazards using a smartphone-type device and a mobile thermal camera. The algorithm works in two stages. First, it analyses the environment of a disabled person for areas with a high or very high temperature. If they are detected, it signals by voice messages the appearance of such an object in the camera field of view. The second stage is the detection of a situation when a visually impaired person brings their hand closer to a hot object. In this situation, the application automatically detects the hand and the hot object and signals by voice messages a higher hazard level. In order to classify the level of thermal hazards, image thresholding methods were used, which enable to detect objects with temperatures above 40, 55, 70 °C. For hand detection in a situation threatening burns, an approach based on sequential thermal image analysis and machine learning was used. Tests were carried out for various algorithm configurations. The accuracy and precision values were as follows: Acc = 0.89, Prec = 0.91. The proposed method allows for quick and completely automatic warning of hazards and can be used for popular Android mobile devices.

Keywords Safety · Hand localization · Thermovision · Image segmentation · Machine learning · Blind and visually impaired people

1 Introduction

Monitoring the environment or vital signs is increasingly used to improve the quality of life and care for the elderly, sick or disabled [1–4]. It is also possible to use similar solutions to increase safety and comfort of life. Various devices, ranging from motion sensors through sensor networks to cameras and vision systems, are

M. Marzec (✉)
Faculty of Science and Technology, Institute of Biomedical Engineering, University of Silesia, ul. Będzińska 39, 41-200 Sosnowiec, Poland
e-mail: mariusz.marzec@us.edu.pl

© The Editor(s) (if applicable) and The Author(s), under exclusive license to Springer Nature Switzerland AG 2021
E. Piętka et al. (eds.), *Information Technology in Biomedicine*, Advances in Intelligent Systems and Computing 1186, https://doi.org/10.1007/978-3-030-49666-1_29

Fig. 1 FLIR One camera
and connection to a
smartphone [6]

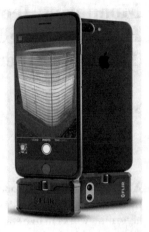

used to observe and record parameters, phenomena or the environment. Common
hazards for disabled or elderly people include: falls, cuts, bruises, burns, etc.

Detection of elevated or dangerous to health or life temperatures can increase
the safety of the visually impaired or blind and protect them against burns. This
is especially important for typical activities related to daily functioning. Burns can
occur already at 42 °C and several hours of exposure, at 55 °C burns occur within
3 min, whereas at 70 °C, 1 s is enough for a burn to occur [5]. The solution proposed
here is based on the Flir One Pro thermal camera [6] cooperating with an Android
mobile phone. The camera used enables to record a thermal and visible image and
transfer this information to a mobile device (Fig. 1).

The Pro version camera offers an optical resolution of 160×120 (images scaled
to 320×240) and a temperature range up to 400 °C. The data from a thermal
camera (in the form of temperatures in degrees Celsius) can be used to monitor
hazards. This will enable the application to react directly, based on the temperature
value in the image, which can also be an indicator of the hazard level. Based on
the above, the paper proposes a system and an image analysis algorithm that allow
for the detection of hazards and protection of a blind or visually impaired person
against burns. Preliminary assumptions and requirements for such a system were
also formulated and possibilities of implementation on the mobile platform were
discussed. A thermal camera mounted at chest height records the thermal image
directly in front of the user and transmits it to the mobile monitoring application,
which determines the hazard level. The algorithm implemented in the application
(discussed below) allows for an appropriate response to the hazard level. When areas
with a temperature above 40, 55, 70 °C appear in the observation area, the user
is warned by a voice message. When the hazard level increases (the temperature
reaches higher values), the intensity of messages increases up to the alarm level,
which should force the user to move away immediately from a dangerous place. The
algorithm has the ability to automatically analyse thermal images based on machine
learning methods, which allows for additional hazard classifications when the user's
hands or arms appear in the observed area.

2 Related Work

The issue of hand detection is widely discussed in the available literature. Most often these solutions are used to create human-computer communication interfaces, to recognize gestures and hand position, to track hands and gestures, to control devices and systems (without additional devices such as a keyboard or mouse) or to manipulate objects in virtual space [7, 8]. The proposed algorithms use image analysis methods (which allow for hand detection) or additional devices in the form of gloves connected to the computer. Due to the appearance of depth sensors, 3D analysis methods are also created [8], which enable to assess the position of hands in space. Most often these solutions are found in visible light systems. Most of these methods are based on analysing the colour in the image. Images in the RGB or YCbCr palette are subjected to appropriate analysis allowing for hand detection or localization, which is the basis for further interpretation. In publication [9], an image was converted to the CbCr palette and subjected to morphological operations to enable edge detection. As a result, the algorithm located areas that matched the colour criteria and separated the hand areas. The authors achieved the following results of the algorithm effectiveness: TP $= 94.6\%$ and FP $= 2.8\%$. However, they did not discuss the set of examined images, hence it is difficult to assess the versatility of the solution. Another publication is also an example of hand segmentation in visible light [10]. The authors note that hand detection in colour images based on colour may be difficult in the case of a complex, coloured background containing areas of similar colours. To solve these problems, an adaptive model of skin and background colour (Gaussian model) in combination with information about the hand surroundings in the image was proposed. Based on the results obtained, the authors suggest that the use of additional information about the background of the examined image can positively affect the effectiveness of hand localization compared to methods based only on skin colour. The segmentation efficiency was assessed by comparing the ratio of the common part of the binary mask determined by the algorithm and marked manually to the sum of the masks of these areas. The results reached the maximum value of Accr $= 90.36\%$. However, the method is difficult to assess in a broader aspect due to the lack of a detailed description of the set of examined images. The solution was used to recognize gestures in cooperation with a computer. Another example of a hand localization method in visible light is the method described in [11]. In this case, the authors proposed a fast real-time hand shape classification method. The algorithm detects the hand area based on the colour, determines the hand orientation in a vertical position and then, in order to determine the shape coefficients and their classification, it uses, among others: shape context analysis, template matching, Hausdorff distance analysis, comparison of the orientation histograms and Hu moments analysis. The examined set contained 499 images. The method was used to recognize gestures. Currently, along with the rapid development of thermovision and lower device prices, hand segmentation and detection in thermovision seems to be an interesting application. It opens up quite different possibilities in this field and allows to extend the previously known functionality to medicine, safety or biometrics. Hand detection in thermal images eliminates typical problems of visible light, i.e. uneven or lack of lighting, skin colour, and coloured background. Solutions can be based on the hand area model (model-based) or information about the brightness in the area (appearance-based). Paper [12] describes a hand segmentation method based on texture statistical features. The features included, among others, mean brightness, standard deviation, entropy, homogeneity, contrast, etc. Image segmentation was carried out using k-means with the assumed number of clusters = 3. The separated areas were then analysed using the above features to classify which regions were in the hand area. An algorithm was used to assess rheumatoid arthritis. An adaptive hand segmentation algorithm was proposed in publication [13]. In the beginning, the hand region—ROI was roughly separated from the background by means of a prepared Gaussian model. Then 5 areas were generated in different places of the hand, on the basis of which temperature distribution models were created. After analysing the image using 5 models, the resulting masks were combined to obtain the resulting mask. Accuracy was assessed by comparing mask surfaces marked by an expert with masks determined by the algorithm, and it was 86%. Hand segmentation in thermovision is also used in biometry [14]. The purpose of the algorithm, in this case, was hand segmentation in order to determine the pattern of vein distribution. The authors proposed different approaches based on segmentation in both visible light and thermovision, as well as in thermovision only. In the case involving only thermovision, ASM (active shape model) was used. It was pre-positioned in the middle of the hand area and after 150 iterations it allowed for segmentation of the hand (pointing thumb down or thumb up). In the case of combining visible light images with thermovision, masks established in visible light were used in thermovision to predict the hand area. In these cases, the best possible fit of the mask obtained from the visible image to the hand shape in the thermal image was important. Another interesting case is the use of thermal images in combination with visible light and depth images [15, 19]. For 3D methods, images containing information about the colour and depth of the scene (RGB-D) were used. According to the authors, the use of a thermal camera increased efficiency by reducing the impact of variable external lighting on segmentation results. A deep neural network (Fast R-CNN) was used for image analysis. It was trained based on a set of several thousand images (2000 RGB images, 1000 thermal images, and 1000 depth images) recorded with 2 cameras and a depth sensor. The test results indicated that RGB, followed by depth images and thermal images, had the greatest impact on detection accuracy. In the light of the studies and examples described above, a hand detection method based on the mask shape and area and SVM classifier has been proposed. The presented algorithm completely automatically and in real time analyses images from a mobile thermal camera and warns of the presence of hot objects and the risk of burning hands. Its task is to increase the safety of visually impaired or blind people during their daily activities. A novelty in relation to the publications described above is the use of image analysis and hand detection methods in thermovision, in applications related to the safety of people with disabilities.

3 Research Material

For the purposes of the study, thermal images covering similar environments and objects were recorded. The images were recorded in several sequences at different times. The set contained over 5,182 thermal images (1,761 without the hand, 3,421 with the left or right hand). The sets included various cases and locations of hot objects and hands. The resolution of the recorded images (transferred to the analysis algorithm) was 240×320 pixels and the temperatures recorded in the images ranged from several dozen to several hundred degrees. The images were recorded in a vertical orientation. Examples of images in the form of thermograms and grey-scale temperature matrices are presented below.

The images represent different hazard levels and typical situations, objects and devices that blind or visually impaired people can come across in their daily activities. In the case of Fig. 2a and b, there is a hot object in the camera field of view (well above 70 °C). The user should be warned of this situation at a level corresponding to the temperature value. However, this situation does not pose a direct risk of burns. In the case of Fig. 2c and d, the situation becomes much more dangerous because it can cause a direct burn. Here the algorithm should alert the user about the situation with messages of much greater intensity.

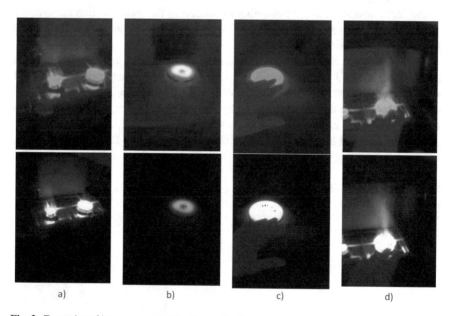

a)   b)   c)   d)

Fig. 2 Examples of images recorded by the application

4 Assumptions of the Proposed Hazard Detection Method

The adopted requirements, which are described below, ensure the proper operation of the independent system and allow for the preparation of the mobile application for automatic detection of an elevated temperature and hazard classification:

- registration of the environment in the field of view of the disabled person,
- camera mounted at chest or head height,
- remote non-contact temperature measurement—localization of places with an elevated or dangerous temperature,
- autonomous scene image analysis directly on a mobile device,
- no need to control and manipulate the device,
- information about the threat, e.g. by means of voice/audio messages, in real time,
- different levels of warnings depending on the hazard,
- detection of arms and hands near a hot object,
- use of fast image processing and analysis algorithms.

Meeting these requirements enabled to prepare an algorithm for a completely independent, mobile system, monitoring and warning of an elevated temperature. The attachment of the devices is illustrated in Fig. 3. Taking into account the user's comfort and the device dimensions, it is better to mount them on the chest. However, taking into consideration the possibility of observing the area at which the eyes are directed, it may be justified to attach the devices to a helmet or headband. The present study used the solution shown in Fig. 3a.

Based on the temperature values described earlier (which cause different burns at different times), 3 warning levels and 1 alarm level have been proposed. Table 1 shows the adopted warning levels generated by the application when a specific heat source is located in the area monitored by the application. The temperature ranges were based on the criteria described above. For the thermal images presented in Fig. 2, the proposed levels should be activated for Fig. 2a, b—High Warning Level,

Fig. 3 Attachment of the thermal camera and smartphone

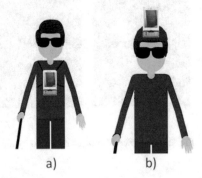

a)   b)

Table 1 Adopted levels of warnings and alarms

Level of warning	Temperature hazard	Voice message
Low	Above 40 °C	Warning: High temperature
Medium	Above 55 °C	Warning: Very high temperature
High	Above 70 °C	Warning: Dangerous temperature
Alarm	Above 70 °C and hands near the heat area	Alarm: High temperature

and c, d— Alarm Level. In the case of the alarm, the risk of burns is very high and immediate action should be taken.

5 Proposed Method

The block diagram of the developed algorithm describing individual stages is presented below—Fig. 4. The thermal camera records images at a frequency of 8 frames per second. The raw data are transformed into a temperature matrix in degrees Celsius. The temperature matrix with a 240 × 320 resolution is passed to the image analysis algorithm. The algorithm detects areas with a dangerous temperature. The highest temperature warning has the highest priority. If areas of different hazardous temperatures appear in the observed area, the algorithm warns of the greatest hazard. In the second block, the algorithm additionally attempts to detect the hand. The classifier analyses the data and returns information whether the image includes hands. Based on the image assessment, the algorithm decides to generate a warning or alarm message. Figure 4, on the left side, shows the case when the algorithm has detected a hot object but there is no risk of burns, and a high temperature message is generated. On the right side, there is a situation when the left hand is near a hot object, and in this case an alarm message should be generated. The individual stages of the algorithm are discussed later in the article.

The main objectives of the developed algorithm were high accuracy under various conditions and high speed, enabling real-time operation. Image acquisition speed is limited by the camera operating frequency (i.e. 8 frames per second). With a faster camera, the image analysis and warning process could be performed more frequently. To detect a hazardous situation, i.e. a potentially dangerous temperature in the field of view, the algorithm uses threshold methods for 3 temperature values. Depending on the threshold, in the binary image after analysis, I_{BW40}, I_{BW55}, I_{BW70}, there appeared area masks representing areas above a certain temperature (1).

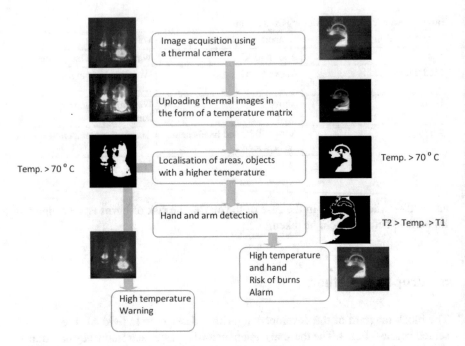

Fig. 4 Block diagram of the algorithm for thermal hazard detection

$$
I_{BW40}(x, y) = \begin{cases} 0 & \text{if } I_{IR}(x, y) < 40 \\ 1 & \text{if } I_{IR}(x, y) >= 40 \end{cases}
$$

$$
I_{BW55}(x, y) = \begin{cases} 0 & \text{if } I_{IR}(x, y) < 55 \\ 1 & \text{if } I_{IR}(x, y) >= 55 \end{cases} \tag{1}
$$

$$
I_{BW70}(x, y) = \begin{cases} 0 & \text{if } I_{IR}(x, y) < 70 \\ 1 & \text{if } I_{IR}(x, y) >= 70 \end{cases}
$$

The algorithm determines the highest temperature that appears in the image and selects the warning level accordingly. When binary masks of areas with an elevated temperature appeared in two resulting images, e.g. I_{BW55}, I_{BW70}, a higher risk was signalled—Table 1—High level. Each time the image detects a temperature higher than 70 °C, the algorithm additionally attempts to detect arms or hands. A set of image features and machine learning methods were proposed to detect the risk of burns. The first step was to determine the temperature range for which the hand area is best visible and the threshold value of the mask surface above which the area is recognized as the hand. The lower threshold $T_1 = 25$ °C and the upper threshold $T_2 = 40$ °C, as well as the mask area threshold $A_{HT} = 1\%$ resolution (320×240) were adopted experimentally (2). These values allowed for the best identification of the hand area in the examined set of images.

$$I_{BW}(x, y) = \begin{cases} 0 & \text{if } I_{IR}(x, y) <= T_1 \\ 1 & \text{if } T_1 < I_{IR}(x, y) <= T_2 \\ 0 & \text{if } I_{IR}(x, y) > T_2 \end{cases} \qquad (2)$$

In the next step, the algorithm analyses the examined thermal image using a sliding window sized 80×80 pixels placed on the left and right side of the image. When it detects an area whose mask is greater than the A_{HT} value, it determines the image and mask features in this place and saves them—Fig. 5. After analysing the whole image (left and right side—for the left and right hand), the algorithm selects the largest area, whose features are passed to the classification block. When analysing the examined images, a set of features including shape and texture parameters was initially proposed [16, 17]:

- W_1—area of the binary mask of the hand in the image (the largest mask)—A_H,
- W_2—ratio of the hand mask area to the smallest convex area—A_H/A_{Convex},
- W_3—ratio of the hand mask area to the bounding box area—A_H / A_{BB},
- W_4—ratio of the length of the image border on the left or right side intersecting the hand area to the perimeter of the hand mask—$L + Border/A_{Perim}$,
- W_5—eccentricity—A_{Ecc},
- W_6—mean pixel temperature—A_{Mean},
- W_7—standard deviation of the pixel temperature in the examined area—A_{Std},
- W_8—ratio of the complement image with binary mask to the bounding box area—A_{HComp}/A_{BB},
- W_9—texture contrast (3),
- W_{10}—texture correlation (3),
- W_{11}—texture energy (3),
- W_{12}—texture homogeneity (3).

$$texContrast = \sum_i \sum_j (i - j)^2 N_g(i, j)$$

$$texCorrelation = \frac{\sum_i \sum_j (i - \mu_i)(j - \mu_j) N_g(i, j)}{\sigma_i \sigma_j}$$

$$texEnergy = \sum_i \sum_j N_g^2(i, j) \qquad (3)$$

$$texHomogeneity = \sum_i \sum_j \frac{N_g(i, j)}{1 + |i - j|}$$

where: i, j are the numbers of the row and column of the co-occurrence matrix N_g, μ_i, μ_j and σ_i, σ_j are the means and standard deviations of the row i and column j.

The proposed features were then assessed for significance in the classification process by comparing their correlation with the class. The highest values of correlation with the class of about 0.70 were obtained by the features W_2, W_3, W_8. Therefore,

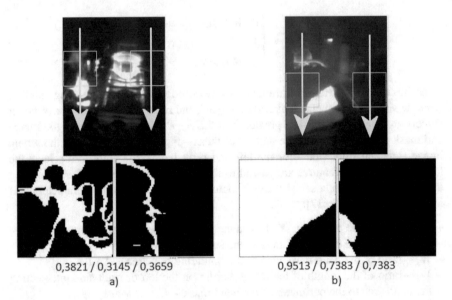

0,3821 / 0,3145 / 0,3659   0,9513 / 0,7383 / 0,7383

a)   b)

Fig. 5 Selection of the analysis window in the image and feature values (for the left window area)

they were selected as the features of the vector passed to the classifier training block (4).

$$W = \{W_2, W_3, W_8\} \tag{4}$$

A popular machine learning method—Support Vector Machine [18], which can easily divide two-class data, was proposed as a classifier. The training set of 5182 images was divided into the training and test sets in the proportion of 75/25 and 90/10% to test the impact of training data on the results. The classifier training time for the set of about 4,600 feature vectors oscillated around 80 s. Figure 5 presents examples of image analysis, sliding windows in the image (left and right hand) and the resulting feature vectors W_2, W_3, W_8 for the biggest mask (left side regions).

Each image is analysed for the left or right hand occurrence. The windows analysing the image, sized 80×80 pixels, move simultaneously from the top of the image down every 10 pixels. If more potential areas appear, the region with the largest surface area is selected (the largest region representing the left or right hand/arm). If, after analysing the left and right sides, the hand or arm area is not detected, the algorithm recognizes that they do not appear in the image. The values of the features from Fig. 5a, b were determined for the left window area. They differ significantly for the images with and without hands. Based on these features, the classifier determines whether or not the image includes hands. On the basis of this information, the algorithm decides whether a high temperature warning or alarm about the possibility of burns is needed.

6 Experimental Results

The results of the detection and classification of the hazard level obtained using the developed algorithm are shown below. Hot object detection is relatively easy. Fast image processing operations based on temperature thresholding allow for 100% effective detection of hazardous areas with a temperature that meets the given criteria. Since the occurrence of a dangerous temperature (and not its characteristics) in the observed area is the most important, image analysis is fast and effective. The second block of the algorithm, i.e. detection of the risk of burns, requires more complex image analysis. Here, based on the proposed features, the algorithm decides whether the hand appears in the field of view of the camera. In order to assess the algorithm effectiveness, its results were compared for several different configurations. Four typical values were proposed, namely Accuracy, Precision, Specificity and Sensitivity, to measure the effectiveness based on a confusion matrix that specifies the number of correct and incorrect hand detections in images. The set was divided into training and test sets in two configurations: 75/25 and 90/100. Finally, 10-fold cross-validation was carried out for the trained classifier [18]. The mean values for 10 cases are presented in Table 2.

Table 2 clearly shows that the results of the algorithm in the examined set of images are very good considering the speed of operation and the low computational complexity of the algorithm. Taking into account the fact that the algorithm will ultimately work in real time, it can be assumed that even in the case of ineffective detection in one of the recorded image frames, the algorithm will correctly classify previous or subsequent images. The algorithm efficiency can be improved by increasing the number of images in the training set, recording them under other conditions, or further development of the algorithm. Some selected cases of correct and incorrect hand detection are presented below. Figure 6a and e show cases when the algorithm correctly reacted to the presence of the hand (TP). The sliding window for the left side of the image (also shown in Fig. 5) indicates the selected area with the largest surface area in the specified temperature range (according to Eq. 2). The mask area representing the left hand is characterized by parameters (W2, W3, W8—Eq. 4) which allow for correct hand detection by SVM trained classifier. Since the image includes the hand and hot area—Fig. 6a the system should activate the Alarm—according to Table 1.

Figure 6b and f show examples when the algorithm incorrectly detected the hand even though it did not actually appear in the image (FP). This situation results from the existence of a warm area of a temperature close to the hand temperature. The

Table 2 Comparison of results for different variants of training and test sets

Case	Accuracy	Precision	Specificity	Sensitivity
Training/Test 75/25	0.86	0.83	0.87	0.87
Training/Test 90/10	0.89	0.92	0.87	0.90

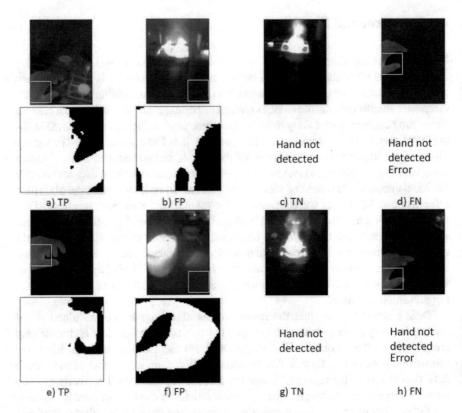

Fig. 6 Examples of algorithm detection and operation. The thermal image and binary mask of the selected area with the result of hand/arm detection

next two images (Fig. 6c, g are examples when the algorithm did not detect the hand correctly (TN), although there was a hot object in the image. Based on image analysis, the algorithm will detect the hot object and activate a lower level warning signal—Table 1. The last two images Fig. 6d, h are false negative (FN) cases—the algorithm did not detect the hand. This is due to the fact that the surface area of the hand mask is too small, it is just appearing in the image. As the algorithm analyses subsequent frames on an ongoing basis, it should be noted that the hand will be detected when most of it appears in the image. In order to eliminate such cases, it is necessary to further increase the effectiveness of the hand detection block, which should positively affect the system operation.

Based on the cited literature, an attempt was made to compare the proposed algorithm with those described above. Because in the methods described in thermovision the authors did not present the obtained efficiency, the results obtained in visible light were included in the comparison. The results presented by the authors are provided for the comparative methods. For the method discussed here, a set of the best parameters obtained during tests for various training and test set configurations is presented Table 3.

Table 3 Comparison of the effectiveness of hand detection methods with the proposed solution

Method	Accuracy	Precision	Specificity	Sensitivity	PR [%]	Images
RGB Visible [9]	ND	ND	ND	ND	94.6	ND
RGB-D [19]	0.97	ND	ND	ND	94.9	1080
Proposed Method IR	0.89	0.91	0.83	0.92	92.4	5181

7 Summary and Conclusions

The presented method, due to its high efficiency and speed of detection, can be used as part of a system warning against thermal hazards. Detection of an elevated or dangerous temperature is carried out with 100% efficiency, whereas the detection of hands and risk of burns reaches the following levels: Acc = 0.89 and Prec = 0.91. The most important features of the proposed solution are a fully automatic detection block, operation speed and classification of various hazard levels. Given that the detection of a dangerous temperature is carried out with 100% efficiency, it can be assumed that a person using the system will be warned sufficiently early about the existing threat. The situation of an immediate risk of burns will therefore only appear when a blind or visually impaired person does not react to previous warnings and approaches a hot object. In this situation, the hand and arm detection block will notice that they are too close to a hot object and alert the user with louder and more intense messages. Methods based on shape descriptors throughout the whole image, image size reduction and data size reduction (PCA), as well as statistical classifiers were tested in the hand detection process. The effectiveness of these methods achieved significantly lower results (Acc below 0.70). Therefore, it was finally decided to analyse the image using a sliding window (for the left and right hand) and the SVM classifier. The results obtained at the current stage of research show that it is possible to effectively monitor and protect against burns using the proposed devices and solutions. Further development of the algorithm and improvement of its capabilities seem to be possible by increasing the set of training images or by expanding and modifying the algorithm. The proposed solution can be used to improve the safety of visually impaired people as well as people performing work under low visibility conditions, where thermal hazards may occur. At this stage, the algorithm is able to independently and autonomously monitor the user's environment and warn of threats. The initial versions of the system and algorithm have been implemented in Java on the Android platform using the OpenCV library. High temperature warning functions have been tested on a mobile device in the form of a mobile phone with a typical, currently available hardware configuration (8 core processor clocked at 2.2 GHz and 6 GB RAM). The image analysis and segmentation functions used at this stage have allowed for continuous monitoring of the environment and their effective and quick operation enables faultless localization of hot objects. At a camera frequency of

8 frames/s, the time taken to analyse a single image cannot exceed 125 milliseconds. For the above-mentioned test hardware configuration, the algorithm analysed the images with sufficient speed 9–15 miliseconds. In the next stages of working on the system, further implementation of the hand detection mechanism will be carried out based on the analysis and classification algorithm proposed above. The equipment capabilities and reserves offered by this type of devices allow for further expansion related to the implementation of more advanced methods of thermal image analysis. They also allow for fast and efficient storage of data obtained from the camera for the purposes of registration.

Acknowledgements This work was supported by the National Centre for Research and Development, "Intelligent system for effective analysis of diagnostic and repair work on industrial installations using mobile units and advanced image analysis— INRED", Project number: POIR.01.01.01-00-0170/17.

References

1. Augustyniak, P., Barczewska, K.: Systemy techniczne formujące inteligentne otoczenie osoby niepełnosprawnej. EXIT, Warszawa (2015)
2. Yazar, A., Erden, F., Enis Cetin, A.: Multi-sensor ambient assisted living system for fall detection. In: Proceedings of the IEEE International Conference on Acoustic, Speech and Signal Processing (2014)
3. Chaaraoui, A.A., Climent-Pérez, P., Flórez-Revuelta, F.: A review on vision techniques applied to human behaviour analysis for ambient-assisted living. Expert Syst. Appl. **39** (2012)
4. Szajewska, A., Rybiński, J.: History of the application of thermovision in the fire protection system in Poland, vol. 63, No. 4, PAK, pp. 124–127 (2017)
5. http://www.medonet.pl/choroby-od-a-do-z/choroby-skory,oparzenia-cieplne-i-chemiczne, artykul,1578469.html. Access 15.09.2019
6. FLIR https://www.flir.eu/flirone. Access 15.09.2019
7. Ibraheem, N.: Survey on gesture recognition for hand image postures. Comput. Inf. Sci. **5**(3) (2012)
8. Hong, C., Yang, L., Zicheng, L.: A survey on 3D hand gesture recognition. IEEE Trans. Circuits Syst. Video Technol. **26**, 1–1 (2015)
9. Dawod, A.Y., Abdullah, J., Alam, M.J.: A new method for hand segmentation using free-form skin color model. In: 3rd International Conference on Advanced Computer Theory and Engineering (ICACTE) (2010)
10. Wang, W., Pan, J.: Hand segmentation using skin color and background information. In: International Conference on Machine Learning and Cybernetics (2012)
11. Nalepa, J., Kawulok, M.: Fast and accurate hand shape classification. In: Kozielski, S., Mrozek, D., Kasprowski, P., Małysiak-Mrozek, B., Kostrzewa, D. (eds.) Beyond Databases, Architectures, and Structures. BDAS 2014. Communications in Computer and Information Science, vol. 424. Springer, Cham (2014)
12. Snehalatha, R., Anburajan, M., Sowmiya, V., Venkatraman, B., Menaka, M.: Automated hand thermal image segmentation and feature extraction in the evaluation of rheumatoid arthritis. In: Proceedings of the Institution of Mechanical Engineers. Part H, J. Eng. Med. **229**, 319–31 (2015)
13. Song, E., Lee, H., Choi, J., Le, S.: AHD: thermal image-based adaptive hand detection for enhanced tracking system. IEEE Access Special Section on Human-Centered Smart Systems and Technologies (2018)

14. Mekyska, J., Font-Aragones, X., Faúndez Zanuy, M., Hernández-Mingorance, R., Morales, A., Ferrer-Ballester, M.: Thermal hand image segmentation for biometric recognition. In: Proceedings of 45th Annual IEEE International Carnahan Conference on Security Technology, pp. 26-30. ISBN: 978-1-4577-0901-2 (2011)
15. Luo, R., Luppescu, G.: Using RGB, Depth, and Thermal Data for Improved Hand Detection. Stanford University, Department of Electrical Engineering (2016)
16. Gonzalez, R.C., Woods, R.E., Eddins Steven, L.: Digital Image Processing Using MATLAB 2e. Gatesmark Publishing (2009)
17. Zieliński, K., Strzelecki, M.: Komputerowa analiza obrazu biomedycznego. Wydawnictwo Naukowe PWN, Warszawa (2013)
18. Osowski, S.: Metody i narzędzia eksploracji danych. Wydawnictwo BTC, Legionowo (2013)
19. Molchanov, P., Yang, X., Gupta, S., Kim, K., Tyree, S., Kautz, J.: Online detection and classification of dynamic hand gestures with recurrent 3D convolutional neural networks. In: IEEE Conference on Computer Vision and Pattern Recognition (CVPR) (2016)

Author Index

A
Adamczyk, Waclaw M., 239
Adamczyk, Wojciech, 255, 265
Affanasowicz, Alicja, 147
Augustyniak, Piotr, 317

B
Badura, Aleksandra, 227
Badura, Dariusz, 147
Badura, Paweł, 3, 41
Bas, Mateusz, 81, 303
Benova, Mariana, 289
Bialecki, Ryszard, 255, 265
Bibrowicz, Karol, 187, 201
Bielecka, Katarzyna, 303
Bieńkowska, Maria, 227
Binkowski, Marcin, 107
Böck, Dominik, 277
Brück, Rainer, 277, 345
Bugdol, Marcin, 175
Bugdol, Monika N., 147, 161, 213

C
Czajkowska, Joanna, 3
Czarlewski, Robert, 227

D
Danch-Wierzchowska, Marta, 175
Danecka, Aneta, 121
Doniec, Rafał, 359
Doroniewicz, Iwona, 147
Dzieciątko, Mariusz, 303
Dziurowicz, Wojciech, 3

E
Eiler, Tanja Joan, 345

F
Forneberg, Tobias, 345

G
Gertych, Arkadiusz, 55
Gethmann, Carl Friedrich, 345
Gouverneur, Philip J., 239
Gracka, Maria, 255
Grünewald, Armin, 345
Grzegorzek, Marcin, 133, 239

J
Jahn, Katharina, 345
Jędzierowska, Magdalena, 107

K
Kania, Damian, 161
Kieszczyńska, Katarzyna, 147
Klucken, Tim, 345
Koprowski, Robert, 107
Korzekwa, Szymon, 3
Kręcichwost, Michał, 41
Kulwa, Frank, 13, 27
Kwaśniok, Ewa, 41

L
Lang, Marta, 359
Ledwoń, Daniel, 147
Li, Chen, 13, 27

Li, Frédéric, 133, 239
Li, Hong, 27
Lipowicz, Anna, 187, 201
Li, Zihan, 13, 27
Luedtke, Kerstin, 239

M
Machulska, Alla, 345
Maćkowski, Michal, 303
Mańka, Anna, 121, 213
Marzec, Mariusz, 369
Masłowska, Aleksandra, 227
Matyja, Małgorzata, 147
Mazur, Patrycja, 71
Melka, Bartlomiej, 255, 265
Michnik, Robert, 121
Miodońska, Zuzanna, 41
Mitas, Andrzej W., 147, 121, 161, 175, 187,
    201, 213
Mocny-Pachońska, Katarzyna, 359
Mydlova, Jana, 289
Myśliwiec, Andrzej, 147, 227

N
Niedzwiedź, Sandra, 121
Niehaves, Björn, 345
Nowak, Marcin, 255, 265
Nowakowska-Lipiec, Katarzyna, 121

O
Obuchowicz, Rafał, 71
Ostrowski, Ziemowit, 255, 265

P
Pająk, Anna, 317
Piaseczna, Natalia, 359
Pietka, Ewa, 227
Piórkowski, Adam, 71
Pollak, Anita, 161
Psenakova, Zuzana, 289
Pyciński, Bartlomiej, 55

R
Rojczyk, Marek, 255
Rojewska, Katarzyna, 303
Romaniszyn, Patrycja, 121, 161, 213

S
Sage, Agata, 41
Shirahama, Kimiaki, 133
Sieciński, Szymon, 359
Smondrk, Maros, 289
Speich, Alexandra, 277
Spinczyk, Dominik, 81, 303
Szajerman, Dominik, 327
Szikszay, Tibor M., 239
Szurmik, Tomasz, 187, 201
Szymczyk, Jacek, 359

T
Takashima, Naoki, 133
Trzaskalik, Joanna, 41
Turner, Bruce, 121
Twardawa, Patrycja, 121

U
Ustinov, Swetlana, 277

V
Viehbeck, Jana, 277

W
Walts, Ann E., 55
Wiehl, Michael, 277
Wojciechowski, Adam, 327
Wróbel, Filip, 327
Wróbel, Zygmunt, 107

X
Xu, Hao, 13, 27

Y
Yagi, Yukako, 55

Z
Zarychta, Piotr, 95
Zhang, Jinghua, 13, 27
Zhao, Xin, 13, 27

Printed in the United States
By Bookmasters